# Advanced Musculoskeletal MR Imaging

*Editors*

ROBERTO CÔRTES DOMINGUES
FLÁVIA MARTINS COSTA

# MAGNETIC RESONANCE IMAGING CLINICS OF NORTH AMERICA

www.mri.theclinics.com

*Consulting Editors*
SURESH K. MUKHERJI
LYNNE S. STEINBACH

November 2018 • Volume 26 • Number 4

**ELSEVIER**

1600 John F. Kennedy Boulevard • Suite 1800 • Philadelphia, Pennsylvania, 19103-2899

http://www.mri.theclinics.com

**MRI CLINICS OF NORTH AMERICA Volume 26, Number 4**
**November 2018 ISSN 1064-9689, ISBN 13: 978-0-323-64161-6**

Editor: John Vassallo (j.vassallo@elsevier.com)
Developmental Editor: Meredith Madeira

*Magnetic Resonance Imaging Clinics of North America* (ISSN 1064-9689) is published quarterly by Elsevier Inc., 360 Park Avenue South, New York, NY 10010-1710. Months of issue are February, May, August, and November. Business and Editorial Offices: 1600 John F. Kennedy Blvd., Ste. 1800, Philadelphia, PA 19103-2899. Customer Service Office: 3251 Riverport Lane, Maryland Heights, MO 63043. Periodicals postage paid at New York, NY and additional mailing offices. Subscription prices are $395.00 per year (domestic individuals), $701.00 per year (domestic institutions), $100.00 per year (domestic students/residents), $437.00 per year (Canadian individuals), $913.00 per year (Canadian institutions), $545.00 per year (international individuals), $913.00 per year (international institutions), and $275.00 per year (international and Canadian students/residents). International air speed delivery is included in all *Clinics* subscription prices. All prices are subject to change without notice. **POSTMASTER:** Send address changes to *Magnetic Resonance Imaging Clinics*, Elsevier Health Sciences Division, Subscription Customer Service, 3251 Riverport Lane, Maryland Heights, MO 63043. Customer Service (orders, claims, online, change of address): Elsevier Health Sciences Division, Subscription **Customer Service, 3251 Riverport Lane, Maryland Heights, MO 63043. Tel:1-800-654-2452 (U.S. and Canada); 314-447-8871 (outside U.S. and Canada). Fax: 314-447-8029. E-mail: journalscustomer service-usa@elsevier.com (for print support); journalsonlinesupport-usa@elsevier.com (for online support).**

*Reprints.* For copies of 100 or more of articles in this publication, please contact the Commercial Reprints Department, Elsevier Inc., 360 Park Avenue South, New York, NY 10010-1710. Tel.: 212-633-3874; Fax: 212-633-3820; E-mail: reprints@elsevier.com.

*Magnetic Resonance Imaging Clinics of North America* is covered in the *RSNA Index of Imaging Literature, MEDLINE/PubMed (Index Medicus),* and *EMBASE/Excerpta Medica.*

# Contributors

## CONSULTING EDITORS

**SURESH K. MUKHERJI, MD, MBA, FACR**
Professor and Chairman, Walter F. Patenge
Endowed Chair, Department of Radiology,
Michigan State University, Chief Medical
Officer and Director of Health Care Delivery,
Michigan State University Health Team, East
Lansing, Michigan, USA

**LYNNE S. STEINBACH, MD, FACR**
Professor of Radiology and Orthopaedic
Surgery, Department of Radiology and
Biomedical Imaging, University of California,
San Francisco, San Francisco, California,
USA

## EDITORS

**ROBERTO CÔRTES DOMINGUES, MD**
Imaging Medical Director, DASA - Rio de
Janeiro, Centro Médico BarraShopping,
CDPI, Rio de Janeiro, Rio de Janeiro,
Brazil

**FLÁVIA MARTINS COSTA, MD, PhD**
Radiologist, Clínica de Diagnóstico por
Imagem (CDPI)/DASA, Centro Médico
BarraShopping, CDPI, Rio de Janeiro, Rio de
Janeiro, Brazil

## AUTHORS

**SHIVANI AHLAWAT, MD**
Assistant Professor, The Russell H. Morgan
Department of Radiology and Radiological
Science, Johns Hopkins School of Medicine,
Baltimore, Maryland, USA

**ELIE BARAKAT, MD**
Department of Radiology, Institut de Recherche
Expérimentale et Clinique (IREC), Cliniques
universitaires Saint-Luc, Université catholique
de Louvain (UCL), Brussels, Belgium

**MATTHEW BLACKLEDGE, PhD, BSc, MSc**
Cancer Research UK Cancer Imaging Centre,
The Institute of Cancer Research, Sutton,
United Kingdom

**MARCELO BORDALO-RODRIGUES, MD,
PhD**
Head of the Diagnostic Imaging Center, Institute
of Orthopedics and Traumatology, Diagnostic
Center, Head of Musculoskeletal Radiology,
Radiology Institute, Faculty of Medicine, Clinics
Hospital, University of São Paulo Medical School,
Head of Musculoskeletal Radiology, Sirio-
Libanese Hospital, São Paulo, São Paulo, Brazil

**CLARISSA CANELLA, MD, PhD**
Radiologist at Radiology Department of Clínica
de Diagnóstico por Imagem (CDPI)/DASA,
Rio de Janeiro, Rio de Janeiro, Brazil; Adjunct
Professor at Radiology Department of
Universidade Federal Fluminense, Niterói, Rio
de Janeiro, Brazil

**FLÁVIA MARTINS COSTA, MD, PhD**
Radiologist, Clínica de Diagnóstico por
Imagem (CDPI)/DASA, Centro Médico
BarraShopping, CDPI, Rio de Janeiro, Rio de
Janeiro, Brazil

**RÔMULO DOMINGUES, MD**
Brazilian Olympic Radiology Manager at
Rio 2016, Medical Director of Clínica de
Diagnóstico por Imagem (CDPI)/DASA,
Consultant Radiologist at Clínica de
Diagnóstico por Imagem (CDPI)/DASA,
Rio de Janeiro, Rio de Janeiro, Brazil

**RICARDO DONNERS, MD**
Department of Radiology, University Hospital
Basel, Basel, Switzerland

**LAURA M. FAYAD, MD**
Professor of Radiology, Orthopaedic Surgery
and Oncology, Chief of Musculoskeletal
Imaging, Director of Translational Research for
Advanced Imaging, The Russell H. Morgan
Department of Radiology and Radiological
Science, Johns Hopkins School of Medicine,
Baltimore, Maryland, USA

**CHRISTINE GALANT, MD**
Department of Pathology, Institut de Recherche
Expérimentale et Clinique (IREC), Cliniques
universitaires Saint-Luc, Université catholique
de Louvain (UCL), Brussels, Belgium

**BRUNO HASSEL, MD**
Radiologist at Clínica de Diagnóstico por
Imagem (CDPI)/DASA e Alta Excelência
Diagnóstico/DASA, Fellowship Coordinator of
Radiology at DASA, Rio de Janeiro, Rio de
Janeiro, Brazil

**JACOB L. JAREMKO, MD, PhD, FRCPC**
Associate Professor, Department of Radiology
and Diagnostic Imaging, University of Alberta,
Edmonton, Alberta, Canada

**MARTIN KAISER, MD**
Clinician Scientist, Myeloma Group, The
Institute of Cancer Research, Honorary
Consultant Haematologist, The Royal Marsden
Hospital, Sutton, United Kingdom

**THOMAS KIRCHGESNER, MD**
Department of Radiology, Institut de Recherche
Expérimentale et Clinique (IREC), Cliniques
universitaires Saint-Luc, Université catholique
de Louvain (UCL), Brussels, Belgium

**DOW-MU KOH, MD, MRCP, FRCR**
Cancer Research UK Cancer Imaging Centre,
The Institute of Cancer Research, Department
of Radiology, Royal Marsden Hospital, Sutton,
United Kingdom

**ROBERT G.W. LAMBERT, MB BCh, FRCR,
FRCPC**
Professor, Department of Radiology and
Diagnostic Imaging, University of Alberta,
Edmonton, Alberta, Canada

**FREDERIC E. LECOUVET, MD, PhD**
Radiology Department, Institut de Recherche
Expérimentale et Clinique, Université
Catholique de Louvain, Cliniques Universitaires
Saint-Luc, Brussels, Belgium

**FLÁVIA PAIVA PROENÇA LOBO LOPES,
MD, PhD**
Clinical Research Coordinator at Clínica de
Diagnóstico por Imagem (CDPI)/DASA e Alta
Excelência Diagnóstica/DASA, Invited
Professor at Radiology Department of Federal
University of Rio de Janeiro (UFRJ), Rio de
Janeiro, Rio de Janeiro, Brazil

**PEDRO HENRIQUE MARTINS, MD**
Radiologist at Radiology Department of Clínica
de Diagnóstico por Imagem (CDPI)/DASA,
Rio de Janeiro, Rio de Janeiro, Brazil

**ELMAR M. MERKLE, MD**
Department of Radiology, University Hospital
Basel, Basel, Switzerland

**CHRISTINA MESSIOU, MD, BMedSci,
BMBS, MRCP, FRCR**
Consultant Radiologist, Department of
Radiology, Cancer Research UK
Cancer Imaging Centre, The Royal
Marsden Hospital, Honorary Faculty,
The Institute of Cancer Research,
Sutton, United Kingdom

**JOÃO GRANGEIRO NETO, MD, MS**
Brazilian Olympic Committee Chief Medical
Officer Rio 2016, Chief of Sports Trauma Group
at Instituto Nacional de Traumato-Ortopedia,
Rio de Janeiro, Rio de Janeiro, Brazil

**RENATA NOGUEIRA, MD, MSc**
Radiologist at Clínica de Diagnóstico por
Imagem (CDPI)/DASA e Alta Excelência
Diagnóstica/DASA, Rio de Janeiro, Rio de
Janeiro, Brazil

**MIKKEL ØSTERGAARD, MD, PhD, DMSc**
Professor, Copenhagen Center for Arthritis
Research, Center for Rheumatology and Spine
Diseases, Rigshospitalet, Glostrup, Denmark;
Department of Clinical Medicine, Faculty of
Health and Medical Sciences, University of
Copenhagen, Copenhagen, Denmark

**ANWAR R. PADHANI, MBBS, MRCP, FRCR**
MR unit, Paul Strickland Scanner Centre,
Mount Vernon Hospital, Middlesex, United
Kingdom; Consultant Radiologist, Mount
Vernon Cancer Centre, Professor of Cancer
Imaging, The Institute of Cancer Research,
London, United Kingdom

**GIUSEPPE PETRALIA, MD**
Deputy Director, Department of Radiology,
IEO - European Institute of Oncology IRCCS,
Researcher, Department of Oncology and
Hematology, University of Milan, Milan,
Italy

**MARIA STOENOIU, MD, PhD**
Department of Rheumatology, Institut de
Recherche Expérimentale et Clinique (IREC),
Cliniques universitaires Saint-Luc, Université
catholique de Louvain (UCL), Brussels,
Belgium

**HUASONG TANG, MD**
Resident Physician, The Russell H. Morgan
Department of Radiology and Radiological
Science, Johns Hopkins School of Medicine,
Baltimore, Maryland, USA

**PERRINE TRIQUENEAUX, MSc**
Department of Radiology, Institut de
Recherche Expérimentale et Clinique (IREC),
Cliniques universitaires Saint-Luc, Université
catholique de Louvain (UCL), Brussels,
Belgium

**NINA TUNARIU, MD, MRCP, FRCR**
Cancer Research UK Cancer Imaging Centre,
The Institute of Cancer Research, Department
of Radiology, Royal Marsden Hospital, Royal
Marsden NHS Foundation Trust, Sutton,
United Kingdom

**HERON WERNER, MD, PhD**
Coordinator of Fetal Medicine at Clínica de
Diagnóstico por Imagem (CDPI)/DASA e Alta
Excelência Diagnóstica/DASA, Rio de Janeiro,
Rio de Janeiro, Brazil

# Contents

Whole-body diffusion-weighted MRI has emerged as a powerful diagnostic tool for disease detection and staging mainly used in systemic bone disease. The large field-of-view functional imaging technique highlights cellular tumor and suppresses normal tissue signal, allowing quantification of an estimate of total disease burden, summarized as the total diffusion volume (tDV), as well as global apparent diffusion coefficient (gADC) measurements. Both tDV and gADC have been shown to be repeatable quantitative parameters that indicate tumor heterogeneity and treatment effects, thus potential, noninvasive, imaging biomarkers informing on disease prognosis and therapy response.

Whole-body MRI (WB-MRI) has emerged as a radiation-free method for the diagnosis, staging, and therapy response assessments in cancer patients. This article reviews the current roles for WB-MRI in the clinical context of limitations of currently used techniques, focusing on bone marrow disease applications. Indication for broader clinical use are discussed, including guideline recommendations. The emerging screening role of WB-MRI in subjects at high risk of cancer is discussed, as is normal population screening.

This article outlines current international guidance for the role of imaging in myeloma and summarizes evidence regarding the role of whole-body MR imaging in diagnosis and response assessment. Whole-body MR imaging protocols, including diffusion-weighted MR imaging, are suggested as well as notes on pearls, pitfalls, and variants.

Whole-body MR imaging incorporating diffusion-weighted imaging is increasingly recommended as a radiation-free imaging method for assessing bone and soft tissue pathology, and for evaluating response to therapy. Metastasis Reporting and Data System for prostate cancer provides the minimum standards for whole-body MR imaging with diffusion imaging regarding image acquisitions, interpretation, and reporting of baseline and follow-up monitoring examinations of patients with advanced, metastatic cancers, focusing on prostate cancer. This article summarizes and illustrates Metastasis Reporting and Data System using a case-based approach in patients with advanced prostate cancer.

This article discusses the features of multiparametric MR imaging as an accurate method to evaluate soft tissue tumors and pseudotumors. The discussion also considers conventional and advanced sequences providing both functional tissue and anatomic information to improve the diagnostic accuracy of this method and assess pretreatment staging, treatment response focused on the extent of necrosis, and recurrence.

Although radiography is a first-line test for the assessment of bone lesions, MR imaging is needed for defining the extent of a bone tumor. In addition, MR imaging provides features and metrics for the characterization of bone lesions as well as for the evaluation a tumor following treatment. There are several noncontrast and contrast-enhanced sequences available for clinical use that collectively provide valuable information for tumor evaluation, and include conventional T1-weighted imaging, fluid-sensitive sequences, chemical shift imaging, and diffusion-weighted imaging with ADC mapping, as well as postcontrast sequences, including static postcontrast imaging and dynamic contrast-enhanced MR imaging.

Neoplastic musculoskeletal lesions are heterogeneous tumors with variable outcomes that require a precise diagnosis and delivery of optimal, specific treatment. Advanced MR imaging techniques can help differentiate and characterize musculoskeletal soft tissue tumors and are the method of choice for detection, evaluation, local staging, and surgical planning. MR imaging–ultrasound fusion is the process of combining relevant information from 2 methods into a single image that is more informative than the images obtained separately. This article assesses the potential of fusing real-time ultrasound spatial registration with previously acquired musculoskeletal MR imaging to guide tumor tissue biopsies and procedures.

Whole-body magnetic resonance (MR) imaging techniques and protocols have been evolving continuously for the last 20 years, resulting in a powerful and mature tool for the detection, staging, and treatment monitoring of many oncologic and musculoskeletal disorders. The unique contrast resolution of MR imaging makes this imaging modality highly sensitive to pathologic alterations in bones, muscles, entheses, joints, and soft tissues, enabling this method to be expanded to the whole musculoskeletal system. Whole-body MR imaging is now used in numerous rheumatic, bone, and muscle disorders, and a full range of developing applications for this method have been emerging.

Robert G.W. Lambert, Mikkel Østergaard, and Jacob L. Jaremko

Magnetic resonance (MR) imaging has traditionally only played a small role in the clinical care of most patients with arthritis. However, with modern therapeutic strategies, early diagnosis is now more important than ever before. Consequently, advanced MRI techniques and applications now play a crucial role in managing an increasing proportion of rheumatology patients. This article reviews MR imaging techniques that are in widespread use and in development for detection and quantification of inflammation and structural damage in arthritis. It focuses on the role of MR imaging for diagnosis, management, and research in inflammatory arthropathies. Osteoarthritis and gout are briefly reviewed.

Marcelo Bordalo-Rodrigues

Magnetic resonance neurography is defined by direct visualization of nerves with MR imaging. Technical advancements enabled high-resolution protocols, and clinical interest has increased. The author discusses basics of magnetic resonance neurography protocols and review clinical magnetic resonance neurography applications in the musculoskeletal system.

Heron Werner, Renata Nogueira, and Flávia Paiva Proença Lobo Lopes

This article outlines the main findings in prenatal musculoskeletal disorders. Three main technologies are generally used to obtain images within the uterus during pregnancy: ultrasound (US), MR imaging, and computed tomography (CT). Currently, the primary imaging method used for fetal assessment during pregnancy is US because it is patient friendly, useful, cost-effective, and (considered) safe. MR imaging is generally performed when US yields equivocal results because it offers additional information about fetal abnormalities and conditions in situations in which US is unable to provide high-quality images.

Rômulo Domingues, Bruno Hassel, João Grangeiro Neto, and Flávia Paiva Proença Lobo Lopes

A facility with ultimate imaging technology was established to provide diagnostic care for the athletes during the 2016 Olympic and Paralympic Games, two of the world's most prestigious sports events. The Imaging Center featured 3.0-T and 1.5-T wide-bore MRI scanners. High-end, wide-bore 3.0-T and 1.5-T MRI systems with dedicated coils provided high-quality imaging solutions, enabling diagnoses of even minor injuries with the utmost accuracy during the games. This article outlines the authors' experience using 3.0-T and 1.5-T wide-bore MRI during the Rio 2016 Olympic and Paralympic Games, including the advantages and potential applications of this diagnostic method in sports medicine.

# MAGNETIC RESONANCE IMAGING CLINICS OF NORTH AMERICA

---

---

VISIT THE CLINICS ONLINE!
Access your subscription at:
www.theclinics.com

## PROGRAM OBJECTIVE

The goal of *Magnetic Resonance Imaging Clinics of North America* is to keep practicing physicians up to date with current clinical practice by providing timely articles reviewing the state of the art in patient care.

## TARGET AUDIENCE

All practicing physicians and healthcare professionals who provide patient care utilizing findings from Magnetic Resonance Imaging.

## LEARNING OBJECTIVES

Upon completion of this activity, participants will be able to:
1. Review advanced MRI and ultrasound fusion in musculoskeletal procedures
2. Discuss whole-body MRI in rheumatic and systemic diseases, as well as in oncology.
3. Recognize multiparametric MRI of soft-tissue tumors and pseudotumors, as well as benign and malignant bone lesions.

## ACCREDITATION

The Elsevier Office of Continuing Medical Education (EOCME) is accredited by the Accreditation Council for Continuing Medical Education (ACCME) to provide continuing medical education for physicians.

The EOCME designates this enduring material for a maximum of 15 *AMA PRA Category 1 Credit*(s)™. Physicians should claim only the credit commensurate with the extent of their participation in the activity.

All other healthcare professionals requesting continuing education credit for this enduring material will be issued a certificate of participation.

## DISCLOSURE OF CONFLICTS OF INTEREST

The EOCME assesses conflict of interest with its instructors, faculty, planners, and other individuals who are in a position to control the content of CME activities. All relevant conflicts of interest that are identified are thoroughly vetted by EOCME for fair balance, scientific objectivity, and patient care recommendations. EOCME is committed to providing its learners with CME activities that promote improvements or quality in healthcare and not a specific proprietary business or a commercial interest.

**The planning committee, staff, authors and editors listed below have identified no financial relationships or relationships to products or devices they or their spouse/life partner have with commercial interest related to the content of this CME activity:**

Shivani Ahlawat, MD; Elie Barakat, MD; Matthew Blackledge, PhD, BSc, MSc; Marcelo Bordalo-Rodrigues, MD, PhD; Clarissa Canella, MD, PhD; Flávia Martins Costa, MD, PhD; Rômulo Domingues, MD; Ricardo Donners, MD; Laura M. Fayad, MD; Christine Galant, MD; Bruno Hassel, MD; Jacob L. Jaremko, MD, PhD, FRCPC; Martin Kaiser, MD; Alison Kemp; Thomas Kirchgesner, MD; Dow-Mu Koh, MD, MRCP, FRCR; Pradeep Kuttysankaran; Frederic E. Lecouvet, MD, PhD; Flávia Paiva Proença Lobo Lopes, MD, PhD; Pedro Henrique Martins, MD; Elmar M. Merkle, MD; Christina Messiou, MD, BMedSci DMDO, MROP, FROP, Ouresh K. Mukherji, MD, MDA, FAOR, João Orangeiro Neto, MD, MO, Renata Nogueira, MD, MSc, Anwar R. Padhani, MBBS, MRCP, FRCR; Giuseppe Petralia, MD; Lynne S. Steinbach, MD, FACR; Maria Stoenoiu, MD, PhD; Huasong Tang, MD; Perrine Triqueneaux, MSc; Nina Tunariu, MD, MRCP, FRCR; John Vassallo; Heron Werner, MD, PhD.

**The planning committee, staff, authors and editors listed below have identified financial relationships or relationships to products or devices they or their spouse/life partner have with commercial interest related to the content of this CME activity:**

**Robert G.W. Lambert, MB BCh, FRCR, FRCPC:** is a consultant/advisor for AbbVie, Inc., Bioclinica, PAREXEL International Corporation, and UCB, Inc.

**Mikkel Østergaard, MD, PhD, DMSc:** is a consultant/advisor for and/or receives research support from AbbVie, Inc., Bristol-Myers Squibb Company, Boehringer Ingelheim International GmbH, Celgene Corporation, Eli Lilly and Company, GlaxoSmithKline, Johnson & Johnson Services, Merck & Co., Inc., Mundipharma International, Novartis AG, Novo Nordisk A/S, Orion Corporation, Pfizer Inc., Regeneron, F. Hoffmann-La Roche Ltd, Takeda Pharmaceutical Company Limited, UCB, Inc.

## UNAPPROVED/OFF-LABEL USE DISCLOSURE

The EOCME requires CME faculty to disclose to the participants:
1. When products or procedures being discussed are off-label, unlabelled, experimental, and/or investigational (not US Food and Drug Administration [FDA] approved); and
2. Any limitations on the information presented, such as data that are preliminary or that represent ongoing research, interim analyses, and/or unsupported opinions. Faculty may discuss information about pharmaceutical agents that is outside of FDA-approved labelling. This information is intended solely for CME and is not intended to promote off-label use of these medications. If you have any questions, contact the medical affairs department of the manufacturer for the most recent prescribing information.

## TO ENROLL

To enroll in the *Magnetic Resonance Imaging Clinics of North America* Continuing Medical Education program, call customer service at 1-800-654-2452 or sign up online at http://www.theclinics.com/home/cme. The CME program is available to subscribers for an additional annual fee of USD 260.

## METHOD OF PARTICIPATION

In order to claim credit, participants must complete the following:

1. Complete enrolment as indicated above.
2. Read the activity.
3. Complete the CME Test and Evaluation. Participants must achieve a score of 70% on the test. All CME Tests and Evaluations must be completed online.

## CME INQUIRIES/SPECIAL NEEDS

For all CME inquiries or special needs, please contact elsevierCME@elsevier.com.

# Foreword

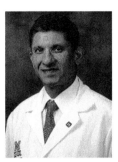

Suresh K. Mukherji, MD, MBA, FACR
*Consulting Editor*

This issue entitled "Advanced Musculoskeletal MR Imaging" focuses on various pathologies involving the musculoskeletal system and skillfully combines common pathologies with advanced imaging. There are specific articles devoted to oncology, inflammatory disorders, multiple myeloma, rheumatology, and MR neurography. There are also some very unique articles devoted to the role of the MR imaging–ultrasound fusion in assessment and intervention, applications of multiparametric MR imaging, MR imaging of fetal musculoskeletal disorders, and an article summarizing the experience of our colleagues using state-of-the-art wide-bore MR imaging scanners on high-performance athletes at the Rio 2016 Olympics and Paralympics Games!

I want to both thank and congratulate our Guest Co-editors. I have known Drs Domingues and Costa for many years and appreciate their numerous contributions to elevating radiological imaging in both Brazil and South America. *Magnetic Resonance Imaging Clinics of North America* has a global outreach, and it is an honor for us to be able to recruit these two outstanding Guest Editors. I also wish to express my gratitude to all of the article authors. Their contributions are extremely well written and beautifully illustrated. Thank you again for all of your tireless efforts in creating such an excellent issue of *Magnetic Resonance Imaging Clinics of North America*.

Suresh K. Mukherji, MD, MBA, FACR
Department of Radiology
Michigan State University
Michigan State University Health Team
846 Service Road
East Lansing, MI 48824, USA

*E-mail address:*
mukherji@rad.msu.edu

Magn Reson Imaging Clin N Am 26 (2018) xiii
https://doi.org/10.1016/j.mric.2018.08.002

mri.theclinics.com

# Preface

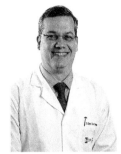

Roberto Côrtes Domingues, MD    Flávia Martins Costa, MD, PhD

*Editors*

## ACKNOWLEDGMENT FROM DR CÔRTES DOMINGUES

In the last few years, we have seen new techniques and approaches introduced into the field of musculoskeletal MR imaging. This issue focuses on topics that have been making a significant impact on the care of patients with pathologies involving the musculoskeletal system. The contributors are all prominent individuals who are actively involved in promoting the advancement of MR imaging, and who have done an excellent job describing the use of whole-body MR imaging for assessing pathologies that can present a systemic involvement of the musculoskeletal system, such as oncologic (metastasis, multiple myeloma), inflammatory, and congenital processes. They approach the application of functional sequences, including diffusion-weighted imaging and dynamic contrast-enhanced sequences, and show further advances in the role of MR imaging, such as an increase in the sensitivity and specificity of oncology lesion detection and characterization; detection and quantification of inflammation and structural damage in inflammatory diseases; therapy response evaluation; and the use of quantitative metrics parameters. There are still other interesting topics, such as the assessment of the potential of fusing of real-time ultrasound spatial registration with previously acquired musculoskeletal MR imaging, in order to guide tumor biopsies and other procedures; MR neurography; MR imaging of fetal musculoskeletal disorders, when ultrasound yields equivocal results; as well as the experience of our colleagues using state-of-the-art wide-bore MR imaging scanners on high-performance athletes at the Rio 2016 Olympics and Paralympics Games.

Besides all that, the articles are beautifully illustrated and will certainly encourage radiologists to utilize these tools in their daily practice.

I would like to express my thankfulness to Suresh Mukherji for the privilege of having been chosen and of entrusting me with this project.

I look at this with pride and thank my colleagues from DASA, particularly Flávia Costa, MD, PhD, coeditor, and Flávia Paiva Lopes, MD, PhD, who were deeply involved in this making.

I want to dedicate this conquest to my parents, José e Marília, who dedicated their lives to my education and that of my brothers, Romeu Domingues, MD, and Rômulo Domingues, MD, with whom I have had the privilege of working.

I would also like to express my heartfelt thanks to my wife, Marisa Domingues, MD, for her priceless support.

## ACKNOWLEDGMENT FROM DR MARTINS COSTA

MR imaging with advanced techniques has emerged in the last decade owing to the development of high-resolution scanners, specialized coils, variable pulse sequences, and postprocessing techniques that enable the detection of discrete changes that are not routinely seen with other methods.

The development of high-resolution anatomy images with dynamic and functional analyses has proven to be an essential tool to assess many disorders, ranging from sports injuries to oncologic diseases.

This special issue aims to discuss the applicability of these new advances in musculoskeletal imaging and to highlight its potential for precise diagnosis, adequate management, and follow-up treatment of several pathologies in different specialties.

I hope that these articles can be of special use not only by musculoskeletal radiologists but also by orthopedists, oncologists, obstetricians, rheumatologists, and hematologists.

I thank and congratulate the partnership of authors involved, and especially Dr Roberto Domingues and Dr Flávia Paiva, who provided the opportunity to highlight advanced diagnostic imaging methods in musculoskeletal.

Toward this goal, the reader will find valuable and enough information to appreciate the utility behind advanced imaging techniques as well as the current application and navigate into the future directions of MR imaging in musculoskeletal disorders.

Roberto Côrtes Domingues, MD
Clínica de Diagnóstico por Imagem (CDPI)/DASA
Centro Médico BarraShopping
CDPI, Avenida das Américas
4666, sala 301B
Barra da Tijuca
Rio de Janeiro
RJ CEP: 22640-102, Brazil

Flávia Martins Costa, MD, PhD
Clínica de Diagnóstico por Imagem (CDPI)/DASA
Centro Médico BarraShopping
CDPI, Avenida das Américas
4666, sala 301B
Barra da Tijuca
Rio de Janeiro
RJ CEP: 22640-102, Brazil

*E-mail addresses:*
roberto.domingues.ext@dasamed.com.br
(R.C. Domingues)
flavia26rio@hotmail.com (F.M. Costa)

# Quantitative Whole-Body Diffusion-Weighted MR Imaging

Ricardo Donners, MD[a], Matthew Blackledge, PhD, BSc, MSc[b],
Nina Tunariu, MD, MRCP, FRCR[b,c],
Christina Messiou, MD, BMedSci, BMBS, MRCP, FRCR[b,c],
Elmar M. Merkle, MD[a], Dow-Mu Koh, MD, MRCP, FRCR[b,c,*]

## KEYWORDS

• Quantitative • Whole body • Diffusion • DWI • MR Imaging

## KEY POINTS

- Whole-body diffusion-weighted MRI has emerged as a powerful diagnostic tool for disease detection and staging mainly used in systemic bone disease.
- The large field-of-view functional imaging technique highlights cellular tumor and suppresses normal tissue signal, allowing quantification of an estimate of total disease burden, summarized as the total diffusion volume (tDV), as well as global apparent diffusion coefficient (gADC) measurements.
- Both tDV and gADC have been shown to be repeatable quantitative parameters that indicate tumor heterogeneity and treatment effects, thus potential, noninvasive, imaging biomarkers informing on disease prognosis and therapy response.

## INTRODUCTION

Whole-body diffusion-weighted MRI (WB-DWI) has emerged as a powerful diagnostic tool. It was first described for clinical imaging in 2004 by Takahara and colleagues[1] and remains a subject of eager research, because its quantitative potential is yet to be fully exploited. The principles of body DWI are discussed in existing literature and are beyond the scope of this review.[2–4] DWI is a functional MRI technique, which visualizes differences in water mobility. Higher cellularity and microstructural organization in tissues are associated with greater impeded movement of water molecules, which is exploited by DWI to generate image contrast between tissues. The degree of impeded water diffusion can be quantified by the apparent diffusion coefficient (ADC), derived from monoexponential fitting of the signal decay observed at increasing diffusion weightings (b-values). The ADC value has been shown to be inversely correlated to cellularity, making it a potentially noninvasive, quantitative imaging biomarker with good measurement repeatability and reproducibility, facilitating multicenter investigations.[5–10]

Disclosure Statement: No disclosures.
[a] Department of Radiology, University Hospital Basel, Spitalstrasse 21, Basel 4031, Switzerland; [b] Cancer Research UK Cancer Imaging Centre, The Institute of Cancer Research, 15 Cotswold Road, Sutton SM2 5NG, UK; [c] Department of Radiology, Royal Marsden Hospital, Downs Road, Sutton SM2 5PT, UK
* Corresponding author. Department of Radiology, Downs Road, Sutton SM2 5PT, UK.
*E-mail address:* dowmukoh@icr.ac.uk

In this article, the authors

- Review the relative merits of quantitative versus qualitative WB-DWI;
- Discuss specific image acquisition technique for quantitative WB-DWI assessment;
- Survey the quantitative parameters that can be derived from a typical WB-DWI study and highlight their applicability for disease assessment; and
- Appraise the current and evolving applications of quantitative WB-DWI.

### Qualitative Versus Quantitative DWI

Although subjective, qualitative visual assessment of the signal intensities on DWI and the contrast between presumed normal and abnormal tissue remains the mainstay for DWI interpretations. Most clinical DWI examinations are optimized to highlight cellular disease while suppressing the signal from normal tissues. Using such qualitative approach, the radiologist arrives at a diagnostic conclusion by the cognitive appraisal of the disease signal intensity and morphology on multiple MRI sequences.

However, there are limitations to qualitative assessment on WB-DWI:

1. The observed tissue signal intensity depends on both water mobility and the T2-relaxation time of tissue. Lesions with very long T2 relaxation times (eg, cystic or necrotic tissue) may demonstrate high signal intensity on the DWI and are mistaken for cellular disease.
2. The signal intensity of different solid lesions on DWI may be similar, making it difficult to characterize lesions based on their signal intensity alone.
3. When performing DWI to assess treatment response, changes in lesion signal intensity may be difficult to appreciate due to differences in machine signal adjustment and display between studies. The human eye may also fail to pick up small, but quantifiable differences in signal intensity as a result of treatment response, despite a significant increase in the quantitative ADC value.
4. Tumors within an individual can be nonuniform and may respond heterogeneously to treatment. Although qualitative assessment can help to identify such differences, it cannot provide objective measurements of such variations.

Applying quantitative WB-DWI can overcome many of these shortcomings. Studies using organ- or region-specific DWI have shown that the quantitative mean or median ADC values are robust and can be applied for disease assessment.[5,6,8,11,12] The roles for ADC measurement will be discussed in detail with other quantitative parameters in the context of WB-DWI.

## IMAGING TECHNIQUE FOR QUANTITATIVE WB-DWI

Hardware requirements and patient set-up are identical between qualitative and quantitative WB-DWI. Both 1.5-T and 3-T scanners may be used. At present, the benefits of imaging at 3 T are outweighed by its challenges, namely, increase in artifacts due to eddy and dielectric currents, as well as inhomogeneous fat suppression, making 1.5 T the field strength of choice.[13,14] MRI scanner hardware should support the range of table movement required for anatomic whole body coverage. Strategies to minimize bulk patient movement (eg, emptying of urinary bladder before examination and careful patient instructions) should be used to guarantee optimal data quality for quantification.

For WB-DWI acquisition, a free-breathing fat-suppressed single-shot echo-planar imaging technique is most commonly used. Axial DWI is performed with 5-mm slices as a "vertex-to-toe" examination or, more commonly, as a "skull-vault to mid-thigh" study analogous to the coverage on PET-computed tomography (CT) with fludeoxyglucose F 18. The diffusion-weighted images are acquired as contiguous 20- to 50-cm stacks, each taking approximately 4 to 6 minutes, depending on stack length, protocol, and MR platform. In contrast to single-area DWI, inversion recovery fat suppression is preferred over chemical saturation for more homogenous results over the large field-of-view.[15] The number and scale of $b$-values applied depends on the quantification intended. As a minimum for ADC quantification, two $b$-values should be used, with the lower $b$-value chosen between 50 and 100 s/mm$^2$ (to suppress vascular perfusion effects) and the higher $b$-value between 800 and 1000 s/mm$^2$. However, for optimal quantification of disease before and after treatment, a protocol using three $b$-values is advantageous, with the additional $b$-value in the range of 500 to 600 s/mm$^2$. This allows better characterization of responding posttreatment disease, which typically has higher ADC values.

To ensure reliable and repeatable quantitative measurements from WB-DWI, the imaging acquisition should maximize image signal-to-noise ratio (SNR) within the scan duration and avoid artifacts, such as chemical shift, Nyquist ghosting, eddy currents, image distortion, susceptibility, and motion artifacts. A detailed description of technical optimization is beyond the scope of this review and the reader should refer to prior publications for specific discussions.[15,16]

In most institutions, WB-DWI is combined with conventional anatomic axial T1- and T2-weighted sequences. However, when assessing bone disease, sagittal T1-and T2-weighted images of the spine are also acquired.[17] Gradient-echo DIXON T1-weighted images can supply additional information, allowing the semiquantitative relative water and fat fraction maps to be derived.[18] Typical images from a quantitative WB-DWI study for metastatic bone disease are shown in **Fig. 1**. **Table 1** shows the standard acquisition parameters to achieve this at 1.5 T on current major vendor MR systems.

## QUANTITATIVE MEASUREMENT ON WB-DWI AND WB-MR IMAGING

WB-DWI enables the quantification of the disease volume and associated ADC from the same

examination. When performing WB-DWI, the ADC is usually calculated using monoexponential fitting to 2 or 3 b-value DWI data, which assumes a Gaussian distribution of water displacement. However, water diffusion in the body has been shown to be non-Gaussian and nonmonoexponential. The application of more complex diffusion models taking into account the nonmonoexponential behavior of water diffusion requires multiple b-values with good image SNR.[19] This significantly increases the imaging time, rendering it nonfeasible for wider clinical application, although this has been investigated in research settings.[20] Other semiquantitative measurements, such as relative fat fraction (rFF) and relative water fraction (rWF), are obtained from the contemporaneous DIXON T1-weighted imaging.[21]

## Diffusion Volumes (Including Total Diffusion Volumes)

On high b-value images, cellular tumor shows greater signal than the attenuated surrounding

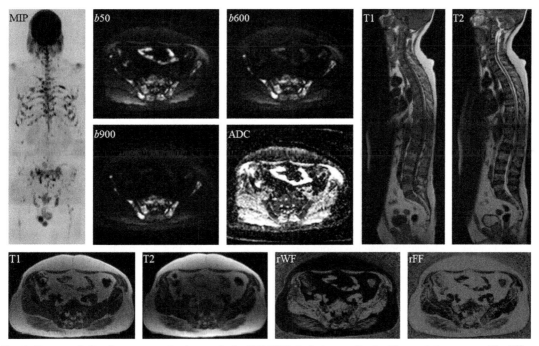

Fig. 1. Representative images acquired as part of a WB-DWI study in a patient with prostate cancer with diffuse bone metastasis. The MIP (maximum intensity projection) image derived from the axial b900 images is inverted to facilitate comparison with PET and bone scans. On the DWI images (b50, b600, b900), cellular lesions show persistent high-signal intensity with increasing b-value indicating impeded water mobility, whereas the increasing suppression of background signal (eg, signal from bowel loops) can be appreciated. The ADC map is calculated from monoexponential fitting of all three b-value images. T1-and T2-weighted axial images are acquired for morphologic assessment. The rFF (relative fat fraction) and rWF (relative water fraction) images are calculated from the DIXON T1-weighted images. The rFF image shows subtotal replacement of fatty marrow of the pelvis, with corresponding nonphysiologic, high water content within skeleton on the rWF image. For the assessment of bone disease, T1 and T2 sagittal images of the spine are also acquired to aid lesion and to assess complications such as vertebral fractures.

**Table 1**
**WB-MR imaging parameters at 1.5 T on MR systems from major vendors**

| Protocol | Siemens Healthcare Avanto | GE Healthcare Signa | Philips Healthcare Intera |
|---|---|---|---|
| FOV (cm) | 380 × 380 | 440 × 440 | 400 × 280 |
| Matrix size | 150 × 256 | 128 × 88 | 128 × 96 |
| TR | 14,000 | 6625 | 8322 |
| TE | 72 | 64.6 | 70 |
| Echo-planar imaging factor | 150 | | 37 |
| Parallel imaging factor | 2 | | 2 |
| Number of signal averaged | 4 | 3 | 4 ($b$ = 0), 2 ($b$ = 1000) |
| Section thickness in mm | 5 | 8 | 5 |
| Direction of motion probing gradients | 3-scan trace | | Tetrahedral encoding |
| Receiver bandwidth | 1800 Hz/pixel | | 7757 (water-fat shift/pixel) |
| Fat suppression | STIR | STIR | STIR |
| b-value (s/mm$^2$) | 0–100 and 600–1000 | Single $b$-value, 600 | 0, 1000 |
| Acquisition time per station | 4 min 30 s | 1 min 28 s | 4 min 2 s |

*Abbreviations:* FOV, field-of-view; STIR, short tau inversion recovery; TE, echo time; TR, repetition time.

normal tissue. The resulting high lesion-to-background contrast facilitates tumor segmentation. The aggregated volume of all segmented high signal intensity disease on high $b$-value DWI is the total diffusion volume (tDV), which reflects the disease burden across the whole body.

Emerging software using a signal intensity–based algorithm allows semiautomated segmentation of the tDV to be undertaken. Such software typically applies computed ultrahigh $b$-values (>1000 s/mm$^2$) exceeding the acquired $b$-values, to maximize lesion-to-background contrast and increase suppression of the background tissue signal.[22,23] This approach increases lesion conspicuity and ultimately facilitates disease segmentation. The multistep image processing to achieve this has been described in detail by Blackledge and colleagues.[23] The multiple volumes of interest (VOIs) defined by this process can be manipulated, corrected, and dismissed by the reporting radiologist to achieve a final tDV that reflects the overall disease burden, excluding erroneous high signal intensity volumes unrelated to disease or due to artifacts. The tDV calculated using semiautomatic WB-DWI segmentation has high inter- and intraobserver agreement.[23,24] Based on repeatability measurements, a 40% to 50% reduction in tDV would indicate response to therapy.[23,25] Pre- and posttreatment tDV can be directly compared: a decrease in tDV is linked to therapy response, because of the associated reduction of high

cellular, hence high signal tumor volume. By contrast, a tDV increase may translate into nonresponding or progressive disease (**Fig. 2**).[23]

However, there are potential drawbacks to defining tDV based on diffusion signal characteristics alone. High signal intensity on the high $b$-value images due to T2 shine-through effect will be part of an automatic segmentation. In contrast, posttherapeutic lesions with normalized signal intensity on high $b$-value images but containing viable, cellular tumor may not be included. For these reasons, image correlation with the ADC maps will aid the reading radiologist in disease interpretation and the final definition of VOI. However, this approach may be associated with greater subjectivity and can result in larger measurement variability than a largely automated process.

A second approach of generating a representative disease volume is by the manual delineation of multiple lesions. This is undertaken by simultaneous assessment of the anatomic T1-and T2-weighted images, $b$-value images, as well as ADC maps. This method may tackle the issue of potential false-positive and false-negative signal representing malignant disease on the high $b$-value images. Obviously, manual segmentation is time-consuming, operator-dependent, and not feasible in daily practice for patients with extensive disease. One approach of compromise is to the perform volume segmentation of 5 target lesions

**Pre-treatment**            **Post-treatment**

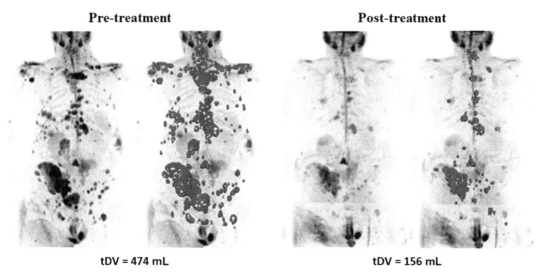

tDV = 474 mL                 tDV = 156 mL

**Fig. 2.** Semiautomatic segmentation of the tDV in a responding 61-year-old patient with prostate cancer with bony, hepatic, and lymphatic metastasis. The left figure demonstrates the tumor burden on a maximum intensity projection WB-DW image and the corresponding, red color–coded semiautomatically segmented tDV before therapy. After effective treatment, a 67% decrease in tDV is observed, shown on the right, indicating treatment response.

across the body instead of total disease volume segmentation. This method has been shown to give a similar assessment of the global treatment response compared with the tDV in patients with metastatic bone disease.[25] Target lesion segmentation can be more readily implemented in clinical practice, because it enables quantitative analyses to be undertaken in centers without access to sophisticated software or significant physics support (**Fig. 3**).

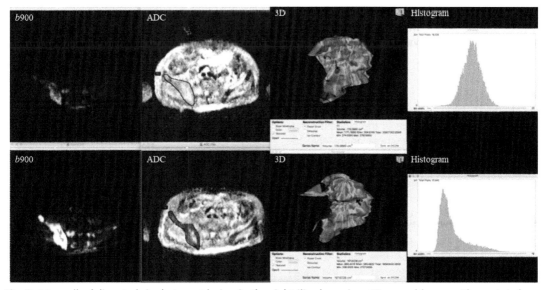

**Fig. 3.** Manually delineated single target lesion in the right iliac bone in a 67-year-old man with prostate bone metastases, with the corresponding 3-dimensional reconstruction of the lesion to derive disease volume and associated ADC histogram. The interface of open-access postprocessing software is shown. The lower row shows the pretreatment and the upper row the posttreatment images. A decrease in lesion signal intensity is observed on the posttreatment b900 images, with a visually perceptible increase in its ADV value. By quantification, the lesion volume has decreased 10% after treatment, associated with an 85% increase in ADC value and a change in the shape of the ADC histogram.

### ADC Values (Including Global ADC Values)

Using the computed tDV or volume of target lesions, the VOIs can be transferred onto the corresponding ADC map to calculate the global ADC (gADC) or target lesion ADC. The gADC specifically refers to the ADC value derived from the tDV. From the histogram distribution of the ADCs, specific histogram parameters such as the mean, median, minimum (min), maximum (max), percentiles, skewness, and kurtosis can be derived and recorded.

### Mean and median ADC

The mean and median ADC values are the most commonly used gADC parameters, the latter being more robust in skewed distributions and with outliers. The mean and median ADC aids disease characterization. Furthermore, an increase in the mean or median ADC value correlates with therapy response in multiple cancer types.[26–28] The mean and median ADC values have also been shown to be highly robust with good measurement repeatability and reproducibility.[6,7,24,29] In a well-conducted serial MRI study, a change in ADC value greater than 30% is unlikely to be due to measurement errors and can be ascribed to treatment effects. Although both parameters provide useful summary values, they do not inform on tumor heterogeneity. In particular, heterogeneous tumors containing significant necrosis, edema, and cystic and hemorrhagic components may mask mean or median ADC increase resulting from treatment response.[19] For these reasons, other ADC histogram parameters described later may provide additional information that informs on tumor and response heterogeneity.

### Minimal ADC value

By hypothesis, intralesional voxels with the lowest ADC value will include areas of the highest cellularity; hence, potentially the most aggressive tumor.[19,30] This association may render the min ADC more sensitive for disease detection and staging.[31,32] In the posttherapeutic setting, the min ADC may indicate remaining viable tumor in treated lesions because residual, high cellular tumor is expected to have a lower ADC than treatment-related cell death or inflammatory changes. A superiority of the min ADC for response assessment compared with the mean ADC has been reported in osteosarcomas.[33] In an interlesion comparison, lesions with higher min ADC showed greater cell kill, whereas lower values identified viable tumor. However, the min ADC is not without limitations, the main one being very poor measurement repeatability due to its sensitivity to image noise and signal variations.[34]

Therefore, it is difficult to recommend its application in the wider clinical setting. In addition, the min ADC is unhelpful for the characterization of bone metastases since the ADC of normal, fatty bone marrow is lower than the ADC in metastasis.[7]

### Maximum ADC value

By contrast to the min ADC value, voxels of the highest ADC may indicate the least cellular tissue within the tumor. Response to therapies translates into cell death, decreased cellularity, and increased water diffusion, thus increasing ADC values. As a result, the max ADC values may help to identify areas within tumors that show a good response to treatment. This might be especially helpful in the first follow-up after initializing a new therapy. Although the min ADC and median ADC may not significantly alter in an early stage of treatment, an increase of the max ADC (especially at values $>1.60–2.00 \times 10^{-3}$ mm$^2$/s) may indicate cell death. This may also be applicable showing cell kill where there is a differential response to treatment (ie, some lesions show cell death as response to treatment while others do not).

One has to keep in mind, however, that some forms of treatment, such as vascular-growth inhibitors, may initially lead to impediment of water diffusion resulting in an ADC decrease.[16] Furthermore, preexisting cystic or necrotic components will raise the max ADC and potentially remain unchanged during the course of treatment, thus masking potential therapeutic effects.

By contrast with min ADC, max ADC shows better measurement repeatability but is still less robust than the mean or median values.[34] Not surprisingly, extremes of the histogram are easily affected by outliers, resulting in higher variability and poorer repeatability. For these reasons, the use of low and high percentiles may improve these shortcomings.[34]

### Percentiles

Percentiles represent ADC values below or above which a proportion of the analyzed voxels are found. For example, 10% of all voxels will be lower than the 10th percentile ADC value. Promising better reproducibility, percentiles can be used analogously to the min ADC and max ADC: low percentiles (eg, 5th percentile) represent low ADC values and high cellularity, whereas high percentiles (eg, 95th percentile) represent high ADC values and low cellularity.[34]

### Skewness

The skewness reflects the asymmetry of the ADC distribution. Positive skewness translates into a histogram with a large left shoulder, with most of the lower ADC values typical for untreated solid disease. Vice versa, a negative skewness translates into a large proportion of higher ADC values, which is often observed in treated or responding disease. In a therapy setting, a decrease in skewness, describing a shift from a "left- to right-shouldered" histogram is associated with cell death, that is, therapy response (**Fig. 4**A). In a mouse model with histologically confirmed disease response of sarcomas, DWI 24 hours posttreatment showed negative skewness, whereas the nontreated control group showed a positive skewness increase.[35] Similar observations have been made in clinical studies including WB-DWI.[23]

### Kurtosis

The kurtosis represents the "peakedness" of the histogram. A large kurtosis resembles a sharp peak of the ADC distribution values. In the course of treatment, a flattening of the peak (decrease of kurtosis) has been observed with response to treatment (**Fig. 4**B).[36]

Kurtosis and skewness are expected to behave in a coherent pattern with treatment response. In lymphoma, both parameters had a better diagnostic performance in response assessment than mean and median ADC.[36] However, kurtosis, as well as skewness, show high inter- and intraobserver variance in repeatability because of its high sensitivity to outliers, which may limit their use in clinical practice.[24] Nonetheless, a decrease in kurtosis and skewness may alert the onset of therapeutic effects, providing insights into early treatment response.

A typical application of quantitative histogram parameters for therapeutic response evaluation is shown in Fig. 5.

### Relative Fat and Water Fractions

Developments in MRI in 1984 introduced the DIXON MRI technique, which uses in and opposed-phase T1-weighted images to calculate the fat- and water-only images. From these, the semiquantitative whole-body rFF and rWF images are obtained.[37] The fat content of normal, adult marrow is circa 80% and increases with age.[38] Infiltrative, usually highly cellular tumor replaces the fat cells and is associated with a reduction in the rFF and increase in the rWF. By comparison with malignancies, red marrow has a higher fat content of circa 40%, thus producing significantly higher rFF and rWF than cancer.[21] Hence, rFF and rWF can be used to detect and characterize bone disease. Furthermore, changes in the rFF and rWF can be observed in treatment response (**Fig. 6**), thus these may also be potential response biomarkers.[39,40]

## CLINICAL APPLICATIONS OF QUANTITATIVE WB-DWI

Quantitative WB-DWI can aid disease detection and characterization, as well as staging and response evaluation in diseases with systemic manifestation. However, because of the potential challenges of implementing the quantitative analysis, the approach is not yet mainstream in clinical practice. Nonetheless, it is increasingly used, particularly at research centers. The published literature provides the largest amount of information on its application in systemic bone and bone marrow diseases.

### Evaluation of Diseases that Affect the Bone Marrow

The mean ADC values of normal, fatty marrow are low, ranging from 0.2 to $0.5 \times 10^{-3}$ mm$^2$/s. Malignant bone marrow typically displays values between 0.7 and $1.0 \times 10^{-3}$ mm$^2$/s. Osteoporotic fractures, as well as inflammatory changes, will produce ADC values larger than

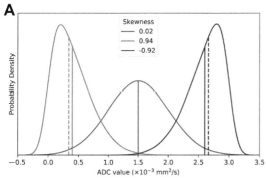
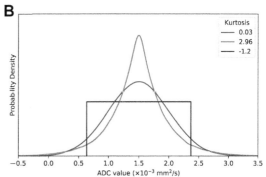

**Fig. 4.** (*A*) Skewness. The green graph is positively skewed, representing a "right-shouldered" histogram; the blue graph is negatively skewed, representing a "left-shouldered" histogram. (*B*) Kurtosis. The green graph shows a leptokurtosis (kurtosis >0), indicating a sharp peak, whereas the blue graph represents a platykurtosis (kurtosis <0). Dotted lines represent the median, continous lines show the mean, the red graph is an example for a graph that is not skewed and shows (almost) no kurtosis.

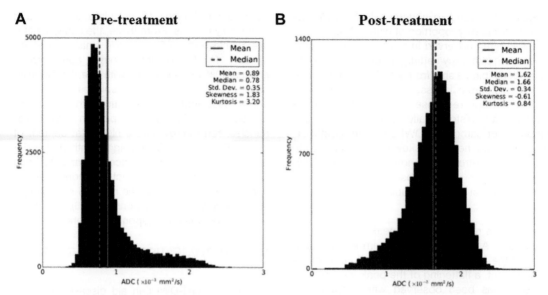

**Fig. 5.** tDV-derived global ADC histograms before and after treatment. The histograms belong to the same patient shown in **Fig. 3.** After treatment, the mean and median gADC increased. This was associated with a decrease in skewness, as seen by the shift from a left- shouldered to a right-shouldered histogram, and also a decrease in the kurtosis value.

$1.0 \times 10^{-3}$ mm²/s.[41] In one study, a cutoff value of $0.77 \times 10^{-3}$ mm²/s was suggested for differentiating normal versus pathologic bone marrow, with higher values indicating pathology.[42] Differences in mean ADC, without statistical significance, were shown between metastatic bone diseases arising from different primary tumors.[7]

### Metastatic bone disease

The skeleton is the most common site of metastatic disease, with prostate and breast cancer accounting for approximately 80% of all cases.[43] Bone metastasis confined to the bone marrow are considered "nonmeasurable" according to the Response Evaluation Criteria in Solid Tumors (RECIST) using conventional imaging.[44,45] WB-DWI can overcome the limitations of conventional CT, MR, and radionuclide imaging, and has been established as one of the most sensitive detection tools.[46,47] Data on quantitative measurements for lesion characterization using WB-DWI are beginning to emerge: a recent article describes a cutoff value of $0.872 \times 10^{-3}$ mm²/s to distinguish hemangiomas from active malignant deposits—the latter showing lower ADC values.[48]

Currently, the most useful emerging application of quantitative WB-DWI is for the assessment of treatment response in metastatic bone disease. In patients with metastatic castration-resistant prostate carcinoma (mCRPC), a significant tDV decrease of 41.1% to 50% was shown

in therapy responders when comparing follow-up and baseline imaging.[23,25] A 40% tDV decrease is currently being investigated as a potential threshold for identifying responders to therapy. The inverse correlation between disease volume and therapy response was also found when analyzing 5 target lesions, instead of the entire volume of skeletal metastasis,[25] an approach that is more easily translatable into current clinical practice. In addition, the pretreatment tDV value was found to be prognostic, with an inverse correlation between tDV and overall survival: patients with higher tDV showed an increased risk of death and shorter overall survival.[49]

Although current guidelines for response assessment in solid tumors fail to address metastatic bone disease, ADC increase in bone metastases responding to treatment was described as early as in 2002.[45,50] More recently, a significant increase in WB-DWI–derived median gADC and decreasing gADC skewness and kurtosis were observed among responders with prostate bone metastases.[23,25] In addition, serum prostate-specific antigen levels decreased with gADC increase in responders.[51] However, when only 5 selected target lesions were used for ADC analysis instead of the gADC measurement, the median ADC derived failed to show a significant inverse correlation with disease response, although a trend was observed ($P = .056$).[25] Nonetheless, this more practical approach is

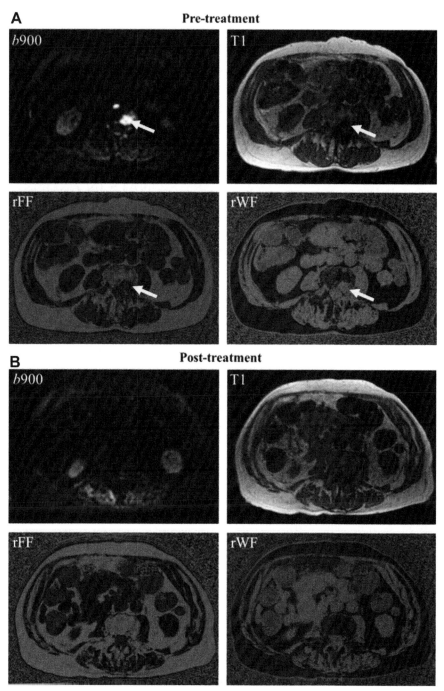

**Fig. 6.** Relative water and fat fractions in a 79-year-old man with advanced prostate cancer and vertebral metastasis responding to treatment. (*A*) Before treatment, the bone lesion (*yellow arrows*) shows impeded diffusion on the −b900 DWI image; it appears hypointense on the T1-weighted image, and shows low relative fat fraction and relatively high water fraction, compared with the adjacent normal yellow bone marrow. (*B*) Following successful therapy, note that the lesion has regressed and there is a return of normal marrow fat to the previous metastatic site.

being investigated in ongoing studies, which aim to provide more accurate segmentation of viable disease within the target lesions to ensure reliable ADC values.

One method used by some radiologists and researchers to evaluate the response of metastatic bone disease is to measure changes in the percentile values with treatment. One approach is to compare the 95th percentile value before and after treatment to observe for a significant increase as a sign of response. Another approach is to use an a priori threshold (eg, ADC of 1.5–1.6 × $10^{-3}$ mm$^2$/s) and quantify the percentage of voxels above this threshold value before and after treatment. The a priori threshold (eg, 1.5–1.6 × $10^{-3}$ mm$^2$/s) is selected as likely associated with cell death but requires further biological and clinical validation.

More recently, histologic validation of DWI, ADC, and rFF measurements has been evaluated in patients with metastatic prostate bone disease who underwent bone biopsies.[52] In this study, the median ADC and normalized DWI signal were found to be significantly higher and the median rFF significantly lower in bone metastases compared with nonmetastatic bone ($P<.001$). Furthermore, the median ADC and rFF were significantly lower and the median normalized DWI signal was significantly higher in the regions where the biopsies revealed tumor cells compared with areas that showed no detectable tumor (0.898 × $10^{-3}$ mm$^2$/s vs 1.617 × $10^{-3}$ mm$^2$/s; 11.5% vs 62%; 5.3 vs 2.3, respectively; $P<.001$). In addition, the tumor cellularity was found to be inversely correlated with ADC and rFF and positively correlated with the normalized DWI signal ($P<.001$).

Although the aforementioned data are largely derived from studies in mCRPC, similar methods may be applied in other entities with metastatic spread such as breast and lung cancers. WB-DWI also allows the evaluation and quantification of any soft tissue component, as currently applied for lymphoma and peritoneal disease.[36,53]

### Multiple myeloma

Multiple myeloma is a plasma cell malignancy potentially involving the whole skeleton. WB-MRI, which includes DWI, has become the diagnostic gold standard for lesion detection and disease surveillance, with a reported sensitivity and specificity of 90% and 93%, respectively. This is also linked to the quantitative potential of DWI.[54,55]

WB-DWI allows quantification of the total number of focal lesions, which is the strongest adverse prognostic factor in smoldering multiple myeloma.[56] In comparison to metastatic bone disease, disseminated marrow infiltration is common and may occur in isolation or in combination with focal lesions. In patients with only diffuse marrow infiltration, the gADC may offer greater potential than tDV as a response biomarker (**Fig. 7**).

An increase in ADC has been associated with therapy response in myeloma marrow.[57] The mean ADC is the most promising parameter, showing a 19.8% to 69.3% increase in responding and 3.3% to 7.8% decrease in nonresponding patients.[29,40,58] The wide range of ADC increase may be related to differences in study population, treatment administered, DWI technique, and imaging time points. A significant increase between pre- and posttreatment imaging in responders was also demonstrated for the median and the 75th and 90th percentiles. The 10th and 25th percentiles also increased during treatment while the skewness decreased, but each without statistical significance. In nonresponders, all percentiles decreased, while skewness and kurtosis increased.[29] An inverse correlation between ADC and prognostic laboratory serum markers (namely the M-gradient) pre- and posttreatment was shown, verifying ADC as an imaging biomarker.[54,58] Furthermore, in one study, the rFF was shown to significantly increase in focal, responding myeloma lesions with excellent repeatability and was found to be superior to the mean ADC for assessing treatment response.[40]

### Disease Screening

Patients with neurofibromatosis type I (NFI) and type II (NFII), as well as those with schwannomatosis, have a high risk for developing multiple peripheral nerve sheath tumors (PNST), which can undergo malignant transformation. Prior studies have shown the benefit of whole-body MRI for evaluating total disease burden in patients with NFI und NFII, using fat-suppressed T2-weighted sequences,[59] suggesting a similar result for a WB-DWI-derived tDV. Although qualitative WB-DWI interpretation allows lesion identification lacking specificity, quantitative min and mean ADC values can differentiate PNST from cystic lesions using min ADC and mean ADC.[60] However, PNST values showed a large variance, most likely due to different levels of cellularity, that is, tumor heterogeneity. The potential benefits of tDV and gADC in further musculoskeletal settings are yet to be explored.

### FUTURE DEVELOPMENT

Although disease detection will continue to largely rely on qualitative DWI image assessment, quantitative WB-DWI for disease characterization, therapy response evaluation, and disease prognostication is likely to become increasingly important. The current thresholds for significant changes in tDV and gADC are informed by

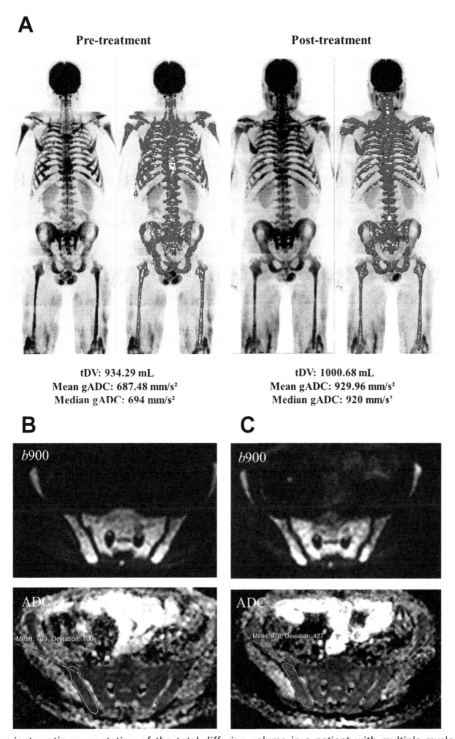

Fig. 7. Semiautomatic segmentation of the total diffusion volume in a patient with multiple myeloma with diffuse bone marrow infiltration. (A) The left figure demonstrates the tumor burden on a maximum intensity projection WB-DW image and the corresponding, red color–coded semiautomatically segmented total diffusion tDV before therapy. The right figures show the equivalent images obtained after chemotherapy. Note that although there is little relative change in tDV, the calculated gADC parameters have increased substantially in keeping with treatment response. Representative axial b900 and ADC maps from the patient (B) before and (C) after treatment are as shown.

measurement repeatability. However, well-conducted clinical trials are needed to determine the biologically relevant thresholds that will identify patients who will benefit from a specific treatment. Establishing the optimum thresholds for differentiating responders from nonresponders will help to establish tDV and gADC as response biomarkers in malignant bone disease.[49]

At the moment, there is also a lack of sophisticated image processing tools to segment and quantify disease across the body from the WB-DWI examinations. The continuing development of postprocessing software, allowing "one-click" lesion segmentation for tDV and gADC calculations, would address the current time-consuming and tedious image analysis necessary for quantitative analysis, thus making quantitative WB-DWI more widely accessible for patient benefit. Quantitative WB-DWI also offers great potential for artificial intelligence and machine learning principles, and efforts from research institutions and commercial companies are being directed to provide innovative image analysis solutions.

Another advantage of WB-DWI that is yet to be explored is the potential for evaluating intra- and interlesion heterogeneity. In untreated tumors, heterogeneity is caused by genetic plasticity leading to differences in phenotype, which influences their sensitivity to treatments. Information derived from histogram parameters from multiple tumors on WB-DWI can provide insights into inter- and intratumor heterogeneity by identifying regions that deviate from most of the disease within patients.

Differences in tumor response to therapy can lead to further tumor heterogeneity. This may become more important with emerging targeted therapies, which may be expensive and should ideally be discontinued on evidence of drug resistance.[61] The extended use of ADC histogram analysis has the potential to provide insights into the development of drug resistance by the early identification of nonresponding lesions or differential response to treatment (**Figs. 8** and **9**). As WB-DWI is able to visualize multiple sites of disease at the same time, it has the potential to be a noninvasive and potentially therapy-altering, noninvasive "histopathological" method, based on the characterization of the imaging phenotype.[62] Further gains may be made by applying other image analysis techniques (eg, texture analysis) to

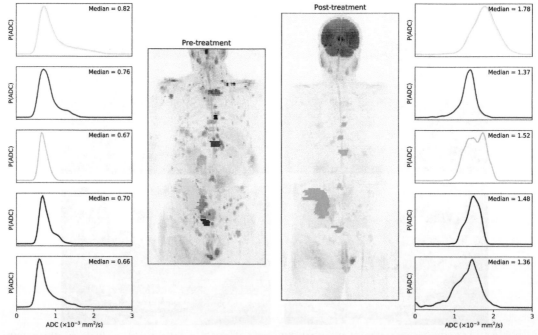

**Fig. 8.** Uniform response of bone metastasis. The left figure shows 5 color-coded target lesions superimposed on an inverted grayscale maximum intensity projection image derived from the *b*900 WB-DW pretreatment images, as well as the individual ADC histograms of each of the color-coded lesions on the far right. This example is taken from the same patient as in **Figs. 3** and **5**. In contrast to **Fig. 9**, all lesions showed a significant increase of median gADC and are all color coded as green and superimposed on the inverted grayscale maximum intensity projection *b*900 WB-DW image obtained posttreatment (*right figure*). The corresponding ADC histograms of the target lesions posttreatment are shown correspondingly on the far right. Also note the decrease in skewness and kurtosis of all 5 target lesions.

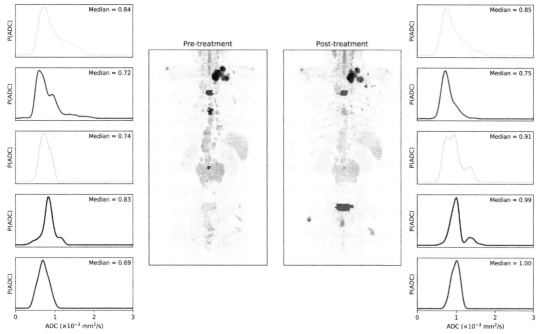

**Fig. 9.** Differential response of bone metastasis. The left figure shows 5 color-coded target lesions superimposed on an inverted grayscale maximum intensity projection image derived from the b900 WB-DW images before treatment. The corresponding gADC histograms of each color-coded lesion are shown on the far left. The right figure is the inverted grayscale maximum intensity projection image obtained following therapy, but the 5 target lesions are color coded as green (for responding) or red (for nonresponding) according to the degree of ADC increase after therapy. The posttreatment ADC histogram of the individual lesions is shown correspondingly in the far right. In this case, 3 of the 5 lesions responded to treatment by ADC measurement, but the other 2 did not, thus demonstrating intertumoral response heterogeneity.

the WB-DWI data to identify more potential imaging biomarkers.

Although WB-DWI has been proved feasible in expert centers, it is important for other centers to adopt best practice available, including establishing the measurement repeatability on their scanners to ensure data consistency and facilitate intercenter comparison.[63] Although the tDV and gADC are shown to be useful in systemic bone disease, the most reliable quantitative parameters across different diseases types need to be further defined.[63]

## SUMMARY

The potential of using DWI-derived biomarkers for evaluating treatment response in malignant bone disease is now driving the use of quantitative WB-DWI in both the clinical and research arenas. Emerging studies have established the duo quantitative parameters of tDV and gADC as potential response biomarkers. Further advances in image postprocessing software, potentially allowing "one-click" lesion segmentation across the whole body, will provide a simple and potentially

repeatable method for disease quantification. This will enable wider application of quantitative WB-DWI for patient disease management.

## ACKNOWLEDGMENTS

The authors would like to acknowledge the NIHR Biomedical Research Centre and NIHR Clinical Research Facility at the Royal Marsden Hospital/Institute of Cancer Research.

## REFERENCES

1. Takahara T, Imai Y, Yamashita T, et al. Diffusion weighted whole body imaging with background body signal suppression (DWIBS): technical improvement using free breathing, STIR and high resolution 3D display. Radiat Med 2004;22(4): 275–82.

2. Patterson DM, Padhani AR, Collins DJ. Technology insight: water diffusion MRI–a potential new biomarker of response to cancer therapy. Nat Clin Pract Oncol 2008;5(4):220–33.

3. Koh DM, Collins DJ. Diffusion-weighted MRI in the body: applications and challenges in oncology. AJR Am J Roentgenol 2007;188(6):1622–35.

4. Morone M, Bali MA, Tunariu N, et al. Whole-body MRI: current applications in oncology. AJR Am J Roentgenol 2017;209(6):W336–49.

5. Sadinski M, Medved M, Karademir I, et al. Short-term reproducibility of apparent diffusion coefficient estimated from diffusion-weighted MRI of the prostate. Abdom Imaging 2015;40(7):2523–8.

6. Koh DM, Blackledge M, Collins DJ, et al. Reproducibility and changes in the apparent diffusion coefficients of solid tumours treated with combretastatin A4 phosphate and bevacizumab in a two-centre phase I clinical trial. Eur Radiol 2009; 19(11):2728–38.

7. Messiou C, Collins DJ, Morgan VA, et al. Optimising diffusion weighted MRI for imaging metastatic and myeloma bone disease and assessing reproducibility. Eur Radiol 2011;21(8):1713–8.

8. Sun Y, Tong T, Cai S, et al. Apparent Diffusion Coefficient (ADC) value: a potential imaging biomarker that reflects the biological features of rectal cancer. PLoS One 2014;9(10):e109371.

9. Lambrecht M, Van Calster B, Vandecaveye V, et al. Integrating pretreatment diffusion weighted MRI into a multivariable prognostic model for head and neck squamous cell carcinoma. Radiother Oncol 2014;110(3):429–34.

10. Cui Y, Zhang XP, Sun YS, et al. Apparent diffusion coefficient: potential imaging biomarker for prediction and early detection of response to chemotherapy in hepatic metastases. Radiology 2008; 248(3):894–900.

11. Wang Y, Chen ZE, Yaghmai V, et al. Diffusion-weighted MR imaging in pancreatic endocrine tumors correlated with histopathologic characteristics. J Magn Reson Imaging 2011;33(5):1071–9.

12. Eiber M, Holzapfel K, Ganter C, et al. Whole-body MRI including diffusion-weighted imaging (DWI) for patients with recurring prostate cancer: technical feasibility and assessment of lesion conspicuity in DWI. J Magn Reson Imaging 2011;33(5): 1160–70.

13. Merkle EM, Dale BM, Paulson EK. Abdominal MR imaging at 3T. Magn Reson Imaging Clin N Am 2006;14(1):17–26.

14. Koh DM, Takahara T, Imai Y, et al. Practical aspects of assessing tumors using clinical diffusion-weighted imaging in the body. Magn Reson Med Sci 2007;6(4):211–24.

15. Koh DM, Blackledge M, Padhani AR, et al. Whole-body diffusion-weighted MRI: tips, tricks, and pitfalls. AJR Am J Roentgenol 2012;199(2):252–62.

16. Padhani AR, Liu G, Koh DM, et al. Diffusion-weighted magnetic resonance imaging as a cancer biomarker: consensus and recommendations. Neoplasia 2009;11(2):102–25.

17. Lecouvet FE, Simon M, Tombal B, et al. Whole-body MRI (WB-MRI) versus axial skeleton MRI (AS-MRI) to detect and measure bone metastases in prostate cancer (PCa). Eur Radiol 2010;20(12):2973–82.

18. Costelloe CM, Madewell JE, Kundra V, et al. Conspicuity of bone metastases on fast Dixon-based multisequence whole-body MRI: clinical utility per sequence. Magn Reson Imaging 2013;31(5): 669–75.

19. Le Bihan D. Apparent diffusion coefficient and beyond: what diffusion MR imaging can tell us about tissue structure. Radiology 2013;268(2):318–22.

20. Filli L, Wurnig MC, Luechinger R, et al. Whole-body intravoxel incoherent motion imaging. Eur Radiol 2015;25(7):2049–58.

21. Lee SH, Lee YH, Hahn S, et al. Fat fraction estimation of morphologically normal lumbar vertebrae using the two-point mDixon turbo spin-echo MRI with flexible echo times and multipeak spectral model of fat: Comparison between cancer and non-cancer patients. Magn Reson Imaging 2016;34(8): 1114–20.

22. Blackledge MD, Leach MO, Collins DJ, et al. Computed diffusion-weighted MR imaging may improve tumor detection. Radiology 2011;261(2): 573–81.

23. Blackledge MD, Collins DJ, Tunariu N, et al. Assessment of treatment response by total tumor volume and global apparent diffusion coefficient using diffusion-weighted MRI in patients with metastatic bone disease: a feasibility study. PLoS One 2014; 9(4):e91779.

24. Blackledge MD, Tunariu N, Orton MR, et al. Inter- and intra-observer repeatability of quantitative whole-body, diffusion-weighted imaging (WBDWI) in metastatic bone disease. PLoS One 2016;11(4): e0153840.

25. Perez-Lopez R, Mateo J, Mossop H, et al. Diffusion-weighted Imaging as a treatment response biomarker for evaluating bone metastases in prostate cancer: a pilot study. Radiology 2017;283(1): 168–77.

26. Pickles MD, Gibbs P, Lowry M, et al. Diffusion changes precede size reduction in neoadjuvant treatment of breast cancer. Magn Reson Imaging 2006;24(7):843–7.

27. Uhl M, Saueressig U, van Buiren M, et al. Osteosarcoma: preliminary results of in vivo assessment of tumor necrosis after chemotherapy with diffusion- and perfusion-weighted magnetic resonance imaging. Invest Radiol 2006;41(8):618–23.

28. Padhani AR, Koh DM, Collins DJ. Whole-body diffusion-weighted MR imaging in cancer: current status and research directions. Radiology 2011; 261(3):700–18.

29. Giles SL, Messiou C, Collins DJ, et al. Whole-body diffusion-weighted MR imaging for assessment of treatment response in myeloma. Radiology 2014; 271(3):785–94.

30. Schnapauff D, Zeile M, Niederhagen MB, et al. Diffusion-weighted echo-planar magnetic resonance imaging for the assessment of tumor cellularity in patients with soft-tissue sarcomas. J Magn Reson Imaging 2009;29(6):1355–9.

31. Pope WB, Kim HJ, Huo J, et al. Recurrent glioblastoma multiforme: ADC histogram analysis predicts response to bevacizumab treatment. Radiology 2009;252(1):182–9.

32. Ahlawat S, Khandheria P, Subhawong TK, et al. Differentiation of benign and malignant skeletal lesions with quantitative diffusion weighted MRI at 3T. Eur J Radiol 2015;84(6):1091–7.

33. Oka K, Yakushiji T, Sato H, et al. The value of diffusion-weighted imaging for monitoring the chemotherapeutic response of osteosarcoma: a comparison between average apparent diffusion coefficient and minimum apparent diffusion coefficient. Skeletal Radiol 2010;39(2):141–6.

34. Jerome NP, Miyazaki K, Collins DJ, et al. Repeatability of derived parameters from histograms following non-Gaussian diffusion modelling of diffusion-weighted imaging in a paediatric oncological cohort. Eur Radiol 2017;27(1):345–53.

35. Foroutan P, Kreahling JM, Morse DL, et al. Diffusion MRI and novel texture analysis in osteosarcoma xenotransplants predicts response to anti-checkpoint therapy. PLoS One 2013;8(12):e82875.

36. De Paepe K, Bevernage C, De Keyzer F, et al. Whole-body diffusion-weighted magnetic resonance imaging at 3 Tesla for early assessment of treatment response in non-Hodgkin lymphoma: a pilot study. Cancer Imaging 2013;13:53–62.

37. Berglund J, Johansson L, Ahlström H, et al. Three-point Dixon method enables whole-body water and fat imaging of obese subjects. Magn Reson Med 2010;63(6):1659–68.

38. Vande Berg BC, Malghem J, Lecouvet FE, et al. Magnetic resonance imaging of the normal bone marrow. Skeletal Radiol 1998;27(9):471–83.

39. Bolan PJ, Arentsen L, Sueblinvong T, et al. Water-fat MRI for assessing changes in bone marrow composition due to radiation and chemotherapy in gynecologic cancer patients. J Magn Reson Imaging 2013;38(6):1578–84.

40. Latifoltojar A, Hall-Craggs M, Bainbridge A, et al. Whole-body MRI quantitative biomarkers are associated significantly with treatment response in patients with newly diagnosed symptomatic multiple myeloma following bortezomib induction. Eur Radiol 2017;27(12):5325–36.

41. Dietrich O, Biffar A, Reiser MF, et al. Diffusion-weighted imaging of bone marrow. Semin Musculoskelet Radiol 2009;13(2):134–44.

42. Padhani AR, van Ree K, Collins DJ, et al. Assessing the relation between bone marrow signal intensity and apparent diffusion coefficient in diffusion-weighted MRI. AJR Am J Roentgenol 2013;200(1): 163–70.

43. Coleman RE. Metastatic bone disease: clinical features, pathophysiology and treatment strategies. Cancer Treat Rev 2001;27(3):165–76.

44. Gandaglia G, Abdollah F, Schiffmann J, et al. Distribution of metastatic sites in patients with prostate cancer: a population-based analysis. Prostate 2014;74(2):210–6.

45. Eisenhauer EA, Therasse P, Bogaerts J, et al. New response evaluation criteria in solid tumours: revised RECIST guideline (version 1.1). Eur J Cancer 2009; 45(2):228–47.

46. Gutzeit A, Doert A, Froehlich JM, et al. Comparison of diffusion-weighted whole body MRI and skeletal scintigraphy for the detection of bone metastases in patients with prostate or breast carcinoma. Skeletal Radiol 2010;39(4):333–43.

47. Nakanishi K, Kobayashi M, Nakaguchi K, et al. Whole-body MRI for detecting metastatic bone tumor: diagnostic value of diffusion-weighted images. Magn Reson Med Sci 2007;6(3):147–55.

48. Winfield JM, Poillucci G, Blackledge MD, et al. Apparent diffusion coefficient of vertebral haemangiomas allows differentiation from malignant focal deposits in whole-body diffusion-weighted MRI. Eur Radiol 2018;28(4):1687–91.

49. Perez-Lopez R, Lorente D, Blackledge MD, et al. Volume of bone metastasis assessed with whole-body diffusion-weighted imaging is associated with overall survival in metastatic castration-resistant prostate cancer. Radiology 2016;280(1): 151–60.

50. Byun WM, Shin SO, Chang Y, et al. Diffusion-weighted MR imaging of metastatic disease of the spine: assessment of response to therapy. AJNR Am J Neuroradiol 2002;23(6):906–12.

51. Reischauer C, Froehlich JM, Koh DM, et al. Bone metastases from prostate cancer: assessing treatment response by using diffusion-weighted imaging and functional diffusion maps–initial observations. Radiology 2010;257(2):523–31.

52. Perez-Lopez R, Nava Rodrigues D, Figueiredo I, et al. Multiparametric magnetic resonance imaging of prostate cancer bone disease: correlation with bone biopsy histological and molecular features. Invest Radiol 2018;53(2):96–102.

53. Gong J, Cao W, Zhang Z, et al. Diagnostic efficacy of whole-body diffusion-weighted imaging in the detection of tumour recurrence and metastasis by comparison with 18F-2-fluoro-2-deoxy-D-glucose positron emission tomography or computed tomography in patients with gastrointestinal cancer. Gastroenterol Rep (Oxf) 2015;3(2):128–35.

54. Messiou C, Kaiser M. Whole body diffusion weighted MRI–a new view of myeloma. Br J Haematol 2015;171(1):29–37.

55. Dimopoulos MA, Hillengass J, Usmani S, et al. Role of magnetic resonance imaging in the management of patients with multiple myeloma: a consensus statement. J Clin Oncol 2015;33(6):657–64.

56. Hillengass J, Fechtner K, Weber MA, et al. Prognostic significance of focal lesions in whole-body magnetic resonance imaging in patients with asymptomatic multiple myeloma. J Clin Oncol 2010;28(9):1606–10.

57. Messiou C, Giles S, Collins DJ, et al. Assessing response of myeloma bone disease with diffusion-weighted MRI. Br J Radiol 2012; 85(1020):e1198–203.

58. Horger M, Weisel K, Horger W, et al. Whole-body diffusion-weighted MRI with apparent diffusion coefficient mapping for early response monitoring in multiple myeloma: preliminary results. AJR Am J Roentgenol 2011;196(6):W790–5.

59. Plotkin SR, Bredella MA, Cai W, et al. Quantitative assessment of whole-body tumor burden in adult patients with neurofibromatosis. PLoS One 2012; 7(4):e35711.

60. Fayad LM, Blakeley J, Plotkin S, et al. Whole body MRI at 3T with quantitative diffusion weighted imaging and contrast-enhanced sequences for the characterization of peripheral lesions in patients with neurofibromatosis type 2 and schwannomatosis. ISRN Radiol 2013;2013:627932.

61. Lin G, Keshari KR, Park JM. Cancer metabolism and tumor heterogeneity: imaging perspectives using MR imaging and spectroscopy. Contrast Media Mol Imaging 2017;2017:6053879.

62. Just N. Improving tumour heterogeneity MRI assessment with histograms. Br J Cancer 2014;111(12): 2205–13.

63. Barnes A, Alonzi R, Blackledge M, et al. UK quantitative WB-DWI technical workgroup: consensus meeting recommendations on optimisation, quality control, processing and analysis of quantitative whole-body diffusion weighted imaging for cancer. Br J Radiol 2017;91(1081):20170577.

# Whole-Body Magnetic Resonance Imaging in Oncology: Uses and Indications

Giuseppe Petralia, MD[a,b,*],
Anwar R. Padhani, MBBS, MRCP, FRCR[c]

## KEYWORDS

- Whole-body-MR Imaging • Response assessment • Bone marrow disease • Breast cancer
- Prostate cancer • Multiple myeloma • Melanoma • Lymphoma

## KEY POINTS

- Whole-body MR Imaging (WB-MR Imaging) is a radiation-free imaging method for detecting bone and soft tissue pathology with application in disease detection (screening, surveillance, and staging).
- WB-MR Imaging is efficacious for overcoming the limitations of bone scintigraphy (BS) and computed tomography (CT) for detection and therapeutic response assessments in patients with bone marrow malignances.
- Established indications include evaluation of metastases in patients with breast and prostate cancers with bone marrow disease and multiple myeloma. Other indications include patients with fluorodeoxyglucose-positron emission tomography/CT-negative malignancies including lobular breast cancer and mucosa-associated lymphoma tissue lymphomas. Screening and surveillance indications can be found for patients with high risk melanoma and Li-Fraumeni syndrome.

## INTRODUCTION

Whole-body MR Imaging (WB-MR Imaging) is increasingly recommended as a radiation-free imaging method for detecting bone and soft tissue pathology, and for evaluating response to therapy in patients with cancer.[1] Specifically, WB-MR Imaging has been found to be efficacious for overcoming the limitations of bone scintigraphy (BS) and computed tomography (CT) for detection and therapeutic response assessments in patients with bone marrow malignances.[2] BS/CT scans are widely used and endorsed by international guidelines as the standard imaging investigations in the staging and follow-up of metastatic breast and prostate cancer with bone involvement.[3]

However, it is becoming clear that BS/CT scans are limited in their effectiveness in directing therapy and may therefore not be fit for that purpose In the era of precision oncology.

Intrinsic diagnostic insensitivity for disease detection is illustrated by the fact that the accepted minimum lymph node diameter (10 mm – short-axis) on CT scan as a measure of disease involvement is poorly correlated with the presence of disease, hence the requirement for a minimum 15 mm short-axis diameter within the RECIST criteria for measurable disease.[4] CT scans cannot accurately evaluate the presence or the therapeutic response in bone disease, the most common disease sites in multiple myeloma, breast and prostate cancer, unless there is a measurable soft tissue component.

Disclosure Statement: The authors have no competing interests to disclose.
[a] Department of Radiology, IEO - European Institute of Oncology IRCCS, Via Ripamonti, 435, Milan 20141, Italy; [b] Department of Oncology and Hematology, University of Milan, Via Festa del Perdono 7, Milan 20122, Italy; [c] MR unit, Paul Strickland Scanner Centre, Mount Vernon Hospital, Rickmansworth Road, Northwood, Middlesex HA6 2RN, UK
* Corresponding author. Department of Radiology, IEO - European Institute of Oncology IRCCS, Via Ripamonti, 435, Milan 20141, Italy.
E-mail address: giuseppe.petralia@ieo.it

Magn Reson Imaging Clin N Am 26 (2018) 495–507
https://doi.org/10.1016/j.mric.2018.06.003
1064-9689/18/© 2018 Elsevier Inc. All rights reserved.

BS is also limited in this regard (eg, in the assessment of multiple myeloma when there is an infrequent osteoblastic reaction to the presence of active disease). Even, when there is an osteoblastic reaction to the presence of malignancy, BS often provides misleading information when attempting to assess therapy effectiveness (eg, in breast and prostate cancer patients). Increased BS uptake in number and extent of lesions can equally occur with the osteoblastic healing (the so-called FLARE reaction) associated with tumor response, but also with osteoblastic progression associated with increasing tumor burden, thus creating confusion between response and progression, in therapy response settings. Patients with metastatic bone superscans are also not evaluable for therapy response, and are therefore excluded from precision oncology developments. Next-generation whole-body imaging tools such as positron emission tomography (PET) with specific tracers and WB-MR Imaging with diffusion-weighted sequences have emerged as powerful alternative assessment tools; however, the challenge remains in validating these newer imaging approaches, so that their use can be justified in wider clinical practice.

WB-MR Imaging has emerged as a powerful tool to address these limitations, because it is able to evaluate both bone and soft tissue disease, reflecting both tissue cellularity and cell viability, thus having clinical applications for disease detection and therapy response. Although increasingly used and recommended by international guidelines,[5–9] WB-MR Imaging usage has been confined mainly to expert centers, causing some concerns about its broader applicability. Important steps in the process of ensuring uniformity in the acquisition, interpretation, and reporting of WB-MR Imaging include the recommendations of UK quantitative WB-DWI technical workgroup[10] and the MET-RADS (METastasis Reporting And Data System) standard.[11] The MET-RADS standard establishes the minimum acceptable technical parameters for imaging acquisitions, built with sequences already available on most modern scanners. Two types of distinct protocols are described (core and comprehensive); the core protocol is designed for bone marrow disease detection, and the comprehensive protocol of other disease site disease detection and response assessments. The MET-RADS standard offers day-to-day reporting guidance, paired with detailed reporting tools that allow the description of the disease phenotype based on anatomic patterns of metastatic spread, thus enabling the systematic collection of analyzable data for research purposes. The upcoming MY-RADS will also set similar standards for use in multiple myeloma (Messiou C, personal communication, 2018). Using

MET-RADS enables (for the first time), the ability to sort metastatic bone disease response into 3 categories (progressive disease, stable disease, and response), rather than the currently employed limited clinically groups of progression and no-progression; this potentially enables the limitations of BS/CT scans to be overcome.[12] Thus, MET-RADS allows bone disease response assessment categorizations to mirror the RECIST criteria used for soft tissue disease. The MET-RADS authors state that this new way of metastatic bone response categorization could lead to a paradigm shift, from the current concept of treating patients with bone disease to documentable progression on CT/BS (when tumor volume could be substantially greater than at baseline), to being guided by the presence or absence of benefit to therapy, thus introducing more nuanced delivery of patient care.

Multiple studies reporting encouraging results for the use of WB-MR Imaging have led to the emergence of a variety of cancer histotypes. These have resulted in guideline endorsement in some cases because of high levels of scientific evidence.[1] This article discusses the use of WB-MR Imaging for a variety of clinical oncology settings.[2]

## CANCER PATIENTS
### Multiple Myeloma

Multiple myeloma (MM) is a hematological cancer characterized by the accumulation of neoplastic plasma cells in the bone marrow space. Symptomatic MM is characterized by the presence of bone fractures, osteolytic lesions, or osteoporosis, which is a significant cause of morbidity and mortality in patients with MM.[13] Ideally, MM should be treated effectively before becoming symptomatic, and accordingly, the International Myeloma Working Group (IMWG) has designated the presence of even asymptomatic bone disease on conventional radiography as a criterion of symptomatic MM that requires treatment.[14] In a series of 611 MM patients, MR Imaging detected more focal lesions compared with lytic lesions detected using radiographs of the spine (78% vs 16%; P=.001), pelvis (64% vs 28%; P=.001), and sternum (24% vs 3%; P=.001)[15] (Fig. 1). Moreover, WB-MR Imaging was found to be superior to conventional whole-body CT for detecting lesions of the skeleton in a study with 41 patients with newly diagnosed MM[16] (Fig. 2). According to recent IMWG guidelines on the use of WB-MR Imaging in MM,[6] which were recently endorsed and expanded by the British Society of Haematology (BSH),[5] the presence of more than 1 lesion, greater than 5 mm in size, unequivocally caused by plasma cell infiltration is an MM defining event, for the purpose of

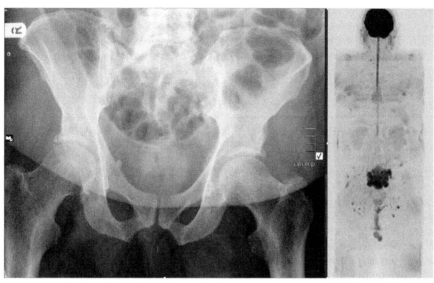

Fig. 1. A 55-year-old man with solitary plasmacytoma for systemic staging. Note how bowel gas obscures visualization of the sacral mass. The b900 s/mm$^2$ maximum intensive projections (MIP) image (inverted scale) confirms a solitary lesion in the sacrum.

identifying symptomatic MM. Note that PET scan positivity without corresponding CT osteolysis is not an MM-defining event in this context. WB-MR Imaging is recommended for staging all form of multiple myeloma (grade of recommendation A; level of evidence (LoE) GR A[17]). The BSH also recommends the use of WB-MR Imaging for the monitoring therapy response of oligosecretory and nonsecretory disease, noting an increasing prevalence of this disease subtype after multiple therapies (LoE 1B[5]), as well as for extramedullary/paramedullary disease (LoE 1B[5]). With a grade A recommendation, WB-MR Imaging is also indicated for the staging of solitary bone plasmacytoma (SBP), an early stage of the malignancy with a clinical course that lies between smoldering myeloma and symptomatic MM. However, it should be noted that not all cases of MM are identifiable on WB-MR Imaging, and that the osteoporotic variant of MM may not be MR Imaging visible because of

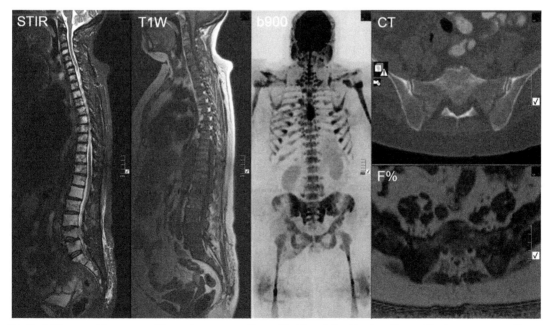

Fig. 2. A 65-year-old woman with myeloma presenting with L4 vertebral body collapse. The bone marrow disease on MR Imaging sequences, including the b900 s/mm$^2$ MIP (inverted scale) images, is not visible on CT scans.

increased BM fat, which has been ascribed to the excessive production of a myeloma protein called DKK-1,[18] which diverts mesenchymal stem cells away from osteoblastic differentiation toward adipocytic morphology.

## Prostate Cancer

The presence of metastatic disease on imaging in prostate cancer is a game changer for patients, helping to define the advanced disease state, and the presence of metastases on metastases outside the true pelvis is highly prognostic, determining therapy choices. For example, at initial staging, metastatic disease precludes all curative therapy options and for patients experiencing biochemical recurrence precludes local salvage therapy. Even in the advanced prostate cancer (APC), the imaging depicted metastatic disease presence, distribution, and volume sub-categorise the disease: no imaging depicted metastases (M0), early/oligometastases (M+), late polymetastatic (M++); these subcategories have therapy decision-making implications. For example, in M0 or M+ castrate naïve disease, there are opportunities to postpone the onset of androgen deprivation treatment (ADT) in oligo-metastatic disease with local salvage treatments and metastasis direct therapies. This ability to treat locally first can help to delay the onset of ADT, thus postponing adverse effects and delaying the inevitable castrate resistance also. Even in the advanced polymetastatic state, the volume, distribution, and response to therapy of disease are highly prognostic, affecting therapy choices for both castrate-naïve and castrate-resistant states.[19–21]

For high-risk patients, guidelines of the European Association of Urology (EAU) recommend at least cross-sectional abdominopelvic imaging and a bone scan (grade A, LoE 2A[22]). These EAU guidelines recognized that WB-MR Imaging is more sensitive (97%) than choline PET/CT (91%) and bone scan (78%) for detecting bone metastasis from prostate cancer, as confirmed in a recent meta-analysis conducted by Shen and colleagues[23] on 18 studies who compared the diagnostic accuracy of these 3 imaging techniques (**Fig. 3**). However, current recommendations still emphasize CT/BS assessments when APC beyond the pelvis is being considered. However, for early disease detection, there is a move toward choline/PSMA PET/CT.

A recent review has identified the potential of WB-MR Imaging to address the unmet need for robust imaging that allows monitoring the response of prostate cancer bone metastases to treatment.[24] The Advanced Prostate Cancer Consensus Conference (APCCC) expressed the need for imaging assessments in castrate-resistant patients, stating that clinical and PSA assessments may not reliable enough for monitoring disease activity in all patients with mCRPC[12] (**Fig. 4**). Indeed, it has been noted that with androgen axis-directed therapies, 21% to 30% of cases can develop radiographic progression without clinical/PSA progression to abiraterone and enzalutamide[25] and that 40% of cases starting off with bone -only disease at baseline before therapy, do develop soft tissue disease at radiographic

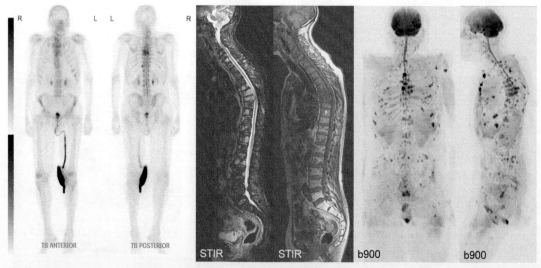

**Fig. 3.** A 79-year-old man with high-risk prostate cancer treated with radical radiotherapy, with rising serum PSA and thoracic back pain for 5 weeks. Planar bone scans are reported as showing uptake in T7/T8 with non-specific uptake at T11 and right 10th rib. WB-MR Imaging reported extensive polymetastatic disease with relative sparing of the irradiated bony pelvis with no nodal or visceral metastases. There is spinal canal narrowing at T7.

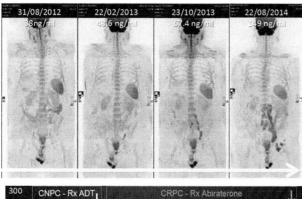

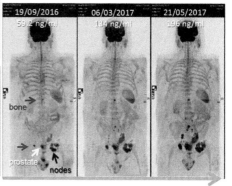

**Fig. 4.** A 73-year-old man with metastatic prostate cancer undergoing serial therapy monitoring using PSA levels and WB-MR Imaging. WB-MR Imaging scans were performed at the time points indicated on the graph of PSA changes. Only the b900 s/mm$^2$ MIP (inverted scale) images are shown here. During androgen deprivation therapy (ADT) for castrate naïve prostate cancer (CNPC), rising PSA levels are associated with the emergence of left-sided pelvic lymphadenopathy. In this case, biochemical relapse is associated with concordant disease relapse. In the castrate-resistant state (CRPC), he received abiraterone therapy with good PSA response. Note that biochemical failure on abiraterone was associated with the emergence of disease at the primary tumor site (slanting yellow *arrow*) in the bones and enlargement of left groin lymph nodes. Note that the retroperitoneum nodes have not re-emerged. This is an example of discordant pattern of disease relapse commonly observed in metastatic CRPC.

progression.[26] Furthermore, when patients are treated with radium-223, PSA monitoring is known to be ineffective. Asymptomatic nonbone disease progression occurs in 46% of patients within 3 to 6 months of radium-223 therapy start.[27] As a result, multiple guidelines now recommend regular imaging monitoring with CT/BS for mCRPC.[28] However, even these guidelines affirmed that "disease monitoring in the bone is especially difficult with well-described bone lesion flare phenomena both on CT and bone scans, ...... and it is recognized that planar bone scintigraphy has short-comings and is less sensitive than other newer imaging technologies such as MR Imaging of the whole body." Finally, even though stating that there is "limited availability of these newer imaging technologies," the APCCC confirmed that "advanced spinal/whole body MR Imaging techniques are also better able to identify and gauge the extent of bone disease than planar bone scans."

## Melanoma

Although there have been significant develops in clinical management of advanced melanoma, most patients with advanced, metastatic melanoma will still die of their disease. For these reasons, multiple guidelines recommend imaging-based surveillance for high-risk patients using combination of PET/CT, CT body scans, and brain MR Imaging scans. Several meta-analysis and systematic reviews have established WB-MR Imaging as a valid alternative method to PET/CT in oncology.[29,30] Further studies confirmed that WB-MR Imaging has promising sensitivity in detecting extracranial metastases in melanoma patients including the liver (**Fig. 5**).[31] Recent developments using ultra-short TE (UTE) MR Imaging sequences have extended the ability of lung metastasis detection using WB-MR Imaging[32] to provide a viable, radiation-free alternative to PET/CT and body CT scans for the detection of small lung metastatic lesions. Pflugfelder and colleagues,[7] on behalf of the German Dermatologic Society and the Dermatologic Cooperative Oncology Group, suggested WB-MR Imaging as highly recommended for cross-sectional imaging of advanced melanoma (stage III or worse), stating the equivalence of this method compared with whole-body CT and PET/CT. Moreover, WB-MR Imaging is also recommended the follow-up of patients with melanoma staged from IIC to IV.[8]

## Breast Cancer

Bone metastasis development is common in women diagnosed with primary invasive breast

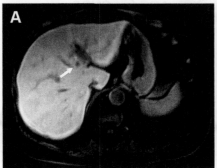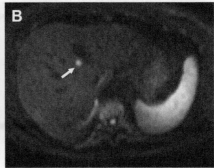

Fig. 5. A patient with a stage III melanoma undergoes WB-MR Imaging with hepatobiliary-specific contrast agent (gadoxetic acid, disodium, Gd-EOB-DTPA). (*A*) The late hepatobiliary phase, 20 minutes after intravenous injection, reveals the presence of a 9 mm metastasis in segment 4 (*white arrow*). (*B*) The same lesion is clearly detectable (*white arrow*) in the high b-value (900 s/mm$^2$) diffusion-weighted image performed in the same session.

cancer.[33] Morphologic MR Imaging has been shown to be highly efficacious for imaging of the bone marrow.[34] In a meta-analysis conducted by Yang and colleagues[35] of 145 studies comprising 15,221 patients with bone metastasis, morphologic WB-MR Imaging was found to have comparable diagnostic performance (90%) to PET (91%) and superior to CT (77%) and bone scan (75%) for bone lesions detection. Furthermore, as already discussed, MR Imaging is also able to assess response to therapy. However, morphologic MR Imaging has shortcomings when assessing response to therapy, including the inability to depict success of response in sclerotic metastases and the so-called T1 pseudo-progression phenomenon. The latter occurs when a strong response to therapy induces bone marrow edema due to profound tumor cell kill related to necroptosis.[36] T1 pseudoprogression is visualized as T1 hypointensity and can be confused with progression using morphologic sequences alone. In such cases, the addition of DWI sequences allows the successful distinction between bone marrow edema and the presence of active bone marrow disease, thus avoiding misdiagnoses[37] (**Fig. 6**). In this case, increases in apparent diffusion coefficient (ADC) values are indicative of tumor cell death. However, readers should note that primary sclerotic response also happens. That is, after successful treatment, bone metastases may remain unchanged on morphologic T1 images, but increases in ADC values may be minimal or not observed at all.

The improved diagnostic performance of WB-MR Imaging compared with conventional imaging methods and the clinical impact on patient care are under investigation. In a recent study, Kosmin and colleagues[38] compared 210 paired WB-MR Imaging and CT performed contemporaneously (within 14 days) for the follow-up of metastatic breast cancer patients. They observed an increased extent of metastatic disease between the imaging modalities, and more importantly differences in response assessments. They noted that systemic anticancer therapy changes caused by progressive disease (PD) occurred in 46 pairs; in 16 out of these pairs (34.7%), PD was only visible at WB-MR Imaging, going undiagnosed by CT (reported stable). This observation highlights the potential value of WB-MR Imaging for patient decision making in the clinic (**Fig. 7**).

Multiple uses of WB-MR Imaging for detection and characterization of disease have emerged in breast cancer patients. These include the need to clarify the nature of equivocal BS or CT scans in newly diagnosed patients, particularly with high-risk presentations such as inoperable locally advanced disease, inflammatory tumors, and more than 4 positive lymph nodes or in those experiencing early locoregional relapse. Other indications include patients at low suspicion for relapse who are developing likely aromatase inhibitor arthralgia; these reassurance scans can provide diagnostic certainty without exposing patients to radiation risks. Another key use is the detection and staging of breast cancer occurring during pregnancy. In these women, breast cancer often presents at an advanced stage in 40% of cases, which is 2.5 times greater than the rate in general population with breast cancer. Accurate staging assessment is mandatory for planning therapy of pregnant women. Recognizing that there is an overwhelming clinical need to avoid the use of imaging techniques that utilize ionizing radiations, and the need to also avoid administration of intravenous contrast agents, WB-MR Imaging represents the imaging technique of choice for systemic staging in pregnant women with breast cancer[39] (**Fig. 8**).

A key use of WB-MR Imaging in breast cancer patients has recently emerged for invasive lobular

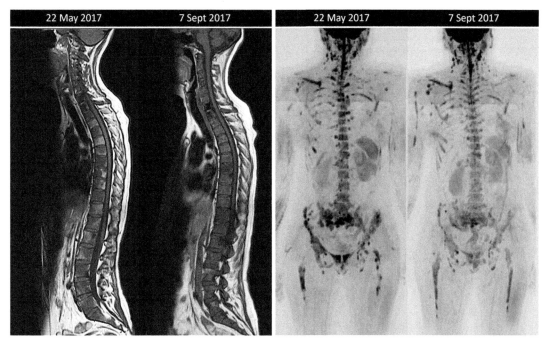

**Fig. 6.** A 45-year-old woman with metastatic breast cancer undergoes WB-MR Imaging before and after capecitabine and vinorelbine chemotherapy. On T1 weighted sagittal images, a diffuse reduction in signal intensity is identified in the whole spine after chemotherapy. However, it is impossible to assess whether this is because of progressive disease or in response to therapy (T1 pseudoprogression). T1 pseudoprogression can be observed after cytotoxic chemotherapy and is related to increases in extracellular water in the bone marrow. MIP of b900 s/mm$^2$ Images (inverted scale) reveals decreases in signal intensity after therapy and rises in apparent diffusion coefficient (ADC) values confirm therapy response.

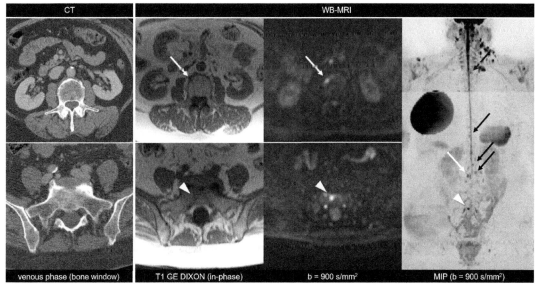

**Fig. 7.** A 69-year-old woman was operated on for a multifocal invasive ductal and lobular breast carcinoma (pT2N2aM0), followed by chest wall radiation therapy and adjuvant chemotherapy. She represented while on adjuvant hormone therapy after 14 months with a ring in serum tumor marker (Ca15.3 = 139 U/mL), for which contrast-enhanced CT scans and WB-MR Imaging were undertaken. Two bone metastases are highlighted in the body of the second lumbar vertebra (*white arrow*) and in the sacrum (white *arrowhead*), visible on T1 DIXON images and on high b-value (900 s/mm$^2$) diffusion-weighted images. Both lesions were not detected in the corresponding CT images. On the b900 s/mm$^2$ MIP projections (inverted scale), other bone metastases are visible in the cervical, dorsal, and lumbar spine (*black arrows*); left supraclavicular and cervical pathologic lymph nodes are also visible. Bone WB-MR Imaging findings were confirmed by follow-up studies, and lymph node metastases were confirmed by ultrasound-guided biopsy.

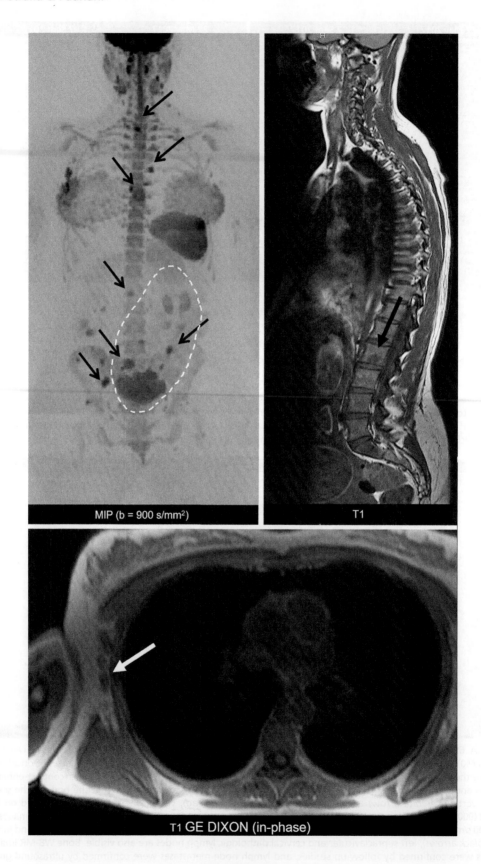

MIP (b = 900 s/mm²)

T1

T1 GE DIXON (in-phase)

breast cancer (ILC). ILC is a common histologic subtype, characterized by a different pattern of metastatic spread compared with the more common invasive ductal breast cancer (IDC). ILC is disposed to spread to the gastrointestinal (GI) organs, peritoneum and retroperitoneum, gynecologic system, and pleura. These features are related to the characteristic histologic pattern of spread of ILC, the so-called Indian file neoplastic growth pattern, where neoplastic cells infiltrating the parenchyma around non-neoplastic ducts of GI organs, blood vessels, or spreading to peritoneum or retroperitoneum.[33] This distinct method of spread is difficult to assess by CT scans. Note also that ILCs are less glucose consuming than IDC and therefore less visible on fluorodeoxyglucose (FDG)-PET/CT scans. WB-MR Imaging can depict the presence of neoplastic spread into the GI tract or peritoneum/retroperitoneum earlier and better than CT scans and FDG/PET-CT for ILC (**Fig. 9**).

### Lymphoma

FDG-PET/CT is the recommended imaging technique for the most common lymphomas, including DLBCL, follicular lymphoma, and Hodgkin lymphoma.[40] However, its diagnostic performances are related to glucose metabolism, and patients without altered glucose metabolism may not be ideal candidates for FDG-PET/CT.[41] Non-FDG avid histotypes include cutaneous T-cell lymphoma, peripheral T-cell lymphoma, follicular B-cell lymphoma, small lymphocytic lymphoma, DCLC B-cell and MALT lymphomas. In contrast, WB-MR Imaging can evaluate almost the entire range of histotypes (except for mucosal disease) because of its ability to depict hypercellularity. In a prospective study conducted on 140 patients, WB-MR Imaging showed better diagnostic performance than FDG-PET/CT and contrast-enhanced CT scans for multiple lymphoma subtypes that show a variable FDG avidity (most were MALT lymphoma).[42]

Another emerging use of WB-MR Imaging is in younger patients with lymphoma. Because survival rates have steadily improved, there is a need to minimize radiation exposure in the follow-up of those patients. Note that current National Comprehensive Cancer Network (NCCN) guidelines suggest

repeated CT or PET/CT examinations at multiple follow-up time points, even for lower stages of disease.[43] WB-MR Imaging shows diagnostic performance comparable to those of PET/CT for staging and follow-up. In order to comply with ALARA principles,[44] radiation doses are minimized for younger patients treated with a curative intent. In these patients, WB-MR Imaging could be considered as an reasonable substitute to PET/CT and CT, particularly in the follow-up period.[45]

## CANCER SCREENING
### Li-Fraumeni Syndrome

Li-Fraumeni (LFS), first described in 1969, is a highly penetrant cancer-prone syndrome,[46] caused by germline mutations of the TP53 tumor suppressor gene. This rare, autosomal-dominant, hereditary disorder predisposes carriers to the development of a wide variety of cancer types including sarcomas, breast cancer, leukemia, and adrenal gland, the so-called SBLA syndrome. These patients are sensitive to the mutagenic effects of ionizing radiation, thus precluding normal radiography-based screening procedures. A recent meta-analysis validated the clinical utility of WB-MR Imaging in screening TP53 mutation carriers,[47] and results from the UK SIGNIFY study in these subjects suggested the need to adopt WB-MR Imaging for baseline assessments.[48] Furthermore, the MD Anderson Cancer Center, jointly with LFCA, the world largest LFS patients' association, produced the first screening guidelines. The LFAD guidelines (Li Fraumeni Syndrome Education and Early Detection) suggested WB-MR Imaging be undertaken in children from 1 to 10 years of age affected by LFS-related sarcomas, as well as older patients with sarcoma, brain, or adrenocortical tumors.[9] Moreover, the recently updated guidance from NCCN suggested annual screening of LFS patients with WB-MR Imaging as the reference standard.[49]

### Neurofibromatosis

Neurofibromatosis is a genetic disorder that causes tumors to form on nerve tissue. These tumors can develop anywhere across nervous system, including brain, spinal cord, and peripheral nerves.

**Fig. 8.** A 37-year-old woman in 31st week of gestation underwent a WB-MR Imaging for systemic staging for a locally advanced breast cancer. Several bone metastases (*black arrows*) are visible on the MIP image (inverted scale), as well as on morphologic T1-weighted sagittal images of the spine. Multiple, abnormal lymph nodes (*white arrow*) are visible in the right axilla on T1 gradient-echo in-phase DIXON images. Areas of high signal intensity are visible in the pelvis and in the left abdomen, corresponding to the brain and kidneys of the fetus (*dotted line*). Based on the outcome of the WB-MR Imaging, cesarean section was undertaken at the 38th week of gestation, after which chemotherapy and hormone therapy were started.

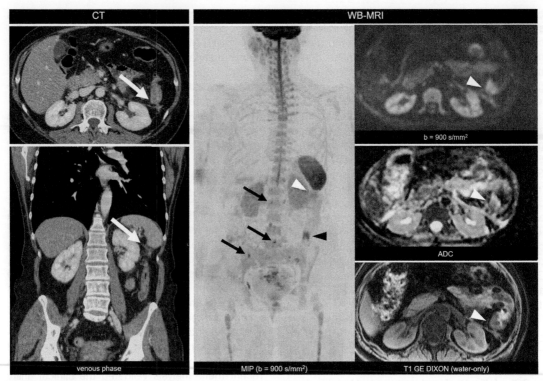

**Fig. 9.** A persistent rise in serum tumor marker (Ca15.3 = 660 U/mL) in a 51-year-old woman with gastric metastases from invasive lobular breast carcinoma, during third-line chemotherapy. A contrast-enhanced CT revealed no measurable disease. Thickening of the left renal and lateroconal fascia (*white arrow*) was interpreted as the result of a prior oophorectomy for benign disease (serous cystadenoma). The WB-MR Imaging showed pathologic tissue extending from the left renal fascia into the wall of the descending colon (white *arrowheads*); this finding is visible on high b-value (900 s/mm²) images, on the ADC map and on T1 gradient-echo water-only DIXON images. In the coronal MIP image, multiple other metastatic lesions are visible in the lumbar spine and in the pelvis (*black arrows*), as well as in the distal descending colon (black *arrowhead*). Based on the imaging evidence of progressive disease, the patient started systemic treatment with everolimus and exemestane. All findings were reconfirmed on subsequent WB-MR Imaging examinations.

Neurofibromatosis is usually diagnosed in childhood or early adulthood. Identifying premalignant and malignant tumors is essential for the clinical management of patients with neurofibromatosis, yet this goal has remained challenging because of the heterogeneity of neurofibromas. Diffusion-weighted imaging is particularly promising in children, because tumors in childhood are often small and round and well detected by DWI. WB-MR Imaging has proven effective for detecting and staging the 3 main clinical manifestations of neurofibromatosis: neurofibromatosis type 1 (NF1), neurofibromatosis type 2 (NF2), and schwannomatosis (SWN).

The US National Cancer Institute has already recommended the development of practical guidelines to introduce WB-MR Imaging for MPNST (malignant peripheral nerve sheath tumors) detection.[50] About half of MPNSTs are detected in people with NF, and the lifetime risk for developing this malignancy in patients with NF1 lies between 8% and 13%. A study by Cashen and colleagues[51] showed an overall survival rate of 84% among treated patients; the authors emphasized the impact of advanced imaging on early diagnosis and management. Recommendations for the use of WB-MR Imaging in NF by The Response Evaluation in Neurofibromatosis and Schwannomatosis International Collaboration (REiNS) are under development.[52] Moreover, the largest NF patient foundation in the United Kingdom, the Neuro Foundation, has already suggested the use of MR Imaging to investigate preliminary signs of NF across the whole body spectrum.[53]

## Asymptomatic Subject Cancer Screening

Early detection of subclinical disease may enable the initiation of preventive measures and early treatments for detected disease, while remembering that overdiagnosis and overtreatment may

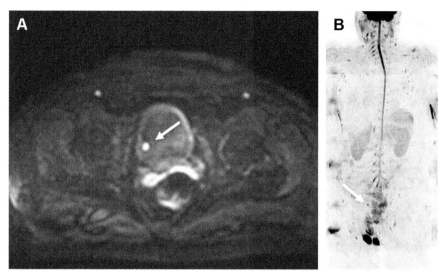

Fig. 10. A 57-year-old man, asymptomatic and with no previous history of cancer, who underwent WB-MR Imaging for cancer screening. A 4 mm bright lesion is visible on the (*A*) high b value (b 900 s/mm$^2$) image and the (*B*) MIP image (inverted scale), located in the right wall of the bladder. Biopsy revealed a small low-grade transitional carcinoma.

also cause harm. The largest ongoing multipart MR Imaging study in 30,000 asymptomatic subjects is the German National Cohort.[54]

Several studies have reported on the use of WB-MR Imaging for cancer screening. The first study evaluated 132 doctors in Hong Kong.[55] Some other studies have been published in the last decade, the largest including 666 asymptomatic subjects, in whom a rate of 1,05% malignant cancers was found.[56]

The authors have also noted similar observations at the Advanced Screening Centers (ASC, Italy), where 394 asymptomatic subjects have been evaluated. At least 1 abnormality was detected in 382 subjects; however, no additional investigations were needed for 80% of them. Seventy-five subjects were re-examined, and with further testing, 4 subjects (1% of the total population screened) had histologically confirmed malignant cancer (**Fig. 10**).

However, there is still a long way to go before WB-MR Imaging can be considered suitable for general population screening. It must be demonstrated that WB-MR Imaging screening is an economically effective use of advanced technologies. WB-MR Imaging interpretations and performance are strongly related to the experience of readers, with a learning curve, requiring the development of suitable quality standards.

## SUMMARY

WB-MR Imaging has significant advantages compared with other whole-body imaging procedures, including its high soft tissue contrast, spatial resolution, and lack of radiation exposure. The demand for WB-MR Imaging in oncologic applications is increasing with the emergence of validated clinical indications for patients with known or suspected malignancy. WB-MR Imaging uses within current indications and guidelines is mainly related to its ability to improve detection of disease. However, the abilities of WB-MR Imaging extend into other areas, including therapy assessments, where quantitative assessments of water diffusivity are helpful, particularly for the evaluation of bone marrow malignancy. This allows WB-MR Imaging to be a comprehensive, noninvasive imaging technique with the ability to diagnose, stage, and assess therapeutic response for multiple neoplastic diseases.

## REFERENCES

1. Wu LM, Gu HY, Zheng J, et al. Diagnostic value of whole-body magnetic resonance imaging for bone metastases: a systematic review and meta-analysis. J Magn Reson Imaging 2011;34:128–35.
2. Koh DM, Blackledge M, Padhani AR, et al. Whole-body diffusion-weighted MRI: tips, tricks, and pitfalls. AJR Am J Roentgenol 2012;199:252–62.
3. Cardoso F, Harbeck N, Fallowfield L, et al, ESMO Guidelines Working Group. Locally recurrent or metastatic breast cancer: ESMO clinical practice guidelines for diagnosis, treatment and follow-up. Ann Oncol 2012;23(Suppl 7):vii11–9.
4. Eisenhauer EA, Therasse P, Bogaerts J, et al. New response evaluation criteria in solid tumours: revised

RECIST guideline (version 1.1). Eur J Cancer 2009; 45:228–47.

5. Chantry A, Kazmi M, Barrington S, et al. Guidelines for the use of imaging in the management of patients with myeloma. Br J Haematol 2017; 178:380–93.

6. Dimopoulos MA, Hillengass J, Usmani S, et al. Role of magnetic resonance imaging in the management of patients with multiple myeloma: a consensus statement. J Clin Oncol 2015;33:657–64.

7. Pflugfelder A, Kochs C, Blum A, et al. Malignant melanoma S3-guideline "diagnosis, therapy and follow-up of melanoma". J Dtsch Dermatol Ges 2013; 11(Suppl 6):1–116, 1–126.

8. Dummer R, Siano M, Hunger RE, et al. The updated Swiss guidelines 2016 for the treatment and follow-up of cutaneous melanoma. Swiss Med Wkly 2016; 146:w14279.

9. Bojadzieva J, Amini B, Day SF, et al. Whole body magnetic resonance imaging (WB-MRI) and brain MRI baseline surveillance in TP53 germline mutation carriers: experience from the Li-Fraumeni Syndrome Education and Early Detection (LEAD) clinic. Fam Cancer 2018;17(2):287–94.

10. Barnes A, Alonzi R, Blackledge M, et al. UK quantitative WB-DWI technical workgroup: consensus meeting recommendations on optimisation, quality control, processing and analysis of quantitative whole-body diffusion-weighted imaging for cancer. Br J Radiol 2018;91:20170577.

11. Padhani AR, Lecouvet FE, Tunariu N, et al. Metastasis reporting and data system for prostate cancer: practical guidelines for acquisition, interpretation, and reporting of whole-body magnetic resonance imaging-based evaluations of multiorgan involvement in advanced prostate cancer. Eur Urol 2017; 71:81–92.

12. Gillessen S, Attard G, Beer TM, et al. Management of patients with advanced prostate cancer: the report of the advanced prostate cancer consensus conference APCCC 2017. Eur Urol 2018;73:178–211.

13. Kristinsson SY, Minter AR, Korde N, et al. Bone disease in multiple myeloma and precursor disease: novel diagnostic approaches and implications on clinical management. Expert Rev Mol Diagn 2011; 11:593–603.

14. Kumar S, Paiva B, Anderson KC, et al. International Myeloma Working Group consensus criteria for response and minimal residual disease assessment in multiple myeloma. Lancet Oncol 2016;17:e328–46.

15. Walker R, Barlogie B, Haessler J, et al. Magnetic resonance imaging in multiple myeloma: diagnostic and clinical implications. J Clin Oncol 2007;25: 1121–8.

16. Baur-Melnyk A, Buhmann S, Becker C, et al. Whole-body MRI versus whole-body MDCT for staging of multiple myeloma. AJR Am J Roentgenol 2008;190: 1097–104.

17. Oxford Centre for Evidence-based Medicine. Levels of evidence (March 2009). Available at: www.cebm. net.

18. Pinzone JJ, Hall BM, Thudi NK, et al. The role of Dickkopf-1 in bone development, homeostasis, and disease. Blood 2009;113:517–25.

19. Halabi S, Lin CY, Kelly WK, et al. Updated prognostic model for predicting overall survival in first-line chemotherapy for patients with metastatic castration-resistant prostate cancer. J Clin Oncol 2014;32:671–7.

20. Cookson MS, Lowrance WT, Murad MH, et al, American Urological Association. Castration-resistant prostate cancer: AUA guideline amendment. J Urol 2015;193:491–9.

21. Gandaglia G, Karakiewicz PI, Briganti A, et al. Impact of the site of metastases on survival in patients with metastatic prostate cancer. Eur Urol 2015;68:325–34.

22. Mottet N, Bellmunt J, Bolla M, et al. EAU-ESTRO-SIOG guidelines on prostate cancer. Part 1: screening, diagnosis, and local treatment with curative intent. Eur Urol 2017;71:618–29.

23. Shen G, Deng H, Hu S, et al. Comparison of choline-PET/CT, MRI, SPECT, and bone scintigraphy in the diagnosis of bone metastases in patients with prostate cancer: a meta-analysis. Skeletal Radiol 2014; 43:1503–13.

24. Padhani AR, Lecouvet FE, Tunariu N, et al. Rationale for modernising imaging in advanced prostate cancer. Eur Urol Focus 2017;3:223–39.

25. Morris MJ, Molina A, Small EJ, et al. Radiographic progression-free survival as a response biomarker in metastatic castration-resistant prostate cancer: COU-AA-302 results. J Clin Oncol 2015;33:1356–63.

26. Bryce AH, Alumkal JJ, Armstrong A, et al. Radiographic progression with nonrising PSA in metastatic castration-resistant prostate cancer: post hoc analysis of PREVAIL. Prostate Cancer Prostatic Dis 2017;20:221–7.

27. Keizman D, Fosboel MO, Reichegger H, et al. Imaging response during therapy with radium-223 for castration-resistant prostate cancer with bone metastases-analysis of an international multicenter database. Prostate Cancer Prostatic Dis 2017;20: 289–93.

28. Fitzpatrick JM, Bellmunt J, Fizazi V, et al. Optimal management of metastatic castration-resistant prostate cancer: highlights from a European Expert Consensus Panel. Eur J Cancer 2014;50:1617–27.

29. Li B, Li Q, Nie W, et al. Diagnostic value of whole-body diffusion-weighted magnetic resonance imaging for detection of primary and metastatic malignancies: a meta-analysis. Eur J Radiol 2014;83: 338–44.

30. Ciliberto M, Maggi F, Treglia G, et al. Comparison between whole-body MRI and Fluorine-18-Fluorodeoxyglucose PET or PET/CT in oncology: a systematic review. Radiol Oncol 2013;47:206–18.

31. Petralia G, Padhani A, Summers P, et al. Whole-body diffusion-weighted imaging: is it all we need for detecting metastases in melanoma patients? Eur Radiol 2013;23:3466–76.

32. Grodzki DM, Jakob PM, Heismann B. Ultrashort echo time imaging using pointwise encoding time reduction with radial acquisition (PETRA). Magn Reson Med 2012;67:510–8.

33. Kwast AB, Groothuis-Oudshoorn KC, Grandjean I, et al. Histological type is not an independent prognostic factor for the risk pattern of breast cancer recurrences. Breast Cancer Res Treat 2012;135:271–80.

34. Mehnati P, Tirtash MJ. Comparative efficacy of four imaging instruments for breast cancer screening. Asian Pac J Cancer Prev 2015;16:6177–86.

35. Yang HL, Liu T, Wang XM, et al. Diagnosis of bone metastases: a meta-analysis comparing (1)(8)FDG PET, CT, MRI and bone scintigraphy. Eur Radiol 2011;21:2604–17.

36. Ntuli TM. Cell Death - Autophagy, apoptosis and necrosis. London: Intech Open Limited; 2015.

37. Padhani AR, Makris A, Gall P, et al. Therapy monitoring of skeletal metastases with whole-body diffusion MRI. J Magn Reson Imaging 2014;39:1049–78.

38. Kosmin M, Makris A, Joshi PV, et al. The addition of whole-body magnetic resonance imaging to body computerised tomography alters treatment decisions in patients with metastatic breast cancer. Eur J Cancer 2017;77:109–16.

39. Peccatori FA, Codacci-Pisanelli G, Del Grande M, et al. Whole body MRI for systemic staging of breast cancer in pregnant women. Breast 2017;35:177–81.

40. NCCN Guidelines, Version 3.2018, Hodgkin Lymphoma. Available at: www.NCCN.org.

41. Weiler-Sagie M, Bushelev O, Epelbaum R, et al. (18)F-FDG avidity in lymphoma readdressed: a study of 766 patients. J Nucl Med 2010;51:25–30.

42. Mayerhoefer ME, Karanikas G, Kletter K, et al. Evaluation of diffusion-weighted MRI for pretherapeutic assessment and staging of lymphoma: results of a prospective study in 140 patients. Clin Cancer Res 2014;20:2984–93.

43. Hoppe RT, Advani RH, Ai WZ, et al. Hodgkin lymphoma, version 2.2012 featured updates to the NCCN guidelines. J Natl Compr Canc Netw 2012;10:589–97.

44. Hendee WR, Edwards FM. ALARA and an integrated approach to radiation protection. Semin Nucl Med 1986;16:142–50.

45. Mayerhoefer ME, Karanikas G, Kletter K, et al. Evaluation of diffusion-weighted magnetic resonance imaging for follow-up and treatment response assessment of lymphoma: results of an 18F-FDG-PET/CT-controlled prospective study in 64 patients. Clin Cancer Res 2015;21:2506–13.

46. Li FP, Fraumeni JF Jr. Soft-tissue sarcomas, breast cancer, and other neoplasms. A familial syndrome? Ann Intern Med 1969;71:747–52.

47. Ballinger ML, Best A, Mai PL, et al. Baseline surveillance in Li-Fraumeni syndrome using whole-body magnetic resonance imaging: a meta-analysis. JAMA Oncol 2017;3:1634–9.

48. Saya S, Killick E, Thomas S, et al. Baseline results from the UK SIGNIFY study: a whole-body MRI screening study in TP53 mutation carriers and matched controls. Fam Cancer 2017;16:433–40.

49. NCCN Guidelines, Version 2.2019, Genetic/Familial High-Risk Assessment: Breast and Ovarian. Available at: www.NCCN.org.

50. Reilly KM, Kim A, Blakely J, et al. Neurofibromatosis type 1 associated MPNST state of the science: outlining a research agenda for the future. J Natl Cancer Inst 2017;109. https://doi.org/10.1093/jnci/djx124.

51. Cashen DV, Parisien RC, Raskin K, et al. Survival data for patients with malignant schwannoma. Clin Orthop Relat Res 2004;426:69–73.

52. Widemann BC, Blakeley JO, Dombi E, et al. Conclusions and future directions for the REiNS international collaboration. Neurology 2013;81:S41–4.

53. The Neuro Foundation. Available at: www.nfauk.org.

54. Bamberg F, Kauczor HU, Weckbach S, et al. Whole-body MR imaging in the German national cohort: rationale, design, and technical background. Radiology 2015;277:206–20.

55. Lo GG, Ai V, Au-Yeung KM, et al. Magnetic resonance whole body imaging at 3 Tesla: feasibility and findings in a cohort of asymptomatic medical doctors. Hong Kong Med J 2008;14:90–6.

56. Cieszanowski A, Maj E, Kulisiewicz P, et al. Non-contrast-enhanced whole-body magnetic resonance imaging in the general population: the incidence of abnormal findings in patients 50 years old and younger compared to older subjects. PLoS One 2014;9:e107840.

# Whole-Body Imaging in Multiple Myeloma

Christina Messiou, MD, BMedSci, BMBS, MRCP, FRCR[a],*, Martin Kaiser, MD[b]

## KEYWORDS

- Myeloma • MR imaging myeloma • MR imaging • Imaging • Functional

## KEY POINTS

- Bone marrow involvement is a myeloma-defining event, and the extent and pattern of myeloma infiltration impact treatment decisions following updated diagnostic criteria by the International Myeloma Working Group (IMWG).
- Whole-body MR imaging is recognized as the gold standard for the imaging diagnosis of bone marrow involvement in myeloma.
- Whole-body MR imaging is particularly recommended for the workup of patients with smoldering or asymptomatic myeloma or those with solitary plasmacytoma.
- The IMWG classifies MR imaging bone involvement as greater than 1 focal lesion with a diameter greater than 5 mm.

## INTRODUCTION

Myeloma is the most common primary malignancy affecting the skeleton, with an incidence of approximately 10 per 100,000.[1] It is a clinically and biologically heterogeneous cancer arising from bone marrow plasma cells that evolves from a premalignant precursor condition (monoclonal gammopathy of undetermined significance) into asymptomatic myeloma and, finally, symptomatic disease.[2] Uncontrolled myeloma frequently causes significant morbidity, which typically includes immunosuppression, kidney impairment, and lytic bone destruction. The pathogenesis of myeloma bone disease starts with expansion of malignant myeloma cells in the bone marrow where they interact with stromal cells and shift the balance toward an excess of osteoclast-activating factors and suppression of osteoblast activity. Unchecked osteoclastic activity promotes the production of various cytokines from stromal cells, which leads directly or indirectly to further multiple myeloma clone proliferation. A vicious cycle is set in motion, with bone destruction feeding tumor growth and multiple myeloma cells promoting bone destruction.[3–5]

Modern therapies can disrupt this vicious cycle and limit other disease morbidity, increasingly mandating sensitive and specific diagnostic tools to identify patients who will benefit from treatment.

## DEFINITION AND ROLE OF IMAGING IN MYELOMA

The International Myeloma Working Group's (IMWG) updated criteria for the diagnosis of multiple myeloma include[6]

- Clonal bone marrow plasma cells greater than 10% or biopsy-proven bony or extramedullary

Disclosure: The authors acknowledge National Health Service funding to the National Institute for Health Research Biomedical Research Center, Clinical Research Facility in Imaging, and the Cancer Research Network. The views expressed in this publication are those of the authors and not necessarily those of the National Health Service, the National Institute for Health Research, or the Department of Health.
[a] Department of Radiology, The Royal Marsden Hospital, The Institute of Cancer Research, Downs Road, Sutton SM2 5PT, UK; [b] Myeloma Group, The Institute of Cancer Research, The Royal Marsden Hospital, Downs Road, Sutton SM2 5NG, UK
* Corresponding author.
*E-mail address:* Christina.Messiou@rmh.nhs.uk

Magn Reson Imaging Clin N Am 26 (2018) 509–525
https://doi.org/10.1016/j.mric.2018.06.006
1064-9689/18/© 2018 The Royal Marsden Hospital. Published by Elsevier Inc. This is an open access article under the CC BY-NC-ND license (http://creativecommons.org/licenses/by-nc-nd/4.0/).

plasmacytoma and any one or more of the following myeloma-defining events:

- Evidence of end-organ damage
  - Hypercalcemia
  - Renal insufficiency
  - Anemia
  - Bone lesions
- Any one or more of the following biomarkers of malignancy:
  - Clonal bone marrow plasma cell percentage of 60% or greater
  - Involved: uninvolved serum free light chain ratio of 100 or greater
  - Greater than 1 focal lesions on MR imaging studies greater than 5 mm

In light of the diagnostic criteria, the major indication for imaging is establishing bone involvement as a myeloma-defining event. However, skeletal complications, such as fractures and spinal cord compression, are highly morbid and imaging is critical for risk assessment, detection, and management guidance. As the therapeutic options for patients with myeloma become more sophisticated, the role of imaging in risk stratification, restaging, and detecting minimal residual disease is also evolving.

Myeloma is primarily a disease of bone marrow that can occur anywhere in the skeleton; therefore, wide skeletal coverage is mandatory. Until very recently, bone destruction was necessary to confirm a diagnosis of bone involvement; thus, cheap and readily available skeletal surveys served as the most commonly used imaging tool. However, plain films offer limited sensitivity; up to 50% of bone demineralization can occur before lesions become evident.[7] Even when MR imaging is limited to the spine, it will upstage one-third of the patients thought to have solitary plasmacytoma on skeletal surveys[8]; whole-body MR imaging has been shown to upstage all patients thought to have solitary disease on skeletal surveys.[9] Whole-body computed tomography (CT) techniques have been used as a more sensitive alternative and can lead to therapy change in between 18% and 61% of the patients compared with skeletal surveys (**Fig. 1**).[10–12] Radiation doses can be minimized using dedicated low-dose CT protocols, but they remain 2 to 4 times greater than those used in plain film skeletal surveys.[12] Despite improved sensitivity, CT also remains inherently limited to primarily imaging the secondary effects of myeloma on cortical bone rather than bone marrow itself. Consequently, plain film and skeletal surveys should not be used for restaging at disease relapse, as cortical bone defects can represent old inactive treated sites of disease. The addition of quantitative information on tumor metabolism in the form of [18]F fluorodeoxyglucose (FDG) PET/CT provides a highly attractive combination of anatomic and functional information albeit at radiation doses 4 to 5 times higher than those used in low-dose CT alone. The IMWG accepts FDG PET/CT as a possible choice of staging tool, particularly for patients with smoldering myeloma. However, MR imaging has greater sensitivity and specificity than FDG PET/CT, its greatest advantage being in assessment of diffuse marrow infiltration, small disease foci (sensitivity and specificity of 68% and 83% for MR imaging compared with 59% and 75% for FDG PET/CT),[11,13,14] and slowly proliferative disease that is not [18]F-FDG avid.[15] Emerging data suggest further improvements in sensitivity with the addition of diffusion-weighted (DW) sequences (**Figs. 2 and 3**).[16–18] Preliminary data showed 77% sensitivity for DW-MR imaging compared with 47% for FDG PET/CT.[18] Pawlyn and colleagues[16] demonstrated overall significantly increased detection of focal and diffuse infiltration on DW-MR imaging compared with FDG PET/CT (P<.02), with scores higher at all anatomic locations except the pelvis and long bones, where both techniques were equivalent.[16] The reported false-negative rate of

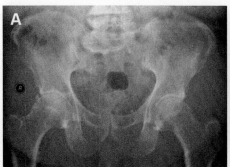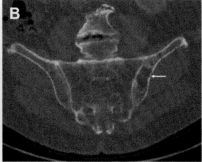

**Fig. 1.** Plain film of the bony pelvis in a patient with suspected myeloma (*A*) shows no focal lytic lesions. However, low-dose CT (*B*) clearly demonstrates a lytic lesion in the left iliac bone (*arrow*).

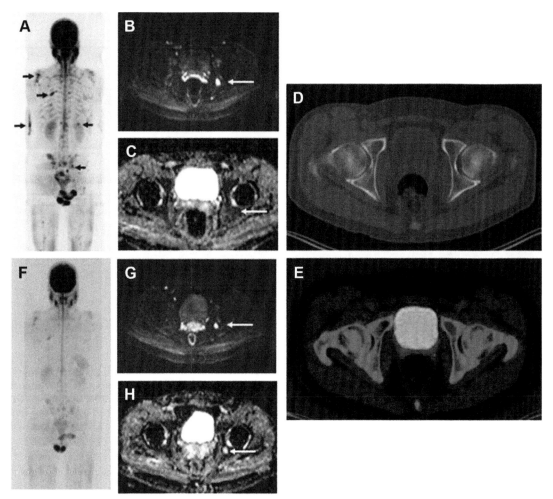

**Fig. 2.** A b900 DW MR Imaging Inverse gray-scale maximum-intensity projection (MIP) (*A*), axial b900 DW MR imaging (*B*), and ADC map (*C*) of a patient with a new diagnosis of myeloma show multifocal bone lesions (*arrows, A*), including a restricted lesion in the posterior left acetabulum (*arrows, B, C*). The posterior acetabular lesion is not evident on corresponding CT (*D*) or FDG PET/CT (*E*) performed on the same day. Following induction chemotherapy, the b900 DW MR imaging inverse gray scale MIP shows reduced burden of disease (*F*). Although the posterior acetabular lesion is only marginally smaller on b900 DW MR imaging (*arrow, G*), the increased ADC (*arrow, H*) indicates a good response.

15% for FDG PET/CT was confirmed by a subsequent larger prospective study, which reported that 10% of the patients would be misclassified using FDG PET/CT as the only functional imaging modality.[10,17] Interestingly, Rasche and colleagues[17] also found that gene expression for hexokinase-2, which is involved in the glycolysis pathway, was significantly lower in false-negative FDG PET/CT cases.

Whole-body MR imaging is recognized as the gold standard for the diagnosis of bone involvement in myeloma and is particularly recommended for the workup of patients with smoldering or asymptomatic myeloma or those with solitary plasmacytoma.[19,20] In some countries, such as the United Kingdom, whole-body MR imaging is now recommended as first-line imaging in all patients with a suspected diagnosis of myeloma.[20,21]

The risk of progression to symptomatic myeloma for patients with smoldering myeloma is about 8% per year after diagnosis.[22] The 2013 landmark study by Mateos and colleagues[23] demonstrated a potential benefit of early therapy for patients with high-risk smoldering multiple myeloma, whereas evidence suggests that MR imaging can be used as a prognostic biomarker in this population.[24–26] The SWOG S0120 study reported that detection of multiple focal lesions on MR imaging conferred an increased risk of progression,[27]

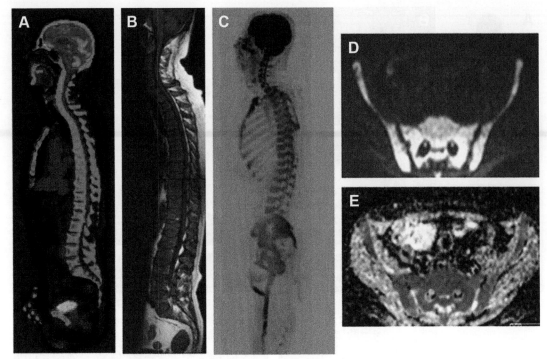

**Fig. 3.** FDG PET/CT (*A*) in a patient with a suspected new diagnosis of myeloma was reported as not showing evidence of marrow disease. Conversely, sagittal T1-weighted MR imaging of the spine (*B*) shows diffuse low signal in vertebral marrow relative to the discs; b900 maximum-intensity projection (*C*), b900 axial DW MR imaging (*D*), and corresponding ADC map (*E*) confirm diffuse abnormal marrow signal. Trephine confirmed 80% plasma cell infiltration of bone marrow.

whereas abnormal signal on MR imaging has been shown to be associated with a very high risk of smoldering myeloma progression with the development of lytic bone lesions.[22] These studies have been highly influential in guiding the IMWG's decision to suggest treatment based on MR imaging focal lesions without confirmation of bone destruction.

### International Myeloma Working Group Definitions of Myeloma Bone Involvement

- CT: one or more osteolytic lesions (≥5 mm)[a]
- [18]F FDG PET/CT: one or more osteolytic lesions (≥5 mm); increased FDG uptake alone is not sufficient; evidence of osteolytic bone destruction is needed on the CT component of the study[a]

- MR imaging: more than one focal lesion of a diameter greater than 5 mm[b]; diffuse marrow abnormality does not qualify

Different patterns of myeloma marrow infiltration are encountered on MR imaging. The presence of focal lesions and more than one focal lesion have been shown to be the strongest adverse prognostic factors for progression followed by diffuse infiltration.[25–28] Conversely, patients with myeloma and normal MR imaging appearances respond better to therapy and survive longer.[29] A micronodular or salt-and-pepper pattern of marrow infiltration is also recognized. Between 3% and 8% of the patients are also thought to have extramedullary sites of disease, although these figures are likely to increase with the growing trend toward the use of cross-sectional imaging.[30,31] Extramedullary

---

[a]Care should be taken to avoid overinterpretation of equivocal or tiny lucencies seen only on CT or PET/CT. For equivocal lesions, a repeat study in 3 to 6 months should be done before a diagnosis of multiple myeloma is established. Such patients might be followed up closely at 1- to 3-month intervals before systemic therapy is started.

[b]In cases of equivocal small lesions, a second MR imaging should be performed after 3 to 6 months; if the MR imaging shows progression, patients should be treated as having symptomatic myeloma.

disease detection is relevant as an independent prognostic factor for progression-free survival.[32]

## DIFFUSION-WEIGHTED MR IMAGING IN MYELOMA

The speed, coverage, and high sensitivity of whole-body DW-MR imaging, with its ability to quantify both the burden of disease and response to treatment, has made it a critical component of whole-body MR imaging for patients with myeloma.

The inverse correlation between cell density in soft tissues and apparent diffusion coefficient (ADC) has been extensively described[33–36] and is supported by indirect evidence that choline, a marker of cell turnover, is inversely correlated with ADC in glioma.[37] However, cellularity is not the sole factor influencing ADC, and the relationship between cellularity and ADC has not been so impressive in all cell types.[33,37] Other factors may influence ADC, for example, cytoplasmic viscosity, capillary bulk flow, active transport, and cell architecture, size and size variability within tissue have been variously implicated in small studies. Therefore, it is likely that ADC is a complex function of tissue microarchitecture that is, influenced by several components.

In response to treatment, the increased extracellular spaces within a tumor manifest as increases in distances of water motion and an increase in ADC.[38] This has been demonstrated in several tumor types including brain, breast, prostate, and liver metastases,[39–41] where it has been used to predict treatment response ahead of conventional imaging and serum markers.[42,43] Some studies have gone further and used DW-MR imaging to detect the emergence of drug resistance during the course of therapy.[44]

However, the presence of fat in marrow necessitates an adapted approach. In normal adult marrow, there is a predominance of fat and a paucity of free water. The motion of the small amount of water that is present is restricted by fat; hence, normal adult marrow has very little signal on DW-MR imaging. As cellularity in marrow increases secondary either to disease or increased hematopoietic tissue, the amount of free water increases and so does the ADC.[45,46] It is thought that the increased vascularity associated with plasma cell infiltration is also influential in this relationship.[46] Hence, in adults, the different microarchitecture of plasma cell–infiltrated marrow results in markedly different signal on DW-MR imaging and contrasts against normal marrow, which returns little signal.

The excellent image contrast between normal and diseased marrow on DW-MR imaging results in superior lesion conspicuity compared with conventional short tau inversion recovery (STIR) and contrast-enhanced MR imaging sequences.[47–49]

Furthermore, unlike extraskeletal tumor types, the ADC value of myeloma-infiltrated marrow is significantly different from that of normal adult marrow, with very little overlap.[28,50] This difference means that qualitative differences in image contrast translate into quantitative differences and the ADC value can be used to separate myelomatous from normal marrow with a sensitivity of 90% and specificity of 93%. The ADC of the marrow of patients in remission and with monoclonal gammopathy of undetermined significance is not significantly different from that of healthy age-matched volunteers, making whole-body DW-MR imaging a promising tool for monitoring of these patients.[51] It should be noted that the IMWG's new guidelines stipulate only focal lesions as an indication to treat patients with asymptomatic myeloma. This stipulation is perhaps because the diagnosis of diffuse infiltration on conventional MR imaging is challenging and is most often a subjective diagnosis based on a comparison of marrow signal with intervertebral discs. There is potential for ADC measurements to reduce this subjectivity, and this should be a priority for future studies. However, whole-body MR imaging can currently be used to make a judgment on whether posterior iliac crest trephine is likely to be representative, which facilitates the diagnosis of diffuse infiltration (**Fig. 4**).

Although whole-body DW-MR imaging is emerging as one of the most sensitive tools for imaging bone marrow with increased lesion conspicuity compared with conventional MR imaging sequences[47,52,53](**Fig. 5**), some debate remains as to its specificity. Although Lecouvet and colleagues[52] presented data to suggest high specificity for detection of metastatic bone disease (98%–100%), a recent meta-analysis showed a pooled specificity of 86.1%.[53] The paucity of specific prospective studies on myeloma and marked heterogeneity in reference standards make current judgments on specificity challenging, and biopsy of all lesions is not feasible. The approach offered by the IMWG of a 3- to 6-month follow-up of equivocal solitary small lesions is a pragmatic solution.[6]

The skull and ribs have historically been difficult sites for interrogation with MR imaging; however, DW imaging has shown increased sensitivity for lesion detection in the ribs compared with skeletal surveys in 2 studies.[54,55] Additionally, a lesion detection in the skull was reduced compared with skeletal surveys in both studies. This finding is possibly because the small volume of marrow in the skull is challenging to interrogate against adjacent high-diffusion signal in the brain. Still, false positives on plain film of the skull secondary to venous lakes and granulations are also possible and difficult to confirm.

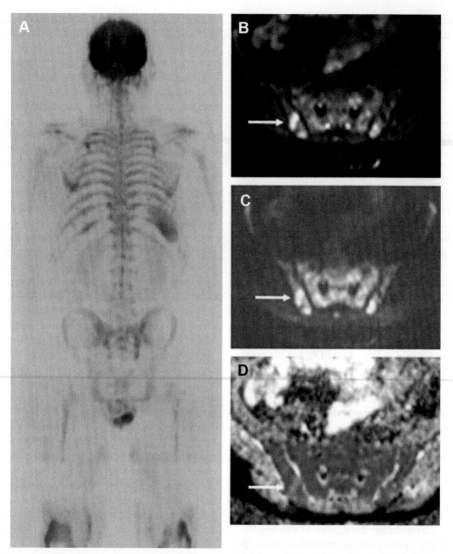

**Fig. 4.** A b900 DW MR imaging inverse gray-scale maximum-intensity projection (*A*) shows subtle alteration in background marrow signal suspicious but not confirmatory for diffuse infiltration. There are no focal lesions. Axial b50 (*B*), b900 (*C*), and ADC map (*D*) of the pelvis confirm suspicion for diffuse abnormal signal. The right-sided trephine tract is clearly seen at b50, b900, and on the ADC map (*arrows*) and suggests that marrow sampled appears similar to marrow elsewhere and should, therefore, be representative. Trephine confirmed 20% plasma cell infiltration.

## WHOLE-BODY MR IMAGING PROTOCOLS

The core whole-body MR imaging protocol, when used alone, is targeted primarily toward imaging bone marrow but can also detect extramedullary disease and should be completed within 45 minutes of table time (**Fig. 6, Table 1**). Sagittal imaging of the spine contributes to disease detection but also provides an essential assessment of mechanical complications, such as vertebral fractures or expansile disease threatening the spinal canal or nerve roots. Particularly for patients with symptoms, it is prudent to perform sagittal spine imaging first, so that essential information is obtained in case of an aborted scan. Axial anatomic detail is provided by Dixon images, but this also facilitates disease detection and quantification in the form of fat-fraction maps. Axial DW-MR imaging is the most sensitive sequence for detecting disease and also provide quantitative capabilities for assessing response. Anatomic correlation is supported by b50 and Dixon imaging. The core protocol can be supplemented with axial T2-weighted (T2W) sequences, but these are not considered mandatory. Regional assessments can be used as clinically indicated, that is, small field-of-view

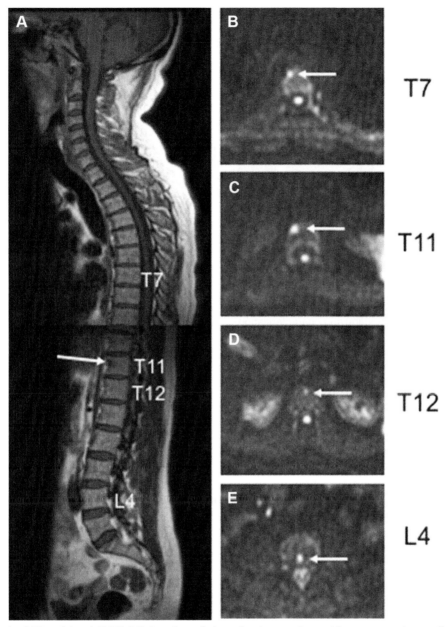

Fig. 5. Sagittal T1-weighted (T1W) MR imaging of the spine in a patient with a suspected new diagnosis of myeloma shows a subtle focal lesion in anterior T11 (*arrow, A*). Axial b900 images confirm the focal lesion in T11 (*C*) but also demonstrate small focal lesions in T7 (*B, arrow*), T12 (*D, arrow*), and L4 (*E, arrow*), which were not evident on T1W imaging.

T2W axial imaging through levels of suspected cord compression. Although 45-minute protocols are generally well tolerated, longer examination times are challenging for some patients.[16]

The evaluation of source b800 to 1000 value images of DW-MR imaging sequences is based on comparing high b-value image intensity to adjacent muscle signal intensity, but ADC maps are quantitative. Inverse gray-scale maximum-intensity projection (MIP) reconstructions are a means of displaying disease distribution and can be useful for identifying sites of disease in the ribs or vertebral spinous processes but should never be interpreted in isolation from source images.

The definitions for hypointense and hyperintense signal on b800 to 1000 value images remains subjective but can be gauged by using adjacent muscle as the reference background tissue.[56]

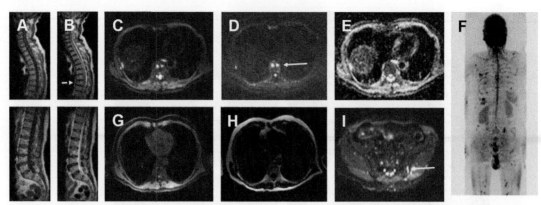

Fig. 6. Core whole-body MR imaging protocol comprises sagittal T1 (*A*) and T2-weighted (*B*) sequences of the spine; axial b50 (*C*), b900 DW MR imaging (*D*), ADC map (*E*), and b900 DW MR imaging inverse gray-scale maximum-intensity projection (*F*); axial water-only (*G*) and fat-only (*H*) Dixon imaging. Two focal lesions within T8 are clearly seen on DW MR imaging (*D, arrow*) but are less well seen on sagittal imaging of the spine (*arrow, B*). The b50 DW MR imaging through the pelvis (*I*) shows the left-sided trephine tract (*arrow*), which suggests that background marrow but not focal lesions are sampled.

The combination of morphologic and functional data also allows for detection and characterization of vertebral fractures. Although morphologic features of diffuse T1 low signal, convex vertebral contour, involvement of pedicles, and a lumbar level are more frequently observed in malignant fractures,[57] the addition of DW-MR imaging to conventional MR imaging sequences has been shown to improve diagnostic accuracy.[58] Theoretically, benign fractures have more edema and free water and, therefore, a higher ADC than malignant fractures, where packed tumor cells lower the ADC. However, there has been conflict in the literature as to whether ADC can reliably be used as a

**Table 1**
**Recommendations for a core whole-body MR imaging protocol for imaging patients with myeloma**

| | Sequence Description | Core Protocol |
|---|---|---|
| 1 | Whole spine: sagittal, T1W, TSE, 4- to 5-mm slice thickness | Yes |
| 2 | Whole spine: sagittal, T2, STIR or fat-suppressed T2W, 4- to 5-mm slice thickness | Yes |
| 3 | Whole-body (vertex to knees): T1W, Dixon technique; fat image reconstructions mandatory<br>A 3D FSE T1W sequence offering multiplanar capability maybe performed as an alternative to replace sequences 1 and 3 | Axial (5 mm) |
| 4 | Whole-body (vertex to knees): axial, DW, STIR fat suppression, 5- to 7-mm contiguous slicing, multiple stations<br>• ADC calculations with mono-exponential data fitting<br>• 3D-MIP reconstructions of highest b-value images | 2 b-values (b50–100 and b800–1000 s/mm$^2$) |
| 5 | Whole-body (vertex to knees): axial, T2W, TSE without fat suppression, 5-mm contiguous slicing, multiple stations, preferably matching the DW images | Optional |
| 6 | Regional assessments, for example, symptomatic/known sites outside the standard field of view, axial T2W through sites of suspected cord compression, para-coronal T1 sacrum for suspected sacral nerve root involvement | Optional |

*Abbreviations:* 3D, 3 dimensional; FSE, fast spin echo; MIP, maximum-intensity projection; T1W, T1 weighted; T2W, T2 weighted; TSE, turbo spin echo.

sole discriminator.[58–60] It seems likely that fracture age and mixed edema and tumor are likely to contribute to overlapping in ADC values of benign versus malignant fracture. Greater understanding of appropriate diffusion protocols and combination with morphologic imaging is likely to move this forward as a useful tool.

The diffusion sequences are also exquisitely sensitive to trephine tracts and, if already performed, whole-body DW-MR imaging can give some indication of the representation of the trephine sample. Alternatively, whole-body DW-MR imaging can be used to select the side for trephine sampling.

## PEARLS, PITFALLS, AND VARIANTS
### T2 Shine Through

T2 shine through refers to a high signal on DW imaging that is not due to restricted diffusion but to high T2 signal shining through. Shine through may be seen on high b-value images and MIPs (**Fig. 7**). To avoid misinterpreting this signal, ADC maps should always be interrogated alongside the source b-value images and MIPs.

### Red Marrow

Red marrow has altered diffusion signal compared with yellow marrow[61]; therefore, detection of marrow disease in younger patients can be challenging. However, this is rarely problematic in myeloma, as its incidence is strongly related to age and nearly half of newly diagnosed patients are 75 years old and older (Cancer Research UK statistics). Granulocyte colony-stimulating factor (G-CSF) given either as part of the preparation for autologous stem-cell transplantation (ASCT) or supportive measures leads to a hypercellular marrow, which can mimic diffuse infiltration (**Fig. 8**). This is also problematic for other imaging techniques, such as conventional MR imaging sequences and FDG PET/CT. Therefore, both DW-MR imaging and FDG PET/CT should be avoided in the days following G-CSF administration; but if this is not possible, diffuse abnormalities should be interpreted with caution.

### Hemangiomas

Vertebral hemangiomas are extremely common, with an incidence of up to 26%. The ADC of hemangiomas is significantly higher than that of focal active myeloma deposits: $1085 \times 10^{-6}\,mm^2s^{-1}$ compared with $682 \times 10^{-6}\,mm^2s^{-1}$.[62] Therefore, the ADC map combined with appearances on sagittal T1 and T2W imaging of the spine should avoid misdiagnosis as active myeloma deposits (**Fig. 9**).

### Trephine Tracts

Although visualization of posterior iliac trephine tracts can allow some estimation of the possibility

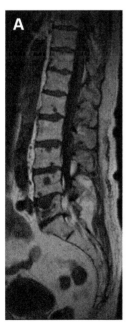
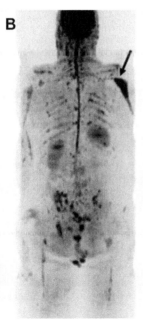
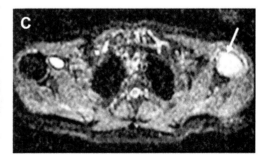

**Fig. 7.** Sagittal T1-weighted MR imaging (*A*) and b900 DW MR imaging inverse gray-scale MIP (*B*) in a patient with treated myeloma suggest the presence of multifocal lesions. However, the ADC map (example left humeral lesion *arrow, B, C*) showed uniformly very high ADC (similar to cerebral spinal fluid) suggesting that these were acellular treated sites of disease. The appearance of multifocal disease on the b900 DW MR imaging inverse gray-scale MIP is an example of T2 shine through.

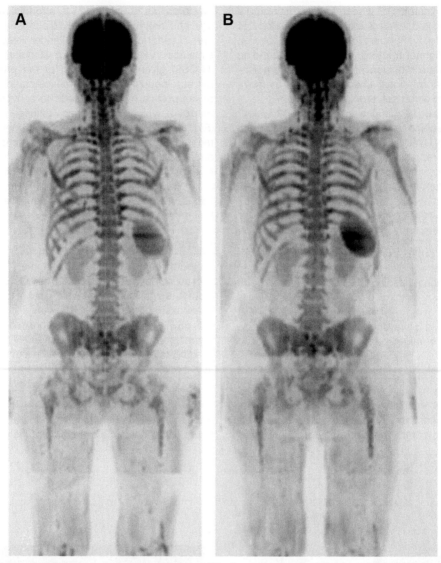

**Fig. 8.** A b900 DW MR imaging inverse gray-scale MIP of a patient with diffuse myeloma marrow infiltration confirmed on trephine, which showed 80% infiltration (*A*). Follow-up b900 DW MR imaging inverse gray-scale MIP (*B*) following induction chemotherapy shows stable imaging appearances of diffuse abnormal signal; but trephine showed no evidence of myeloma, only reactive, regenerative marrow. The diffuse abnormal signal following therapy was secondary to G-CSF administration.

of sampling errors (see **Fig. 6**), on occasion a trephine will cause a hematoma. Blood products can cause restriction of diffusion mimicking disease; therefore, a solitary lesion in the posterior iliac crest, in particular, should be carefully interrogated for the presence of a trephine tract (**Fig. 10**).

### Incidental Findings

Incidental findings on whole-body MR imaging are very common (up to 38%); however, the proposed core protocol allows for characterization of most incidental findings, and reportedly only 3% of the scans will lead to an equivocal finding that requires further investigation.[30] It is important for reporting radiologists to be clear about their level of concern and make recommendations for investigation/management of incidental findings.

## IMAGING RESPONSE

The capability of whole-body MR imaging including DW-MR imaging to demonstrate both focal and diffuse marrow infiltration throughout

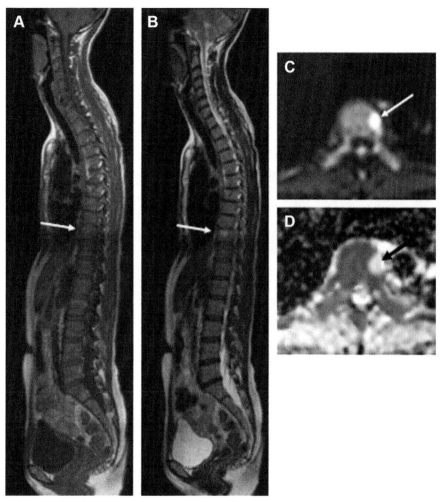

Fig. 9. Sagittal T1-weighted (*A*) and T2W (*B*) MR imaging of the spine in a patient with a suspected new diagnosis of myeloma demonstrates characteristic appearances of a vertebral T10 hemangioma (*arrows*), which is T1 and T2 bright. The corresponding axial b900 image also shows a corresponding focal lesion (*arrow, C*); the ADC map (*arrow, D*) confirms a high ADC, which is more in keeping with a hemangioma than active disease.

the whole skeleton makes this technique extremely promising as a subjective tool for monitoring disease status and assessment of response. For focal lesions, changes in size and number can be easily assessed; for diffuse infiltration, signal changes are evident. However, ADC measurements offer the capability to quantify disease throughout the skeleton. This capability is particularly relevant, as changes in ADC are known to predate changes in the size of focal marrow deposits[51,63] (see **Fig. 2**); dimension-based assessments are not applicable to diffuse infiltration. Advances in data informatics have made semiautomated skeletal segmentation a reality, enabling histogram quantification of a patient's whole marrow. This capability has been demonstrated by Giles and colleagues,[64] who used these

techniques to segment patients' bone marrow on DW-MR imaging to quantify the response to treatment. Reassuringly, the reproducibility was excellent, with a coefficient of variation of 2.8%. The mean ADC increased in 95% of the responding patients and decreased in all nonresponders ($P<.002$). A 3.3% increase in ADC helped identify the response with 90% sensitivity and 100% specificity. Visual assessment was also able to identify the response to treatment with high sensitivity (sensitivity 86%, specificity 95%), with good agreement in posttreatment change between 2 observers. There was a significant negative correlation between change in ADC and change in laboratory markers of response. Conversely, Hillengas and colleagues[28] demonstrated a decrease in ADC following therapy; it is likely that

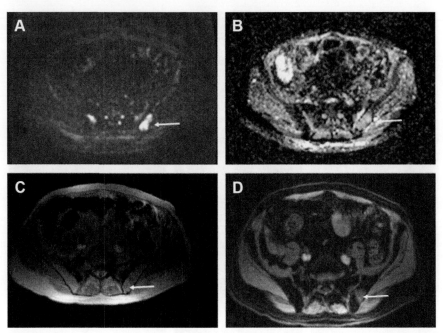

**Fig. 10.** b900 DW MR imaging and ADC map of a patient with a suspected diagnosis of myeloma demonstrates a focal lesion in the left posterior iliac crest (*arrows, A, B*). The intermediate/high ADC is unusual for a new site of focal active disease, which would usually appear restricted. Close interrogation of the corresponding fat-only and water-only images reveals a trephine tract (*arrows, C, D*) through the lesion. The lesion was a hematoma that resolved on follow-up.

the direction of ADC change was influenced by the timing of the measurement. Messiou and colleagues[51] have confirmed that early following treatment, ADC increases presumably due to plasma cell death and resultant increased extracellular spaces. Later follow-up measurements show an ADC decrease when normal marrow architecture including marrow fat is restored (see **Fig. 2; Fig. 11**).

Fat-fraction measurements from Dixon imaging also give insight into the treatment response, as normal marrow fat is restored when the disease is responding[51]; additionally, more recent studies suggest that early fat-fraction measurements may be a potential biomarker of poor response (**Fig. 12**).[65]

### Prognosis

Compelling data from Bartel and colleagues,[66] Zamagni and colleagues,[67] and Moreau and colleagues[32] have shown FDG PET/CT to be prognostic in the postinduction and posttransplant phases. Accurate prognostic information in these settings, where treatment can be both costly and associated with toxicity, is highly desirable for patient selection but also as a tool to stratify treatment intensity, consolidation, or maintenance therapy. Hillengass and colleagues[68] performed

conventional whole-body MR imaging in patients before and after single or double ASCT treatment and found that the number of detected focal lesions on MR imaging significantly correlated with and predicted the overall survival in the patients. Although FDG PET/CT has been shown to be a powerful tool in detecting residual disease, the increased sensitivity of DW-MR imaging and its capability to detect both tiny deposits and diffuse disease gives it a potential advantage, which merits prospective evaluation.

### WHAT THE REFERRING PHYSICIAN NEEDS TO KNOW

The most recent consensus statement from the IMWG[19] recommends whole-body MR imaging in the workup of solitary bone plasmacytoma and patients with smoldering multiple myeloma. In some countries, whole-body MR imaging is recommended as first-line imaging in all patients with a suspected diagnosis of myeloma.[20] Experienced centers have extended the service to monitoring patients with nonsecretory myeloma. On a case-by-case basis, whole-body MR imaging is also used to guide therapeutic decisions and monitor remission status in patients with symptomatic clinically or genetically defined high-risk disease. For patients with previously

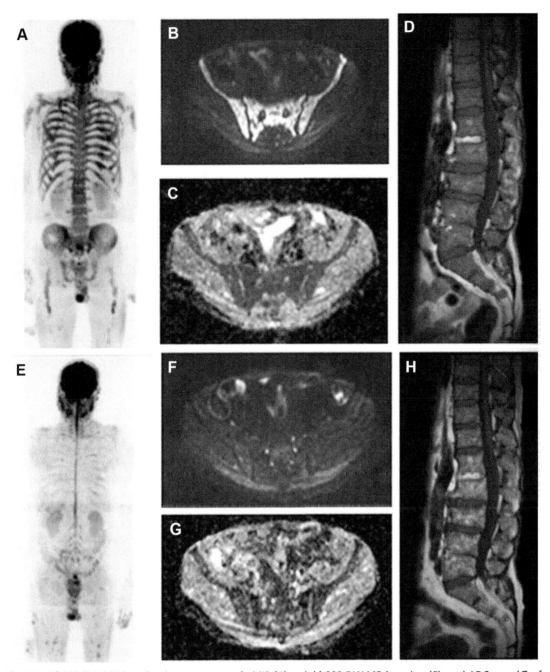

**Fig. 11.** A b900 DW MR imaging inverse gray-scale MIP (*A*), axial b900 DW MR imaging (*B*), and ADC map (*C*) of the pelvis in a patient with a new diagnosis of diffuse myeloma infiltration confirmed on trephine. Corresponding sagittal T1-weighted MR imaging of the spine shows diffuse low signal in vertebral marrow (*D*). Following induction chemotherapy, b900 DW MR imaging inverse gray-scale MIP (*E*), b900 DW MR imaging (*F*), and ADC map (*G*) show normalization of marrow signal. Increased T1 marrow signal (*H*) confirms the return of normal marrow fat.

treated myeloma with borderline remission status or possible recurrence, whole-body DW-MR imaging is also extremely useful in differentiating treated from active sites of disease to guide management.

In many countries, limited MR imaging capacity presents a tangible barrier to providing a whole-body MR imaging service. Clear local referral pathways and guidelines ensure appropriate use of scanner time. Referring physicians should be

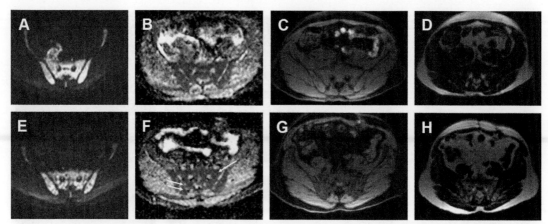

**Fig. 12.** Axial b900 DW MR imaging, ADC map, axial water-only, and fat-only images of the pelvis before (*A–D*) and after treatment (*E–H*) in a patient with a new diagnosis of diffuse myeloma infiltration confirmed on trephine. Following induction chemotherapy, the ADC map shows subtle patchy islands of increasing ADC (*E*), suggesting some response (*arrows, F*). Corresponding water-only images show diffuse reduced water signal (reduced signal *G* compared with *C*), and returning fat signal is seen on fat-only images (increased signal on *H* compared with *D*) in keeping with response.

aware that although 45 minutes of scanning time is well tolerated by most patients,[16] this is not universal. For example, when a patient presents with clinical symptoms and signs of spinal cord compression, the examination may be limited to MR imaging of the spine alone in order to address the acute clinical question. It is imperative that factors such as pain and claustrophobia, which might influence a patient's tolerance for whole-body MR imaging, are communicated to the MR imaging team because, in some circumstances, forward planning, such as arranging analgesia or light sedation, can circumvent an unsuccessful scan attempt.

There is a strong case that the approach of using cross-sectional imaging at the time of diagnosis is a cost-effective strategy for diagnosis in patients with a suspected diagnosis of myeloma. In a recent analysis by the UK National Institute for Health and Care Excellence, the main influence presented was the avoidance of further cross-sectional imaging to guide treatment decisions, following a positive result on a skeletal survey.[20] The cross-sectional approach could be cost saving and health improving. Whole-body MR imaging showed the largest increase in incremental quality-of-life-adjusted life-years, which was heavily influenced by it being assigned as the most sensitive imaging technique. In terms of incremental net monetary benefit, whole-body CT and MR imaging were almost equivalent, followed by MR imaging of the spine. Strikingly, FDG PET/CT was the only imaging modality with a negative incremental net monetary benefit.

## FUTURE DIRECTIONS AND SUMMARY

The advent of whole-body DW-MR imaging has been one of the most significant advances for imaging in oncology patients over the last decade. The high sensitivity, speed, and quantitative capabilities have addressed an unmet need in imaging primary and secondary marrow malignancies.

Combined with anatomic imaging, whole-body DW-MR imaging now forms an imaging tool that has been tailored to detect both focal and diffuse disease and quantify burden and response, while also assessing mechanical complications. This blend of anatomic and functional imaging is well suited to serve the imaging needs of patients with myeloma. The necessity for whole-body imaging of patients with smoldering multiple myeloma and solitary plasmacytoma is now recognized. However, future studies will need to direct positioning of whole-body DW-MR imaging alongside emerging molecular and genetic signals as predictive and prognostic biomarkers. If future studies corroborate the usefulness of whole marrow segmentation techniques, academic and industrial collaborations will be essential to translate this from research to clinical settings. It is also likely that whole-body DW-MR imaging will have an increasing role in stratifying risk; as the number of treatment options continues to grow, it is likely to find its place in guiding therapeutic strategies.

## REFERENCES

1. Cancer Research UK. Myeloma incidence statistics. Available at: http://www.cancerresearchuk.org/health-professional/cancer-statistics/statistics-by-cancer-type/

myeloma/incidence#heading-Three. Accessed March 19, 2018.

2. Landgren O, Kyle RA, Rajkumar SV. From myeloma precursor disease to multiple myeloma: new diagnostic concepts and opportunities for early intervention. Clin Cancer Res 2011;17(6):1243–52.

3. Angtuaco EJ, Fassas AB, Walker R, et al. Multiple myeloma: clinical review and diagnostic imaging. Radiology 2004;231(1):11–23.

4. Lawson MA, McDonald MM, Kovacic N, et al. Osteoclasts control reactivation of dormant myeloma cells by remodelling the endosteal niche. Nat Commun 2015;6:8983.

5. Kovacic N, Croucher PI, McDonald MM. Signaling between tumor cells and the host bone marrow microenvironment. Calcif Tissue Int 2014;94(1): 125–39.

6. Rajkumar SV, Dimopoulos MA, Palumbo A, et al. International myeloma working group updated criteria for the diagnosis of multiple myeloma. Lancet Oncol 2014;15(12):e538–48.

7. Edelstyn GA, Gillespie PJ, Grebbell FS. The radiological demonstration of osseous metastases. Experimental observations. Clin Radiol 1967;18(2): 158–62.

8. Moulopoulos LA, Dimopoulos MA, Weber D, et al. Magnetic resonance imaging in the staging of solitary plasmacytoma of bone. J Clin Oncol 1993; 11(7):1311–5.

9. Fechtner K, Hillengass J, Delorme S, et al. Staging monoclonal plasma cell disease: comparison of the Durie-Salmon and the Durie-Salmon PLUS staging systems. Radiology 2010;257(1):195–204.

10. Kropil P, Fenk R, Fritz LB, et al. Comparison of whole-body 64-slice multidetector computed tomography and conventional radiography in staging of multiple myeloma. Eur Radiol 2008;18(1):51–8.

11. Gleeson TG, Moriarty J, Shortt CP, et al. Accuracy of whole-body low-dose multidetector CT (WBLDCT) versus skeletal survey in the detection of myelomatous lesions, and correlation of disease distribution with whole-body MRI (WBMRI). Skeletal Radiol 2009;38(3):225–36.

12. Hillengass J, Moulopoulos LA, Delorme S, et al. Whole-body computed tomography versus conventional skeletal survey in patients with multiple myeloma: a study of the International Myeloma Working Group. Blood Cancer J 2017;7(8):e599.

13. Dimopoulos M, Terpos E, Comenzo RL, et al. International myeloma working group consensus statement and guidelines regarding the current role of imaging techniques in the diagnosis and monitoring of multiple Myeloma. Leukemia 2009;23(9):1545–56.

14. Shortt CP, Gleeson TG, Breen KA, et al. Whole-body MRI versus PET in assessment of multiple myeloma disease activity. AJR Am J Roentgenol 2009;192(4): 980–6.

15. Durie BG. The role of anatomic and functional staging in myeloma: description of Durie/Salmon plus staging system. Eur J Cancer 2006;42(11):1539–43.

16. Pawlyn C, Fowkes L, Otero S, et al. Whole-body diffusion-weighted MRI: a new gold standard for assessing disease burden in patients with multiple myeloma? Leukemia 2016;30(6):1446–8.

17. Rasche L, Angtuaco E, McDonald JE, et al. Low expression of hexokinase-2 is associated with false-negative FDG-positron emission tomography in multiple myeloma. Blood 2017;130(1):30–4.

18. Sachpekidis C, Mosebach J, Freitag MT, et al. Application of (18)F-FDG PET and diffusion weighted imaging (DWI) in multiple myeloma: comparison of functional imaging modalities. Am J Nucl Med Mol Imaging 2015;5(5):479–92.

19. Dimopoulos MA, Hillengass J, Usmani S, et al. Role of magnetic resonance imaging in the management of patients with multiple myeloma: a consensus statement. J Clin Oncol 2015;33(6):657–64.

20. The National Institute for Health and Care Excellence (NICE). Myeloma: diagnosis and management. Available at: https://www.nice.org.uk/guidance/ng35. Accessed March 19, 2018.

21. Messiou C, Kaiser M. Whole body diffusion weighted MRI–a new view of myeloma. Br J Haematol 2015;171(1):29–37.

22. Kastritis E, Terpos E, Moulopoulos L, et al. Extensive bone marrow infiltration and abnormal free light chain ratio identifies patients with asymptomatic myeloma at high risk for progression to symptomatic disease. Leukemia 2013;27(4):947–53.

23. Mateos MV, Hernandez MT, Giraldo P, et al. Lenalidomide plus dexamethasone for high-risk smoldering multiple myeloma. N Engl J Med 2013; 369(5):438–47.

24. Moulopoulos LA, Dimopoulos MA, Smith TL, et al. Prognostic significance of magnetic resonance imaging in patients with asymptomatic multiple myeloma. J Clin Oncol 1995;13(1):251–6.

25. Moulopoulos LA, Gika D, Anagnostopoulos A, et al. Prognostic significance of magnetic resonance imaging of bone marrow in previously untreated patients with multiple myeloma. Ann Oncol 2005; 16(11):1824–8.

26. Mariette X, Zagdanski AM, Guermazi A, et al. Prognostic value of vertebral lesions detected by magnetic resonance imaging in patients with stage I multiple myeloma. Br J Haematol 1999;104(4): 723–9.

27. Dhodapkar MV, Sexton R, Waheed S, et al. Clinical, genomic, and imaging predictors of myeloma progression from asymptomatic monoclonal gammopathies (SWOG S0120). Blood 2014;123(1):78–85.

28. Hillengass J, Bauerle T, Bartl R, et al. Diffusion-weighted imaging for non-invasive and quantitative monitoring of bone marrow infiltration in patients

with monoclonal plasma cell disease: a comparative study with histology. Br J Haematol 2011;153(6): 721–8.

29. Lecouvet FE, Vande Berg BC, Michaux L, et al. Stage III multiple myeloma: clinical and prognostic value of spinal bone marrow MR imaging. Radiology 1998;209(3):653–60.

30. Wale A, Pawlyn C, Kaiser M, et al. Frequency, distribution and clinical management of incidental findings and extramedullary plasmacytomas in whole body diffusion weighted magnetic resonance imaging in patients with multiple myeloma. Haematologica 2016;101(4):e142–4.

31. Short KD, Rajkumar SV, Larson D, et al. Incidence of extramedullary disease in patients with multiple myeloma in the era of novel therapy, and the activity of pomalidomide on extramedullary myeloma. Leukemia 2011;25(6):906–8.

32. Moreau P, Attal M, Caillot D, et al. Prospective evaluation of magnetic resonance imaging and [(18)F] fluorodeoxyglucose positron emission tomography-computed tomography at diagnosis and before maintenance therapy in symptomatic patients with multiple myeloma included in the IFM/DFCI 2009 trial: results of the IMAJEM Study. J Clin Oncol 2017;35(25):2911–8.

33. Guo AC, Cummings TJ, Dash RC, et al. Lymphomas and high-grade astrocytomas: comparison of water diffusibility and histologic characteristics. Radiology 2002;224(1):177–83.

34. Lyng H, Haraldseth O, Rofstad EK. Measurement of cell density and necrotic fraction in human melanoma xenografts by diffusion weighted magnetic resonance imaging. Magn Reson Med 2000;43(6): 828–36.

35. Sugahara T, Korogi Y, Kochi M, et al. Usefulness of diffusion-weighted MRI with echo-planar technique in the evaluation of cellularity in gliomas. J Magn Reson Imaging 1999;9(1):53–60.

36. Tamai K, Koyama T, Saga T, et al. Diffusion-weighted MR imaging of uterine endometrial cancer. J Magn Reson Imaging 2007;26(3):682–7.

37. Gupta RK, Sinha U, Cloughesy TF, et al. Inverse correlation between choline magnetic resonance spectroscopy signal intensity and the apparent diffusion coefficient in human glioma. Magn Reson Med 1999;41(1):2–7.

38. Chenevert TL, Stegman LD, Taylor JM, et al. Diffusion magnetic resonance imaging: an early surrogate marker of therapeutic efficacy in brain tumors. J Natl Cancer Inst 2000;92(24):2029–36.

39. Charles-Edwards EM, deSouza NM. Diffusion-weighted magnetic resonance imaging and its application to cancer. Cancer Imaging 2006;6: 135–43.

40. Ross BD, Chenevert TL, Kim B, et al. Magnetic resonance imaging and spectroscopy: application to experimental neuro-oncology. Q Magn Reson Biol Med 1994;1(2):89–106.

41. Theilmann RJ, Borders R, Trouard TP, et al. Changes in water mobility measured by diffusion MRI predict response of metastatic breast cancer to chemotherapy. Neoplasia 2004;6(6):831–7.

42. Jennings D, Hatton BN, Guo J, et al. Early response of prostate carcinoma xenografts to docetaxel chemotherapy monitored with diffusion MRI. Neoplasia 2002;4(3):255–62.

43. Moffat BA, Chenevert TL, Meyer CR, et al. The functional diffusion map: an imaging biomarker for the early prediction of cancer treatment outcome. Neoplasia 2006;8(4):259–67.

44. Lee KC, Hall DE, Hoff BA, et al. Dynamic imaging of emerging resistance during cancer therapy. Cancer Res 2006;66(9):4687–92.

45. Nonomura Y, Yasumoto M, Yoshimura R, et al. Relationship between bone marrow cellularity and apparent diffusion coefficient. J Magn Reson Imaging 2001;13(5):757–60.

46. Hillengass J, Fechtner K, Weber MA, et al. Prognostic significance of focal lesions in whole-body magnetic resonance imaging in patients with asymptomatic multiple myeloma. J Clin Oncol 2010;28(9):1606–10.

47. Pearce T, Philip S, Brown J, et al. Bone metastases from prostate, breast and multiple myeloma: differences in lesion conspicuity at short-tau inversion recovery and diffusion-weighted MRI. Br J Radiol 2012;85(1016):1102–6.

48. Squillaci E, Bolacchi F, Altobelli S, et al. Pre-treatment staging of multiple myeloma patients: comparison of whole-body diffusion weighted imaging with whole-body T1-weighted contrast-enhanced imaging. Acta Radiol 2015;56(6):733–8.

49. Dutoit JC, Vanderkerken MA, Anthonissen J, et al. The diagnostic value of SE MRI and DWI of the spine in patients with monoclonal gammopathy of undetermined significance, smouldering myeloma and multiple myeloma. Eur Radiol 2014;24(11):2754–65.

50. Messiou C, Collins DJ, Morgan VA, et al. Optimising diffusion weighted MRI for imaging metastatic and myeloma bone disease and assessing reproducibility. Eur Radiol 2011;21(8):1713–8.

51. Messiou C, Giles S, Collins DJ, et al. Assessing response of myeloma bone disease with diffusion-weighted MRI. Br J Radiol 2012;85(1020): e1198–203.

52. Lecouvet FE, El Mouedden J, Collette L, et al. Can whole-body magnetic resonance imaging with diffusion-weighted imaging replace Tc 99m bone scanning and computed tomography for single-step detection of metastases in patients with high-risk prostate cancer? Eur Urol 2012;62(1):68–75.

53. Wu LM, Gu HY, Zheng J, et al. Diagnostic value of whole-body magnetic resonance imaging for bone

metastases: a systematic review and meta-analysis. J Magn Reson Imaging 2011;34(1):128–35.

54. Giles SL, deSouza NM, Collins DJ, et al. Assessing myeloma bone disease with whole-body diffusion-weighted imaging: comparison with x-ray skeletal survey by region and relationship with laboratory estimates of disease burden. Clin Radiol 2015;70(6): 614–21.

55. Narquin S, Ingrand P, Azais I, et al. Comparison of whole-body diffusion MRI and conventional radiological assessment in the staging of myeloma. Diagn Interv Imaging 2013;94(6):629–36.

56. Padhani AR, Lecouvet FE, Tunariu N, et al. METastasis reporting and data system for prostate cancer: practical guidelines for acquisition, interpretation, and reporting of whole-body magnetic resonance imaging-based evaluations of multiorgan involvement in advanced prostate cancer. Eur Urol 2017; 71(1):81–92.

57. Moulopoulos LA, Yoshimitsu K, Johnston DA, et al. MR prediction of benign and malignant vertebral compression fractures. J Magn Reson Imaging 1996;6(4):667–74.

58. Sung JK, Jee WH, Jung JY, et al. Differentiation of acute osteoporotic and malignant compression fractures of the spine: use of additive qualitative and quantitative axial diffusion-weighted MR imaging to conventional MR imaging at 3.0 T. Radiology 2014; 271(2):488–98.

59. Geith T, Schmidt G, Biffar A, et al. Quantitative evaluation of benign and malignant vertebral fractures with diffusion-weighted MRI: what is the optimum combination of b values for ADC-based lesion differentiation with the single-shot turbo spin-echo sequence? AJR Am ·J Roentgenol 2014;203(3): 582–8.

60. Geith T, Schmidt G, Biffar A, et al. Comparison of qualitative and quantitative evaluation of diffusion-weighted MRI and chemical-shift imaging in the differentiation of benign and malignant vertebral body fractures. AJR Am J Roentgenol 2012; 199(5):1083–92.

61. Lavdas I, Rockall AG, Castelli F, et al. Apparent diffusion coefficient of normal abdominal organs and bone marrow from whole-body DWI at 1.5 T: the effect of sex and age. AJR Am J Roentgenol 2015;205(2):242–50.

62. Winfield JM, Poillucci G, Blackledge MD, et al. Apparent diffusion coefficient of vertebral haemangiomas allows differentiation from malignant focal deposits in whole-body diffusion-weighted MRI. Eur Radiol 2018;28(4):1687–91.

63. Messiou C, Collins DJ, Giles S, et al. Assessing response in bone metastases in prostate cancer with diffusion weighted MRI. Eur Radiol 2011; 21(10):2169–77.

64. Giles SL, Messiou C, Collins DJ, et al. Whole-body diffusion-weighted MR imaging for assessment of treatment response in myeloma. Radiology 2014; 271(3):785–94.

65. Latifoltojar A, Hall-Craggs M, Rabin N, et al. Whole body magnetic resonance imaging in newly diagnosed multiple myeloma: early changes in lesional signal fat fraction predict disease response. Br J Haematol 2017;176(2):222–33.

66. Bartel TB, Haessler J, Brown TL, et al. F18-fluoro-deoxyglucose positron emission tomography in the context of other imaging techniques and prognostic factors in multiple myeloma. Blood 2009;114(10): 2068–76.

67. Zamagni E, Patriarca F, Nanni C, et al. Prognostic relevance of 18-F FDG PET/CT in newly diagnosed multiple myeloma patients treated with up-front autologous transplantation. Blood 2011;118(23): 5989–95.

68. Hillengass J, Ayyaz S, Kilk K, et al. Changes in magnetic resonance imaging before and after autologous stem cell transplantation correlate with response and survival in multiple myeloma. Haematologica 2012;97(11):1757–60.

# Metastasis Reporting and Data System for Prostate Cancer in Practice

Anwar R. Padhani, MBBS, MRCP, FRCR[a],*,
Nina Tunariu, MD, MRCP, FRCR[b]

## KEYWORDS

- Whole-body MR imaging • MET-RADS • Prostate cancer • Imaging standard
- Systematic reporting • Therapy response

## KEY POINTS

- MET-RADS provides the minimum standards for whole-body MR imaging with DWI regarding image acquisitions, interpretation, and reporting of baseline and follow-up monitoring examinations of patients with advanced, metastatic prostate cancers.
- MET-RADS is suitable for guiding patient care in practice (using the regional and overall assessment criteria) but can also be incorporated into clinical trials when accurate lesion size and ADC measurements become more important.
- MET-RADS enables the evaluation of the benefits of continuing therapy to be assessed, when there are signs that the disease is progressing (discordant responses).

## INTRODUCTION

Whole-body MR imaging (WB-MR imaging) incorporating diffusion weighted imaging (DWI) is increasingly recommended as a radiation-free imaging method for assessing bone and soft tissue pathology, and for evaluating response to therapy.[1] DWI is a well-recognized and used sequence in oncologic imaging,[2] with the advantages of being able to offer qualitative (signal intensity) and quantitative assessments (apparent diffusion coefficient [ADC] maps) for disease detection and characterizations. A major strength of WB-MR imaging is the ability of overcoming the limitations of bone scintigraphy (BS) and computed tomography (CT) for detection and therapeutic response assessments in bone metastases,[3] the dominant metastatic site in breast and prostate cancer. Although increasingly used for a variety of cancer types with bone disease predilection and being recommended by international guidelines for multiple myeloma[4] and Li-Fraumeni syndrome,[5] WB-MR imaging usage has been confined mainly to expert centers, causing some concerns about its broader applicability. Although WB-MR imaging is performed on almost all modern MR imaging scanners, inconsistencies in WB-MR imaging acquisition protocols and reporting standards have prevented its widespread testing and implementation.

Recently, a group of oncologic imaging specialists teamed with leading urologists and oncologists, to develop recommendations on the minimum requirements for WB-MR imaging

[a] Paul Strickland Scanner Centre, Mount Vernon Hospital, Rickmansworth Road, Northwood, Middlesex HA6 2RN, UK; [b] Royal Marsden NHS Foundation Trust, Institute of Cancer Research and Cancer Research UK Cancer Imaging Centre, Downs Road, Sutton, Surrey SM2 5PT, UK
* Corresponding author.
E-mail address: anwar.padhani@stricklandscanner.org.uk

Magn Reson Imaging Clin N Am 26 (2018) 527–542
https://doi.org/10.1016/j.mric.2018.06.004
1064-9689/18/© 2018 Elsevier Inc. All rights reserved.

acquisition protocols, and for standardized reporting. They recognized that, for this promising method to become mainstream, it is vital to enforce some uniformity in acquisition, interpretation, and reporting. The authors have named their formulation for metastatic disease response and diagnostic system for prostate cancer as MET-RADS-P (METastasis Reporting And Data System for Prostate cancer).[6]

## Why Metastasis Reporting and Data System Is Needed

BS/CT scans are widely used and endorsed by international guidelines as the standard imaging investigations in the staging and follow-up of metastatic prostate cancer, thereby affecting patient management.[7,8] However, it is well known that currently accepted measurements, such as that the minimum lymph node diameter of 15 mm (short axis) on CT scan as measure of disease involvement, are only modestly correlated with the presence of malignant disease. Also, CT scans cannot accurately evaluate the presence of the therapeutic response in nonlytic bone metastases.[9] Conversely, increase BS uptake in number and extent of lesions can equally occur with the osteoblastic healing (so-called FLARE reaction) associated with tumor response, but also with osteoblastic progression associated with increasing tumor burden, thus creating confusion between response and progression, when response to therapy is being assessed. To overcome the bone scan FLARE limitation, the Prostate Cancer Working Group (PCWG) criteria[10] introduced the need for a confirmatory BS with the demonstration of new lesions. However, there are no BS criteria for assessing progression without the appearance of separate new lesions (enlargement of prior lesions does not count for disease progression). This means that patients with bone superscans are not eligible for bone scan assessments for progression assessments. Furthermore, there are no BS or CT criteria to quantify therapy effectiveness in bone metastases.

Thus, it is becoming increasingly clear that the reduced accuracy of BS/CT in detection of bone metastases and especially in assessing response to therapy in bone metastases diminishes their effectiveness in directing therapy and thus may not be fit for purpose in the era of precision oncology, with a rapidly increasing number of cytostatic and novel therapies becoming available.[3] Next-generation WB imaging tools, such as PET with targeted tracers and WB-MR imaging with DWI, are emerging as powerful alternatives;

however, the challenge remains in validating these newer imaging approaches, so that their use is justified in the clinical routine.

An important step in this process is to ensure uniformity in the acquisition, interpretation, and reporting of next-generation WB imaging methods, so that multicenter trials leading to validation of these methods are more easily performed and evaluated. Important steps for WB-MR imaging standardization include the recommendations of the UK quantitative WB-DWI technical workgroup[11] and the new MET-RADS-P standard for use in patients with advanced prostate cancer.[12] The MET-RADS standard establishes the minimum acceptable technical parameters for imaging acquisitions, built with sequences already available on most modern scanners. Of the sequences recommended, it is acknowledged that WB DWI sequences are the most challenging to implement across imaging platforms. These sequences are grouped to enable fast, high-quality examinations for tumor detection and response assessments (core and comprehensive protocols respectively) (Table 1). Image quality control and quality assurance procedures are also detailed by the standard. The MET-RADS standard is designed to offer day-to-day reporting guidance, paired with a detailed reporting tool that allows the description of the disease phenotype based on anatomic patterns of metastatic spread, thus enabling the systematic collection of analyzable data for research purposes, in line with PCWG3 criteria.[10]

Comprehensive response criteria for bone and soft tissue metastases and local disease are proposed, with the ability to summarize the likelihood of a response to treatment, using a Likert-like 1 to 5 category scale. The summarized likelihood of response in bone uses newly developed MET-RADS criteria, but the response in soft tissues continues to be based on long established standards, prescribed by RECIST v1.1 and PCWG 3[9,10] for clinical research. Discordant/mixed responses in which progressing and responding lesions are seen at same time point are increasing seen with targeted therapy use and are a recognized manifestation of tumor heterogeneity. MET-RADS-P proposes methods to record the presence, location, and extent of spatial discordant responses between and within body parts. The use of MET-RADS-P enables for the first time to categorize bone disease response into three categories (progressive disease, stable disease, and response), rather than the currently used limited clinically categories (progression/no progression) based mostly on BS.[8,9] Thus, MET-RADS allows response assessment

Table 1
MET-RADS core versus comprehensive protocols (including reconstructions)

| Sequence Description | Core Protocol | Comprehensive Assessments |
|---|---|---|
| 1  Whole spine: sagittal, T1W, TSE, 4- to 5-mm slice thickness | Yes | Yes |
| 2  Whole spine: sagittal, STIR (preferred) or fat-suppressed T2W, 4- to 5-mm slice thickness | Yes | Yes |
| 3  Whole body (vertex to mid thighs): T1W, GRE Dixon technique<br>Fat % reconstructions are mandatory<br>• A 3D FSE T1W sequence offering multiplanar capability may be performed as an alternative to replace sequences 1 and 3 | Axial (5 mm[a])<br>Or coronal (2 mm) | Axial and coronal |
| 4  Whole body (skull base to mid-thighs): axial, diffusion-weighted, STIR fat suppression, 5- to 7-mm contiguous slicing, multiple stations<br>• ADC calculations with monoexponential data fitting<br>• Coronal b800–1000 multiplanar reconstructions[b]<br>• 3D-MIP reconstructions of highest b-value images[c] | 2 b-values (b50–100 and b800–1000 s/mm$^2$) | 3 b-values (additional b500–600 s/mm$^2$) |
| 5  Whole body (vertex to mid thighs): axial, T2W, TSE without fat suppression, 5-mm contiguous slicing, multiple stations, preferably matching the diffusion-weighted images | Option | Yes |
| 6  Regional assessments including dedicated lung, pelvis, prostate, small field of view spine, brain studies, and contrast enhancement | No | Option |

*Abbreviations:* 3D, three-dimensional; GRE, gradient-recalled echo; MIP, maximum intensity projection; STIR, short tau inversion recovery; T1W, T1-weighted; T2W, T2-weighted; TSE, turbo spin echo.
  [a] 5–7 mm, axial imaging may be chosen to match section thickness of DWI to facilitate image review.
  [b] b800–1000 images from all diffusion imaging stations are grouped and reconstructed as contiguous, two-dimensional coronal, 5-mm slices.
  [c] Whole-body 3D MIP images, displayed as rotating images (every 3°; 120 images), inverted grayscale.

categorizations that mirror assessments used for soft tissues disease.

The benefits of using a standardized approach include enhanced data collection for outcomes monitoring in clinical trials and from patient registries, enhancing the education of radiologists to reduce variability in imaging interpretations, and for improving communication with referring clinicians. The MET-RADS authors state that the new way of bone response categorization could lead to a paradigm shift, from the current concept of treating patients to documentable progression or no longer clinically benefiting (when tumor volume could be substantially greater than baseline), to being guided by the presence or absence of benefit to therapy thus introducing more precise delivery of patient care.

## METASTASIS REPORTING AND DATA SYSTEM FOR PROSTATE CANCER TEMPLATE FORM
*Response Assessment Categories*

An updated MET-RADS-P template form is found in **Fig. 1**. The use of MET-RADS-P system starts

by allocating the presence of unequivocal identified disease based on morphology and signal characteristics on all acquired images to 14 predefined regions of the body (primary disease, seven skeletal and three nodal regions, lung, liver, and other soft tissue sites) at baseline and on follow-up assessments (MET-RADS-P template form **Fig. 1**).[6]

For follow-up studies, a qualitative response assessment on a scale of 1 to 5 indicating the likely response assessment category (RAC) for each anatomic location is recorded, comparing with the baseline study (RAC-1, indicating highly likely to be responding, up to RAC-5, indicating highly likely to be progressing).

The reporting guideline provides detailed explanations of the imaging criteria to be used to classify the likelihood of response in bones. Thus, RACs that summarize likelihood of response in bone disease use the newly developed MET-RADS criteria (**Table 2**), but RACs for response in soft tissues continues to use established standards already prescribed by RECIST v1.1 and

Name                                    ID                                    DOB

Physician                               Exam date current                     Exam date comparator

| Soft tissues RECIST criteria | MET-RADS Prostate Report | Bones MET-RADS criteria |
|---|---|---|

**Primary**
Involved    Y    N
RAC         1°   2°
Comment

**Pelvic nodes**
Involved    Y    N
RAC         1°   2°
Comment

**Retroperitoneal**
Involved    Y    N
RAC         1°   2°
Comment

**Other nodes**

Involved    Y    N
RAC         1°   2°
Comment

**Liver**
Involved    Y    N

RAC         1°   2°
Comment

**Lungs**
Involved    Y    N
RAC         1°   2°
Comment

**Other sites**
Involved    Y    N
RAC         1°   2°
Comment

**Skull**
Involved    Y    N
RAC         1°   2°
Comment

**Cervical spine**
Involved    Y    N
RAC         1°   2°
Comment

**Dorsal spine**
Involved    Y    N
RAC         1°   2°
Comment

**Lumbosacral spine**
Involved    Y    N
RAC         1°   2°
Comment

**Pelvis**
Involved    Y    N
RAC         1°   2°
Comment

**Thorax**
Involved    Y    N
RAC         1°   2°
Comment

**Limbs**
Involved    Y    N
RAC         1°   2°
Comment

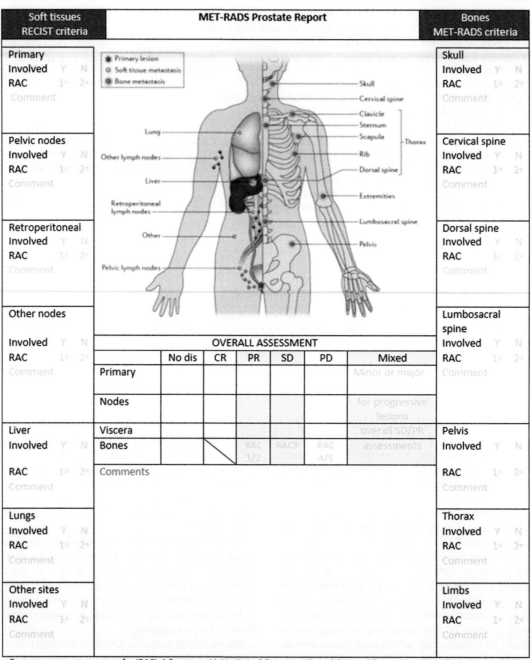

- ★ Primary lesion
- ○ Soft tissue metastasis
- ◉ Bone metastasis

Skull — Cervical spine — Clavicle — Sternum — Scapula — Rib — Dorsal spine — Thorax — Extremities — Lumbosacral spine — Pelvis

Lung — Other lymph nodes — Liver — Retroperitoneal lymph nodes — Other — Pelvic lymph nodes

| OVERALL ASSESSMENT | | | | | | |
|---|---|---|---|---|---|---|
| | No dis | CR | PR | SD | PD | Mixed |
| Primary | | | | | | Minor or major |
| Nodes | | | | | | for progressive lesions |
| Viscera | | | | | | overall SD/PR |
| Bones | | | RAC 1/2 | RAC3 | RAC 4/5 | assessments |
| Comments | | | | | | |

**Response assessment categories (RAC):** 1 Response: highly likely; 2 Response: likely; 3 Stable; 4 Progression: likely; 5 progression: highly likely.  Single lesion 1° RAC only; ≥2 lesions or diffuse disease use both RACs

Radiologist                                                      Date

**Table 2**
**METastasis reporting and data system for prostate cancer regional response assessment categories**

| RAC | Region | MET-RADS-P Descriptions |
|---|---|---|
| 1 Response: highly likely | Local, nodal, and visceral | Consistent with RECIST v1.1/PCWG criteria for unequivocal response (partial/complete) |
| | Bone | Return of normal marrow in areas previously infiltrated by focal/diffuse metastatic infiltration<br>Decrease in number/size of focal lesions<br>Evolution diffuse neoplastic pattern to focal lesions<br>Decreasing soft tissue associated with bone disease<br>Dense lesion sclerosis (edge to edge), sharply defined, very thin/disappearance of hyperintense rim on T2W-FS images<br>The emergence of intratumoral/peritumoral fat within/around lesions (fat dot/halo signs)<br>Previously evident lesion shows increase in ADC from $\leq$1400 µm$^2$/s to >1400 µm$^2$/s<br>$\geq$40% increase in ADC from baseline with corresponding decrease in high b-value signal intensity; and morphologic findings consistent with stable or responding disease |
| 2 Response: likely | Local, nodal, and visceral | Changes depicting tumor response that do not meet RECIST v1.1/PCWG criteria for partial or complete response (see later) |
| | Bone | Evidence of improvement, but not enough to fulfill criteria for RAC 1. For example: previously evident lesions showing increases in ADC from $\leq$1000 µm$^2$/s to <1400 µm$^2$/s<br>>25% but <40% increase in ADC from baseline with corresponding decrease in high b-value signal intensity; and morphologic findings consistent with stable or responding disease |
| 3 Stable | All | No observable change |
| 4 Progression: likely | Local, nodal, and visceral | Changes depicting tumor progression that do not meet RECIST v1.1/PCWG criteria for progression |
| | Bone | Evidence of worsening disease, but not enough to fulfill criteria for RAC 5; equivocal appearance of new lesions<br>No change in size but increasing signal intensity on high b-value images (with ADC values <1400 µm$^2$/s) consistent with possible disease progression<br>Relapse disease: re-emergence of lesions that previously disappeared or enlargement of lesions that had partially regressed/stabilized with prior treatments<br>Imaging depicted bone lesions that might be clinically significant (therefore excludes asymptomatic fractures in noncritical bones)<br>Soft tissue in spinal canal causing narrowing not associated with neurologic findings and not requiring radiotherapy |

*(continued on next page)*

Fig. 1. Updated MET-RADS-P template form and response criteria for bone and soft tissue disease. Updated MET-RADS-P template form allocates the presence of unequivocal identified disease to 14 predefined regions of the body (primary disease, seven skeletal and three nodal regions, lung, liver, and other soft tissue sites) at baseline and on follow-up assessments. At each anatomic location, the presence of disease is indicated (Yes/No) together with the response assessment categories (primary/secondary). The overall response of the primary tumor, nodal, and visceral disease are categorical (no disease, complete response, partial response, stable disease, and progressive disease). However, the overall response of bone disease is on a scale of 1 to 5 indicating the likely overall response category: 1 = highly likely to be responding; 2 = likely to be responding; 3 = stable; 4 = likely to be progressing; 5 = highly likely to be progressing. CR, complete response; No dis, no disease; PD, progressive disease; PR, partial response; RAC, response assessment category; SD, stable disease. (*Courtesy of* A.R. Padhani, MBBS, MRCP, FRCR, Middlesex, United Kingdom.)

**Table 2**
*(continued)*

| RAC | Region | MET-RADS-P Descriptions |
|---|---|---|
| 5 Progression: highly likely | Local, nodal, and visceral | Tumor progression that meet RECIST v1.1/PCWG criteria for unequivocal progression |
| | Bone | New critical fractures/cord compression requiring radiotherapy/surgical intervention → only if confirmed as active malignant by MR imaging signal intensity characteristics |
| | | Unequivocal new focal ($\geq$1 cm)/diffuse metastatic infiltration in regions of prior normal marrow |
| | | Unequivocal increase in number/size of focal lesions |
| | | Evolution of focal lesions to diffuse neoplastic pattern |
| | | Appearance/increasing soft tissue associated with bone disease |
| | | New lesions/regions of high signal intensity on high b-value images with ADC value between 600–1000 $\mu m^2$/s |

RAC allocation rules: compare with relevant prior scan.

Multiple criteria determine RACs; for RAC 1/2, when DWI and morphology are discordant, consideration should be given to pitfalls, such as Tl-pseudoprogression, sclerotic/fibrotic response, and bone marrow fat re-emergence (the latter two may not increase ADC values).
Primary RAC value is based on the predominant response of more than half of the disease within the region; secondary RAC value is for the highest nonpredominant response pattern.
For a single lesion in a region only the primary number category is assessed. Regions with multiple lesions/diffuse disease, all with the same RAC, both the primary and secondary have the same values.
When equal numbers of lesions are of higher and lower RACs then the primary pattern allocation is reserved for the higher RAC.
Mixed response: use when overall assessment is SD/PR but individual lesion progression is detected. Minor/major progression subcategories indicates imaging recommendation on the need to reassess therapy effectiveness.

RECIST v1.1 categories
- CR: disappearance of all target lesions
- PR: at least a 30% decrease in the sum of the longest diameter of target lesions, taking as reference the baseline sum LD
- SD: Neither sufficient shrinkage to qualify for PR nor sufficient increase to qualify for PD, taking as reference the smallest sum LD since the treatment started
- PD: At least a 20% increase in the sum of the LD of target lesions, taking as reference the smallest sum LD recorded since the treatment started or the appearance of one or more new lesions

Progression of local prostate disease: use RECIST v1.1 for progression criteria above applied to local disease
Progression of nodes (short axis)
- <1.0 cm nodes have to have grown by at least 5 mm from baseline or treatment nadir and be $\geq$1 cm to be considered to have progressed
- For nodes that are 1.0–1.5 cm that have grown by at least 5 mm from baseline or treatment nadir and are $\geq$1.5 cm in short axis can be considered to have progressed
- For nodes $\geq$1.5 cm short axis use RECIST v1.1 progression criteria
Progression of visceral disease: use RECIST v1.1 progression criteria above applied to visceral disease

*Abbreviations:* CR, complete response; FS, fat supression; LD, longest diameter; PD, progressive disease; PR, partial response; RAC, response assessment category; SD, stable disease; T2W, T2-weighted.
    Criteria for RACs that summarize likelihood of response in bone disease use the newly developed MET-RADS criteria, but RACs for response in soft tissues uses established standards already prescribed by RECIST v1.1 and PCWG guidance.[9,10] Bone metastases response assessment is indicated on a 1 to 5 scale indicating the likely RAC for each location, comparing with the baseline/best response study (RAC-1, indicates highly likely to be responding, up to RAC-5, indicating highly likely to be progressing). ADC measurements of representative target lesions as necessary.
    *Adapted from* Padhani AR, Lecouvet FE, Tunariu N, et al. METastasis reporting and data system for prostate cancer: practical guidelines for acquisition, interpretation, and reporting of whole-body magnetic resonance imaging-based evaluations of multiorgan involvement in advanced prostate cancer. Eur Urol 2017;71(1):89; with permission.

PCWG guidance.[9,10] In addition to the comprehensively described qualitative RAC criteria for bone metastases, the reporting radiologist can also measure the ADC for representative lesions thus providing additional guidance toward bone RAC classification.

Multiple criteria determine bone RACs; for RAC 1 to 2, when DWI and morphology are discordant, consideration should be given to pitfalls, such as T1-pseudoprogression, sclerotic/fibrotic response, and bone marrow fat re-emergence, all pointing to response[13]; note that the last two mechanisms of response may not increase ADC values.[14]

For each region, only two RACs are needed to account for heterogeneity of responses that may occur in different anatomic areas. The primary RAC value (1–5) is based on predominant pattern of response within the region (ie, the response shown by more than half of the lesions within the region). A secondary RAC value (1–5) is assigned to the second most frequent pattern of response seen within the region (or RAC 4–5 even if minor); that is, the highest predominant RAC. A tertiary RAC value (4–5) may be assigned to the region to illustrate progressing disease (ie, RAC 4–5), if not already captured by the primary or secondary RAC values, but this is not usually necessary in clinical practice.

When assessing a single lesion in a region, only the primary number category is used. Regions with multiple lesions all with the same pattern of response have the same RAC value assigned as both the primary and secondary RACs.

When equal numbers of lesions are of higher and lower RACs then the primary pattern allocation is reserved for the higher RAC. That is, when equal numbers of lesions are category RAC 4/5 (progressing) as RAC 1/2/3 (responding and stable), then the primary pattern allocation is reserved for RAC 4/5 (the higher category). Similarly, when equal numbers of lesions are category RAC 1/2 as RAC 3, then the primary pattern allocation is reserved for RAC 3 (the higher category).

## Overall Response

The final response assessment consists of separately assessing the status of the primary disease, bones, nodes, and viscera without an overall patient response result. The overall patient assessment can instead be summarized in the text report (**Box 1**) that should accompany the MET-RADS-P template report (**Fig. 2**).[6] In summary, the overall response of bone disease should be categorized on a scale of 1 to 5 indicating the likely overall response (RAC) category:

1. Highly likely to be responding
2. Likely to be responding
3. Stable
4. Likely to be progressing
5. Highly likely to be progressing

In contradistinction, the overall response for the primary tumor, nodal, and visceral disease should be categorical, thus following established guidelines,[9,10] to improve communication with clinicians who are already familiar with this format. The following categories should be assigned: no disease, complete response, partial response, stable disease, and progressive disease.

Discordance or mixed response indicates the presence of progressing bone/soft tissue disease, not meeting definite progression criteria in the primary category, that is, when most of disease is stable or responding. Discordant response should also be separately reported for primary, nodal, viscera, and bone; evaluation of regional responses enables the specific identification of the anatomic sites of mixed responses. When discordant response is observed, the degree of discordance should be indicated as major or minor to indicate in the radiologist's on whether alternative therapy options should be considered.

ADC value measurements should be made using a region-of-interest (ROI) technique on ADC images. Because of the lower spatial resolution of WB-MR imaging compared with CT scans, as large as possible ROI is recommended for ADC measurements. ADC measurements in bone disease should only be obtained from lesions that have sufficient signal intensity detected on all b-value images (including low b-value); otherwise the ADC values are erroneous, reflecting only the noise in the images. Note that the mere absence of tissue signal on highest b-value images does not exclude tissues from ADC measurements because signal may be present at lower b-values (thus, low or intermediate b-value images should be chosen instead for ROI placements).

## Research Components

Because of the need to have unequivocally disease and to cope with the lower spatial resolution of WB-MR imaging compared with CT scans, whenever possible, a 1.5-cm diameter threshold is preferred to 1 cm for lesion size assessments. Lesion size should be measured on anatomic

---

**Box 1**
**Original text report for the follow-up examination that accompanies the MET-RADS-P template report**

*30/08/2016 MR imaging whole body*

Clinical details: mCRPC. Restaging posturinary diversion. On abiraterone and zoladez.

Technique: A whole-body MR imaging scan with whole-body diffusion sequences. Comparison is made with the previous whole-body MR imaging scan dated 29/04/2016.

Findings:

Cervical and dorsal spine:

The intervertebral bony alignment is normal. Regrettably, there is marked disease progression. New metastases are seen throughout the cervical and dorsal spine with multifocal lesions. No interval loss of vertebral height. The craniocervical junction is normal. The cervical and dorsal cord outline normally.

Lumbosacral spinei:

The intervertebral bony alignment remains normal with no interval loss of vertebral height. Degenerative spinal stenosis at L3/L4 as noted on the previous occasion. Regrettably, there is marked disease progression in the lumbosacral spine since the previous study.

Body scan:

No skull vault deposits have emerged. Normal sinonasal airways.

No supraclavicular fossa lymphadenopathy. Progressive left axillary lymphadenopathy also.

There is marked disease progression left scapula bone with extraosseous soft tissue disease now visible. Marked disease progression the ribs bilaterally also. There are artifacts, are sternotomy wires.

The central mediastinal and hilar regions are normal. No lung abnormalities are detected.

The liver and spleen are homogeneous. Normal pancreas and adrenal glands. Both kidneys are unobstructed with bilateral renal stents in situ. Small retroperitoneal lymph nodes are also detected.

Extensive metastatic bone disease is present in the sacrum predominantly on the left side, right and left hemipelvis bone disease also.

Nodal disease in the common iliac regions bilaterally. Right obturator region with extranodal tumor spread.

There is large locally advanced prostate carcinoma with bladder and ureteric involvement. No tumor involvement of the rectum or rectosigmoid junction.

Metastatic disease in the right proximal femur also.

Impression:

There is marked disease progression since 29/04/2016. Disease progression is seen locally the prostate gland with extensive bladder invasion. There is disease progression within pelvic and retroperitoneal lymph nodes with extranodal tumor spread. There is disease progression in the left axilla also. Bone disease progression additionally throughout the spine with extraosseous soft tissue disease also visible. No new visceral relapse of disease.

Please see graphical MET-RADS-P report also.

---

T1-weighted images where possible. Note that progression assignments for soft tissues if based on measurements should be from baseline or the treatment-induced summed measurement nadir, whichever is lower as per the RECIST v1.1 guidelines.[7] The type of progression (new disease vs growth of existing lesions) should be separately recorded; the location of progression is accessible from the regional response assessments.

RACs at each time point should be compared with the baseline (pretreatment) study for clinical use, but may be referenced to the immediate prior study for research purposes if needed. WB tumor segmentations and histogram analysis are not part of the MET-RADS-P standard but can be used as ancillary tools if available (and are used in this paper for illustrative purposes only).

**A**

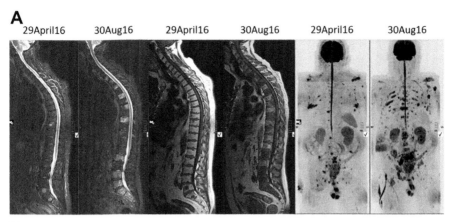

29April16   30Aug16   29April16   30Aug16   29April16   30Aug16

**B**

Physician PO

Exam date (current) 30/8/16

Exam date (comparator) 29/4/16

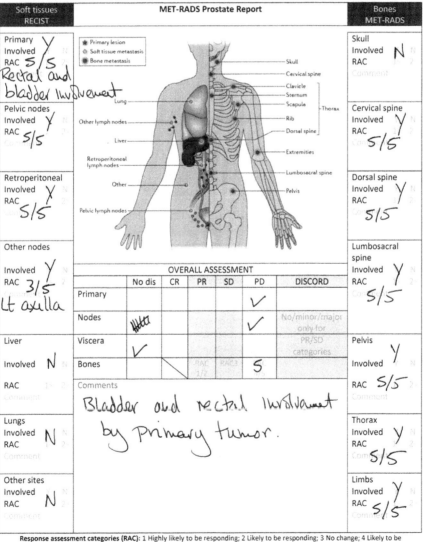

| Soft tissues RECIST | MET-RADS Prostate Report | Bones MET-RADS |
|---|---|---|
| **Primary** Involved Y / N  RAC 5/5  Rectal and bladder Involvement | | **Skull** Involved N / N  RAC |
| **Pelvic nodes** Involved Y / N  RAC 5/5 | | **Cervical spine** Involved Y / N  RAC 5/5 |
| **Retroperitoneal** Involved Y / N  RAC 5/5 | | **Dorsal spine** Involved Y / N  RAC 5/5 |
| **Other nodes** Involved Y / N  RAC 3/5  Lt axilla | | **Lumbosacral spine** Involved Y / N  RAC 5/5 |

**OVERALL ASSESSMENT**

| | No dis | CR | PR | SD | PD | DISCORD |
|---|---|---|---|---|---|---|
| Primary | | | | | ✓ | |
| Nodes | ✓ | | | | ✓ | No/minor/major only for PR/SD categories |
| Viscera | ✓ | | | | | |
| Bones | | | | | S | |

Comments

Bladder and rectal Involvement by Primary tumor.

| Liver Involved N / N  RAC | **Pelvis** Involved Y / N  RAC 5/5 |
|---|---|
| Lungs Involved N / N  RAC | **Thorax** Involved Y / N  RAC 5/5 |
| Other sites Involved N / N  RAC | **Limbs** Involved Y / N  RAC 5/5 |

**Response assessment categories (RAC):** 1 Highly likely to be responding; 2 Likely to be responding; 3 No change; 4 Likely to be progressing; 5 Highly likely to be progressing. Single lesion 1° RAC only; ≥2 lesions/diffuse disease use both RACs

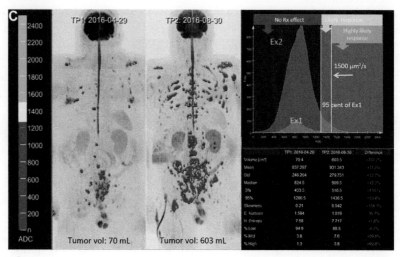

**Fig. 2.** (*continued*)

## WORKED-UP EXAMPLES

An updated MET-RADS-P template form and detailed bone response assessment criteria are found in **Fig. 1** and **Table 2**. **Fig. 2**, **Figs. 3**, and **4** illustrate the use of the MET-RADS-P standard[6] in advanced, metastatic prostate cancer illustrated with examples of disease progression, responding, and discordant responses. The figures also demonstrate the utility of the WB-tumor load segmentation which is

undertaken on work-in-progress software (Siemens Healthineers, Erlangen, Germany). Note that tumor load and ADC histogram analysis is not part of the MET-RADS-P standard, and is included for illustrative and cross-correlations purposes only.

## CONCLUSIONS AND FUTURE DEVELOPMENTS

The MET-RADS-P system provides the minimum standards for WB-MR imaging with DWI image

**Fig. 2.** Primary resistance to hormonal therapy. A 67-year-old man with metastatic castrate-resistant prostate cancer. WB-MR imaging examinations before and on androgen deprivation therapy (abiraterone and goserelin). (*A, C*) There is marked disease progression seen on morphologic T1-weighted and STIR sequences and on WB b900 MIP images (inverted gray-scale) and confirmed by ADC measurements. Disease progression is seen in the prostate gland with extensive bladder invasion together with rectal invasion. There is disease progression in pelvic and retroperitoneal lymph nodes with nodal enlargement in the left axilla. There is bone disease progression throughout the spine with extraosseous soft tissue disease with new and enlarging deposits. No liver or lung disease is seen. The spinal stenosis at L3/l4 is degenerative in nature. (*B*) Completed MET-RADS-P template report indicating sites of disease and RACs at each anatomic location compared with the baseline study. The presence of unequivocal identified disease is indicated together with primary and secondary RACs at each site using the criteria set out in **Table 2**. Short relevant comments are included for clarification purposes where needed. (*C*) WB tumor load segmentation undertaken on work-in-progress software (not part of the MET-RADS-P standard) for illustrative purposes only. The WB b900 images are segmented using computed high b-value images of 1200 s/mm² and signal intensity threshold of approximately 100 AU. Extraneous signals (eg, the brain, kidneys, bowel, gonads) are removed to leave only recognizable disease sites. The color b900 MIP images are overlaid with ADC value classes using the thresholds indicated below. The green voxels are values ≥1500 µm²/s (representing voxels that are highly likely to be responding). The yellow voxels are set to lie between the 95th centile ADC value of the pretreatment histogram (1266 µm²/s) and 1500 µm²/s thus representing voxels likely to be responding. Red voxels represent mostly untreated disease. A total of 70 mL of tumor are segmented before therapy and 603 mL on therapy. Note that there is no significant global increase in ADC values (837 µm²/s and 951 µm²/s) on the corresponding absolute frequency histograms. There is also no increase in the standard deviation of the histogram (248 and 279 µm²/s). Note increased extent and volume of red voxels consistent with disease progression (95% of 70 mL before therapy and 88% of 603 mL after therapy). MIP, maximum intensity projection; STIR, short tau inversion recovery. (*Courtesy of [B, C]* A.R. Padhani, MBBS, MRCP, FRCR, Middlesex, United Kingdom.)

**A**

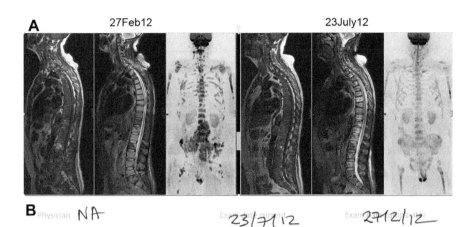

| 27Feb12 | 23July12 |

**B**

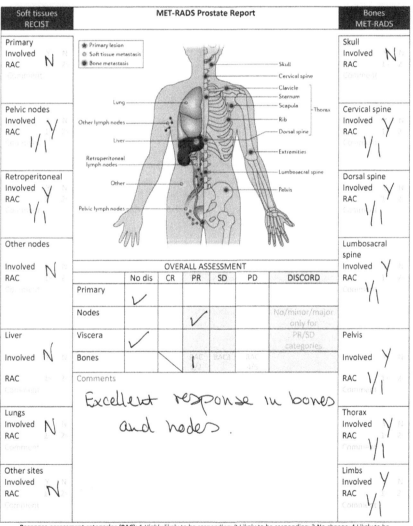

Physician NA    Exam... 23/7/12    Exam... 27/2/12

| Soft tissues RECIST | MET-RADS Prostate Report | Bones MET-RADS |

MET-RADS Prostate Report

Legend:
- ★ Primary lesion
- ◎ Soft tissue metastasis
- ● Bone metastasis

Labels: Skull, Cervical spine, Clavicle, Sternum, Scapula, Thorax, Rib, Dorsal spine, Extremities, Lumbosacral spine, Pelvis, Lung, Other lymph nodes, Liver, Retroperitoneal lymph nodes, Other, Pelvic lymph nodes

**Soft tissues RECIST**

| Primary Involved | N |
| RAC | |
| Pelvic nodes Involved | Y |
| RAC | 1/1 |
| Retroperitoneal Involved | Y |
| RAC | 1/1 |
| Other nodes Involved | N |
| RAC | |
| Liver Involved | N |
| RAC | |
| Lungs Involved | N |
| RAC | |
| Other sites Involved | N |
| RAC | |

**OVERALL ASSESSMENT**

| | No dis | CR | PR | SD | PD | DISCORD |
|---|---|---|---|---|---|---|
| Primary | ✓ | | | | | |
| Nodes | | | ✓ | | | No/minor/major only for PR/SD categories |
| Viscera | ✓ | | | | | |
| Bones | | | 1 | | | |

Comments: Excellent response in bones and nodes.

**Bones MET-RADS**

| Skull Involved | N |
| RAC | |
| Cervical spine Involved | Y |
| RAC | 1/1 |
| Dorsal spine Involved | Y |
| RAC | 1/1 |
| Lumbosacral spine Involved | Y |
| RAC | 1/1 |
| Pelvis Involved | Y |
| RAC | 1/1 |
| Thorax Involved | Y |
| RAC | 1/1 |
| Limbs Involved | Y |
| RAC | 1/1 |

**Response assessment categories (RAC):** 1 Highly likely to be responding; 2 Likely to be responding; 3 No change; 4 Likely to be progressing; 5 Highly likely to be progressing. Single lesion 1° RAC only; ≥2 lesions/diffuse disease use both RACs

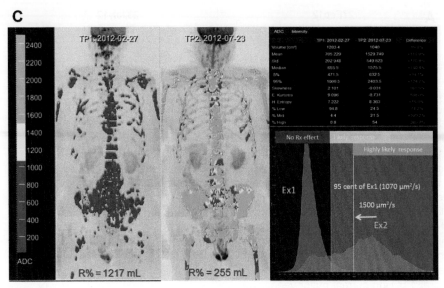

**Fig. 3.** (*continued*)

acquisition, interpretation, and reporting of baseline and follow-up monitoring examinations of men with advanced, metastatic prostate cancer. MET-RADS-P is suitable for guiding patient care in practice (using the regional and overall assessment criteria), but can also be incorporated into clinical trials when accurate lesion size and ADC measurements become more important (thus, recording of measurements is not mandated for clinical practice). MET-RADS-P enables the evaluation of the benefits of continuing therapy to be assessed, when there are signs that the disease is progressing (discordant responses).

**Fig. 3.** Excellent response to chemotherapy. A 65-year-old man with metastatic castrate-naive prostate cancer. WB-MR imaging examinations before and after four cycles of docetaxel, goserelin, and prednisolone therapy. (*A*) There is improvement in the spinal canal narrowing in the mid-dorsal and lumbar spine on the T2-weighted FS images. The T1-weighted images are essentially unchanged or possibly minimally worse. There is also marked improved appearances of the bone and nodal disease on the paired WB b900 MIP images (inverted scale) and (*C*) confirmed by significant increase in ADC values of the bone lesions and reduction in size of the metastatic nodal disease. (*B*) Completed MET-RADS-P template report indicating sites of disease and RACs at each anatomic location compared with the baseline study. Note how the overall response at the primary tumor is indicated as no disease (previous radiotherapy). The overall pelvic nodal and retroperitoneal disease is excellent, indicated as partial response. The bone disease response is indicated by category 1 (highly likely to be responding). (*C*) WB tumor load segmentation undertaken on work-in-progress software (not part of the MET-RADS-P standard) for illustrative purposes only. The WB b900 images are segmented using computed high b-value images of 1000 s/mm² and signal intensity threshold of approximately 30 AU. Extraneous signals (eg, the brain, kidneys, bowel, gonads) are removed to leave only recognizable disease sites. The thresholded masks are overlaid with ADC value classes using the thresholds indicated and superimposed onto the b900 MIP images. The green voxels are values ≥1500 μm²/s (representing voxels that are highly likely to be responding). The yellow voxels are set to lie between the 95th centile ADC value of the pretreatment histogram (1069 μm²/s) and 1500 μm²/s thus representing voxels likely to be responding. Red voxels represent mostly untreated disease. A total of 1283 mL of bone marrow and retroperitoneal nodal disease were segmented before therapy and 1040 mL on therapy. Note that there is marked global increase in ADC values (705 μm²/s and 1530 μm²/s) on the corresponding relative frequency histograms. There is a marked decrease in excess kurtosis of the histograms (9.1 and −0.73). Note decreased extent and volume of red voxels consistent with disease response (95% before therapy and 24% after therapy). The residual red regions on the post-therapy scan are presumed to represent residual active disease with low ADC values, localizable to the lower lumbar spine and in the left proximal femur. (*Courtesy of [B, C]* A.R. Padhani, MBBS, MRCP, FRCR, Middlesex, United Kingdom.)

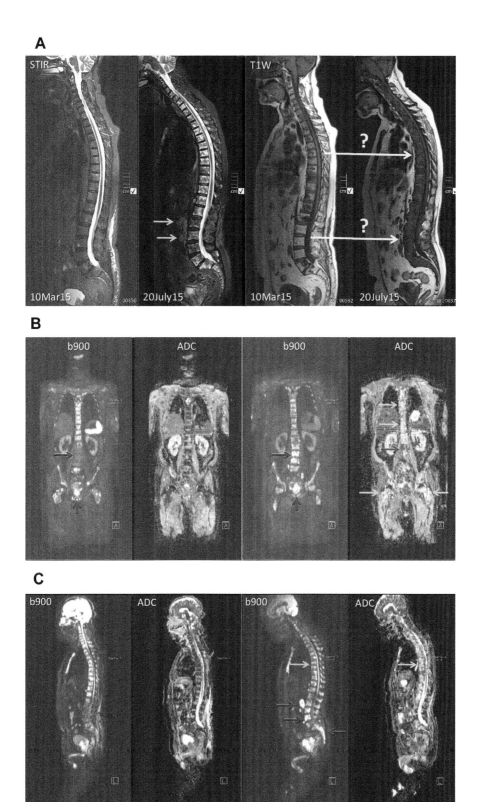

Fig. 4. Discordant response to radium-223 therapy. A 55-year-old man with metastatic castrate-resistant prostate cancer. Previously failed treatments include docetaxel chemotherapy and abiraterone. Previously lumbar spinal radiotherapy. WB-MR imaging scans were obtained before and after radium-223 treatment. Symptomatically the patient is worse with increasing bone pain and has become blood transfusion dependent; however, prostate-specific antigen values are improved from 792 ng/mL to 167 ng/mL thus creating diagnostic confusion on the effectiveness of radium-223 therapy. (A) T1-weighted spine images show increased abnormal signal in the cervical, dorsal, and lumbosacral spine suggestive of disease progression using the criteria in Table 2.

**D**

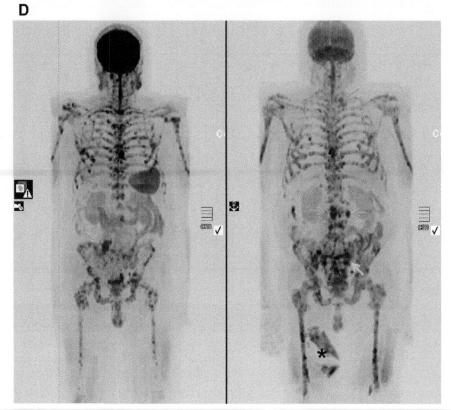

Fig. 4. (*continued*)

However, the STIR sequence shows higher signal intensities in the cervical and dorsal spine indicating increased tissue water. Note increase in size of retroperitoneal nodes (*orange arrows*). Coronal (*B*) and sagittal (*C*) b900 and ADC maps at the corresponding two timepoints. The decreased b900 signal intensities and increases in ADC values in the dorsal spine and proximal femora (*orange arrows*) indicating responding disease (T1-weighted pseudoprogression in the dorsal spine). However, the opposite is seen in the lumbar spine where b900 signal intensity is increased (*red arrows*) and with low ADC values indicating new disease (true progression). Note that there are responding regions in the lumbar spine also. Note some enlargement of the primary prostate tumor also (*vertical red arrows*) and of retroperitoneal lymph nodes. (*D*) Paired b900 MIP images (inverted scale) showing new nodal disease in the left hemipelvis, retroperitoneum, and in the left supraclavicular fossa (*orange arrows*). However, the enlarged lymph nodes in the right common iliac region is improved (*green arrow*). There seems to be an increase in extent of bone marrow signal intensity. The high signal geographic lesion over the right thigh on the follow-up examination is a dipper pad (*asterisks*). Note the lower signal intensity of the brain on follow-up examination caused by the absence of the head coil. (*E*) Completed MET-RADS-P template report indicating sites of disease and RACs at each anatomic location compared with the baseline study. Note how the RAC of response at the primary tumor is mostly stable with some progression (RAC 3/4). The RAC of the pelvic nodes is indicated as 5/2 meaning that (*E*) there is progression in most nodes, although a single lymph node has responded. Overall the bone disease is scored as 2 (likely to be responding in most regions) with major discordance caused by progression in lumbosacral spine and pelvis (both with RAC scores of 5/5). (*F*) WB tumor load segmentation undertaken on work-in-progress software (not part of the MET-RADS-P standard) for illustrative purposes only. The WB b900 images are segmented using computed high b-value images of 1000 s/mm$^2$ and signal intensity threshold of approximately 100 AU. Extraneous signals (eg, the brain, kidneys, bowel, gonads) are removed to leave only recognizable disease sites. The color the b900 MIP images are overlaid with ADC value classes using the thresholds indicated. The green voxels are values $\geq$1500 $\mu$m$^2$/s (representing voxels that are highly likely to be responding). The yellow voxels are set to lie between the 95th centile ADC value of the pretreatment histogram (1230 $\mu$m$^2$/s) and 1500 $\mu$m$^2$/s thus representing voxels likely to be responding. Red voxels represent mostly untreated disease. A total of 584 mL of bone marrow and nodal disease are segmented before therapy and 629 mL on therapy. Note that there is moderate global increase in ADC values (685 $\mu$m$^2$/s and 932 $\mu$m$^2$/s) on the corresponding relative frequency histograms. There is a decrease in excess kurtosis of the histograms (2.3 and 0.03). Note decrease extent and volume of red voxels consistent with disease response (95% before therapy and 73% after therapy). Heterogeneity of response in the spine (more red voxels in the lumbar spine and more green voxels in the dorsal spine) and in the pelvis is appreciable on the color projected images. This heterogeneity of response emphasizes the need to evaluate all the relevant WB-MRI images and to apply regional responses using the MET-RADS-P criteria. (*Courtesy of* [*E, F*] A.R. Padhani, MBBS, MRCP, FRCR, Middlesex, United Kingdom.)

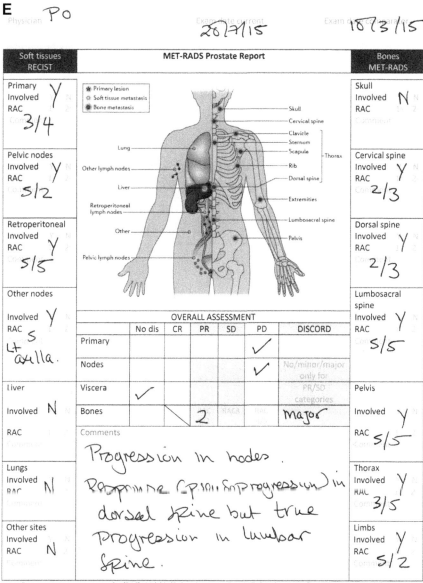

Fig. 4. (continued)

MET-RAD-P requires validation within clinical trials initially in studies that assess the effects of known efficacious treatments, such as those targeting the androgen receptor, cytotoxic chemotherapy, radium-223, and poly ADP ribose polymerase (PARP) inhibitors. MET-RADS-P measures should be correlated to other tumor response biomarkers delineated by PCWG (eg, prostate-specific antigen declines), quality of life measures, rates of skeletal events, radiographic progression-free survival, and overall survival. The latter is needed for the introduction of WB-MR imaging into longer term follow-up studies, which will allow objective assessments of whether WB-MR imaging is effective in supporting patient care. Thus, we recommend that MET-RADS-P be evaluated in clinical care and trials, to assess its impact on the clinical practice of advanced prostate cancer.

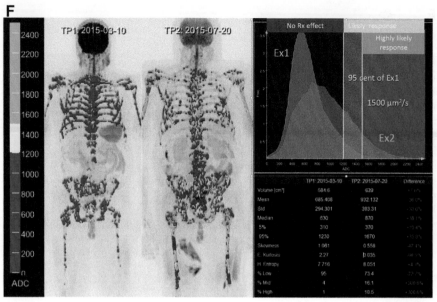

**Fig. 4.** (*continued*)

## REFERENCES

1. Lecouvet FE, Applications M. Whole-body MR imaging: musculoskeletal applications 1. Radiology 2016;279:345–65.
2. Taouli B, Beer AJ, Chenevert T, et al. Diffusion-weighted imaging outside the brain: consensus statement from an ISMRM-sponsored workshop. J Magn Reson Imaging 2016;44:521–40.
3. Padhani AR, Lecouvet FE, Tunariu N, et al. Rationale for modernising imaging in advanced prostate cancer. Eur Urol Focus 2016;44: 198–205.
4. Dimopoulos MA, Hillengass J, Usmani S, et al. Role of magnetic resonance imaging in the management of patients with multiple myeloma: a consensus statement. J Clin Oncol 2015;33:657–64.
5. Ballinger ML, Best A, Mai PL, et al. Baseline surveillance in Li-Fraumeni syndrome using whole-body magnetic resonance imaging: a meta-analysis. JAMA Oncol 2017;3:1634–9.
6. Padhani AR, Lecouvet FE, Tunariu N, et al. METastasis reporting and data system for prostate cancer: practical guidelines for acquisition, interpretation, and reporting of whole-body magnetic resonance imaging-based evaluations of multiorgan involvement in advanced prostate cancer. Eur Urol 2017;71:81–92.
7. Mottet N, Bellmunt J, Bolla M, et al. EAU-ESTRO-SIOG guidelines on prostate cancer. Part 1: screening, diagnosis, and local treatment with curative intent. Eur Urol 2017;71:1–12.
8. Cornford P, Bellmunt J, Bolla M, et al. EAU-ESTRO-SIOG guidelines on prostate cancer. Part II: treatment of relapsing, metastatic, and castration-resistant prostate cancer. Eur Urol 2017;71: 630–42.
9. Eisenhauer EA, Therasse P, Bogaerts J, et al. New response evaluation criteria in solid tumours: revised RECIST guideline (version 1.1). Eur J Cancer 2009; 45:228–47.
10. Scher HI, Morris MJ, Stadler WM, et al. Trial design and objectives for castration-resistant prostate cancer: updated recommendations from the prostate cancer clinical trials working group 3. J Clin Oncol 2016;34:1–38.
11. Barnes A, Alonzi R, Blackledge M, et al. UK quantitative WB-DWI technical workgroup: consensus meeting recommendations on optimisation, quality control, processing and analysis of quantitative whole-body diffusion-weighted imaging for cancer. Br J Radiol 2018;91:20170577.
12. Padhani AR, Lecouvet FE, Tunariu N, et al. Questions that teach. Nurs outlook. Eur Assoc Urol 1966;14:57.
13. Lecouvet FE, Larbi A, Pasoglou V, et al. MRI for response assessment in metastatic bone disease. Eur Radiol 2013;23:1986–97.
14. Padhani AR, Makris A, Gall P, et al. Therapy monitoring of skeletal metastases with whole-body diffusion MRI. J Magn Reson Imaging 2014;39: 1049–78.

# Multiparametric MR Imaging of Soft Tissue Tumors and Pseudotumors

Flávia Martins Costa, MD, PhD[a,b,]*,
Pedro Henrique Martins, MD[a],
Clarissa Canella, MD, PhD[a,b,c],
Flávia Paiva Proença Lobo Lopes, MD, PhD[a,b,d]

## KEYWORDS

- MR imaging • Soft tissue sarcoma • Soft tissue tumors • Pseudotumors
- Diffusion-weighted imaging • Magnetic resonance spectroscopy imaging
- Dynamic contrast-enhanced perfusion imaging • Chemical shift imaging

## KEY POINTS

- Preventing an inadequate approach to soft masses is crucial for successful treatment of soft tissue sarcomas, minimizing oncological sequelae and extensively mutilating surgical procedures of these tumors, and increasing the survival and quality of life of the patients presenting with these tumors.
- Appropriate evaluation and treatment planning are required along with an integrated and multidisciplinary approach by specialists using standard diagnostic methods and adequate techniques.
- The use of multiparametric MR imaging along with conventional and advanced MR sequences provide additional information on the detection, characterization, staging, and treatment follow-up of soft tissue tumors.

## INTRODUCTION

Soft tissue tumors are a heterogeneous group of benign, intermediate (locally aggressive), and malignant subtypes of neoplasms arising from 9 different categories of tumors according to the World Health Organization (WHO).[1] These tumors are routinely found in clinical practice and often impose a substantial diagnostic challenge to radiologists and pathologists.

The initial approach to a patient with a soft tissue mass includes an evaluation of clinical history and radiologic findings. Soft tissue masses may be classified as neoplastic tumors or pseudotumors, the latter including benign conditions that are not neoplastic in nature but have the potential to mimic their malignant counterparts. The ability to recognize the different characteristics of these lesions is essential for their appropriate treatment.

Of various imaging modalities, MR imaging is the method of choice to evaluate soft tissue masses due to this method's multiplanar capabilities, high resolution, and tissue contrast.

Disclosure Statement: The authors have nothing to disclose

[a] Radiology Department, Clínica de Diagnóstico por Imagem (CDPI)/DASA, Avenida das Américas, 4666, sala 301B, Centro Médico BarraShopping, CDPI, Barra da Tijuca, Rio de Janeiro, RJ CEP: 22640-102, Brazil; [b] Radiology Department, Alta Excelência Diagnóstica/DASA, Avenida das Américas, 4666, sala 301B, Centro Médico BarraShopping, CDPI, Barra da Tijuca, Rio de Janeiro, RJ CEP: 22640-102, Brazil; [c] Radiology Department, Universidade Federal Fluminense (UFF), Av Marques do Paraná, 303, Centro, Niterói, RJ CEP: 24020-071, Brazil; [d] Radiology Department, Federal University of Rio de Janeiro (UFRJ), Rua Rodolpho Paulo Rocco, 255, Cidade Universitária, Ilha do Fundão, Rio de Janeiro, RJ CEP: 21941-913, Brazil
* Corresponding author. Centro Médico Barrashopping, Clínica de Diagnóstico por Imagem (CDPI), Avenida das Américas, 4666, sala 301B, Barra da Tijuca, Rio de Janeiro, RJ 22640-102, Brazil.
*E-mail address:* flavia26rio@hotmail.com

Magn Reson Imaging Clin N Am 26 (2018) 543–558
https://doi.org/10.1016/j.mric.2018.06.009

Conventional MR imaging uses morphologic and anatomic parameters to characterize and determine the extent of a soft tissue tumor, but is limited with regard to distinguishing benign from malignant lesions.

Advanced techniques have emerged as additional tools to improve the role of MR imaging, including dynamic contrast-enhanced MR imaging (DCE-MR imaging), diffusion-weighted imaging (DWI), MR spectroscopy (MRS), susceptibility-weighted imaging (SWI), and 3-dimensional (3D) Dixon quantitative chemical shift imaging (Dixon QCSI). Sequences obtained with these techniques combine information of tumor morphology and tissue characteristics using different biomarkers, providing functional information and analyzing the tumor's anatomy, cellularity, vascularity, and metabolism.

## MR IMAGING PROTOCOL
### Conventional and Anatomic Magnetic Resonance Sequences

Conventional MR imaging can evaluate and stage soft tissue tumors by analyzing morphologic parameters, involvement of adjacent vital structures, homogeneity of signal intensity, and measurement of relaxation time. According to these criteria,

malignancy can be predicted with the following parameters[2–4]:

- Heterogeneous signal intensity in T1-weighted images
- Tumor necrosis
- Bone or neurovascular involvement
- Mean diameter of more than 66 mm

However, conventional MR imaging has a limited role, providing low specificity in the differential diagnosis of soft tissue masses.[3]

### Advanced Magnetic Resonance Sequences

#### Proton magnetic resonance spectroscopy: "metabolic technique"
Proton MRS is a noninvasive advanced metabolic technique useful for molecular characterization of musculoskeletal tumors through the detection of several metabolites, including malignancy markers (increased choline peak).[5] Choline is a precursor of acetylcholine, a constituent of the phospholipid metabolism of cell membranes. As choline, along with glycerophosphocholine and phosphocholine, is involved in the synthesis and degradation of cell membranes, increased choline peak detected at 3.2 ppm reflects a high cell membrane turnover

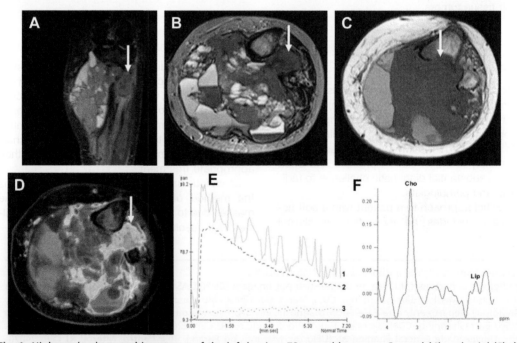

Fig. 1. High-grade pleomorphic sarcoma of the left leg in a 78-year-old woman. Coronal (A) and axial (B) short tau inversion recovery (STIR)-weighted image demonstrating a highly heterogeneous soft tissue lesion with multiple fluid-fluid level in the distal leg (white arrows). On the axial T1-weighted image, the tumor erodes the proximal tibial metaphysis (C) (white arrow). Axial DCE-perfusion imaging color map (D) shows early enhancement of the anterior and lateral aspects of the lesion (solid component) (white arrow), with type IV curve (dotted line) in (E), an adequate region for biopsy. MRS of the tumor demonstrates an increase choline peak (Cho) and a small lipid peak (Lip), suggesting a high potential of malignancy (F).

with cellular proliferation, which correlates with malignant activity (**Fig. 1**).[6]

MRS can map metabolite signal intensity in tissues by obtaining signals from water, choline, creatine, and lipids, acquired from a specific region of interest using both multivoxel and single-voxel techniques. The voxel should be positioned in solid areas with early and high contrast uptake, avoiding bone structures, blood, calcification, fat, and muscles.[7]

Previous reports have demonstrated false-positive choline peaks in nonmalignant musculoskeletal tumors (giant cell tumors of the bone) and other inflammatory and benign neoplastic processes with high metabolic activity.[8,9]

### Susceptibility-weighted imaging

SWI differs substantially from T2*-weighted images because it is based on a long echo time high-resolution, flow-compensated, 3D imaging technique with filtered-phase information in each voxel.[10] The combination of magnitude and phase data produces an enhanced contrast magnitude image that is particularly sensitive to hemorrhage, calcium, iron storage, and slow venous blood, thus allowing a significant improvement compared with T2* sequences.

Hemosiderin, melanin, and calcification appear easily recognized as hypointensity on SWI images and can be useful to improve the differential diagnosis of soft tissue tumors (**Figs. 2–4**).

### Three-dimensional Dixon quantitative chemical shift imaging

Dixon sequences can automatically generate 4 image sets (in-phase, opposed-phase, water-only, and fat-only), from which T1 with fat% and non-fat% images can be calculated.[11]

Chemical shift MR imaging (in-phase and opposed-phase) can evaluate the relationship between the amount of fat and water within the same tissue voxel. The presence of lipid components inside or surrounding the soft tissue tumor is identified as signal intensity reduction on the opposed-phase image, commonly seen in lipomatous and vascular tumors (**Fig. 5**).

The T1 with fat% (fat fraction) may be used as a parameter for evaluation of yellow marrow in the mature ossification of myositis ossificans, usually evaluated with T1 spin-echo sequences (**Fig. 6**).

### Diffusion-weighted imaging

DWI is useful in clinical practice to improve disease assessment, especially in the oncological setting, providing functional information for tumor detection and characterization, including staging and follow-up imaging in malignant tumors.

**Technical aspects** The diffusion sequence derives its images from intravoxel incoherent motion, which includes Brownian motion of extracellular,

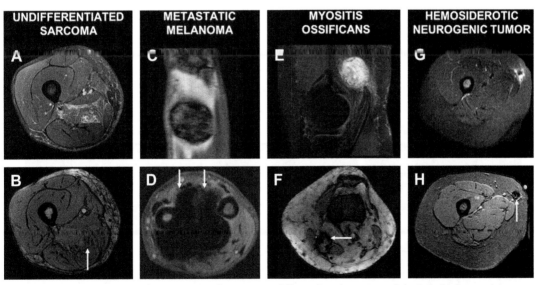

**Fig. 2.** Different applications of SWI-weighted images. Undifferentiated sarcoma of the left thigh on axial proton density–weighted image with fat saturation (*A*) and axial SWI (*B*) demonstrating hemorrhagic foci within the lesion (*white arrow*). Metastatic melanoma of the right forearm on coronal proton density–weighted image with fat saturation (*C*) and axial SWI (*D*) demonstrating melanin areas within the lesion (*white arrows*). Myositis ossificans of the left knee on sagittal proton density–weighted image with fat saturation (*E*) and axial SWI (*F*) demonstrating peripheral calcified areas within the lesion (*white arrow*). Hemosiderotic neurogenic tumor of the left thigh on axial proton density–weighted image with fat saturation (*G*) and axial T2* (*H*) demonstrating hemorrhagic foci within the lesion (*white arrow*).

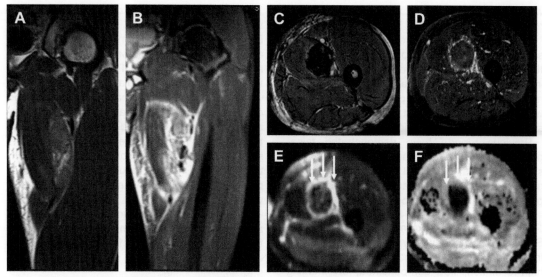

**Fig. 3.** Hematoma of the left thigh in a 19-year-old man. Coronal T1-weighted (*A*) and short tau inversion recovery (STIR)-weighted images (*B*) demonstrating a heterogeneous lesion in the adductor longus muscle. Note the hypointense signal within the lesion on SWI images (*C*) suggesting hemosiderin. Axial DCE-perfusion imaging color map (*D*) does not demonstrate important areas of enhancement of the lesion, just slight peripheral contrast enhancement. Axial DWI (*E*) and ADC map (*F*) reveal magnetic susceptibility artifact within the lesion (*white arrows*).

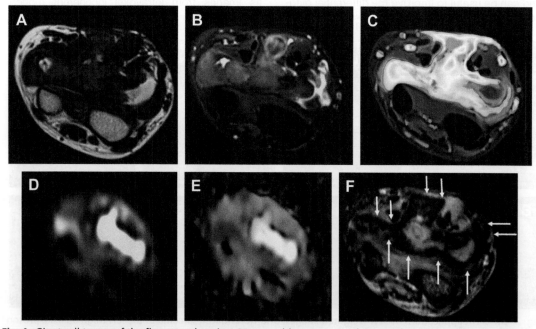

**Fig. 4.** Giant cell tumor of the flexor tendons in a 34-year-old woman. Axial T2-weighted (*A*) and proton density–weighted (*B*) images demonstrating a heterogeneous lesion infiltrating the flexor muscle compartment in the right arm, simulating a malignant lesion. Axial DCE-perfusion color map imaging (*C*) shows early enhancement of the lesion. Axial DWI (*D*) and ADC map (*E*) reveal areas with restriction (ADC value of $0.87 \times 10^3$ mm$^2$/s) and the central portion of the lesion with facilitated diffusion (ADC value of $2.2 \times 10^3$ mm$^2$/s). Axial SWI (*F*) demonstrates peripheral hemorrhagic area (*white arrows*), suggesting the diagnosis of giant cell tumor of the flexor tendons.

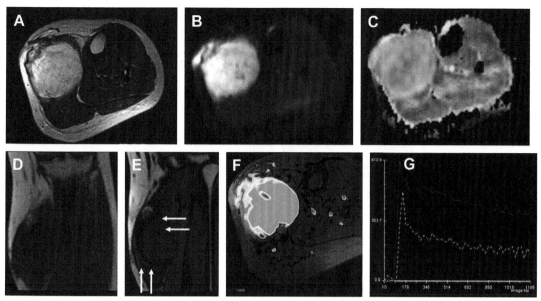

**Fig. 5.** Hemangioma in a 19-year-old woman. Axial T2-weighted image (*A*) demonstrating a high signal intensity lesion in the medial aspect of the right leg. Axial DWI (*B*) and ADC map (*C*) reveal areas of facilitated diffusion (ADC = $1.9 \times 10^3$ mm$^2$/s). In-phase (*D*) and out-phase images (*E*) demonstrate a peripheral hypointense halo surrounding the lesion in the out-phase image (*white arrows*), suggesting fat. Axial color perfusion map (*F*) shows high perfusion with type IV curve in (*G*), of a highly vascularized hemangioma.

intracellular, and transcellular individual water molecules (true diffusion), as well as microcirculation of blood (perfusion). The DWI sequence yields both qualitative and quantitative (by measurement of apparent diffusion coefficient [ADC]) information reflecting tumor cell density and membrane integrity.[12] This sequence should be performed with at least 2 b-values for an adequate interpretation and to calculate the ADC map.[13] There is no consensus in the literature with regard to the best ADC to differentiate adequately benign from malignant soft tissue tumors. However, because it is a fast, noninvasive technique that does not

require intravenous contrast, ADC could serve to characterize these tumors when combined with conventional images, contributing to narrow the differential diagnosis (**Fig. 7**).

**Diffusion-weighted imaging of soft tissue tumors** Most malignant tumors tend to have lower true diffusion measurements due to increased cellularity and cell packing, resulting in restriction of Brownian motion in the extracellular space (**Fig. 8**). Some investigators have reported overlapping ADC values in benign and malignant soft tissue tumors, hindering the differentiation

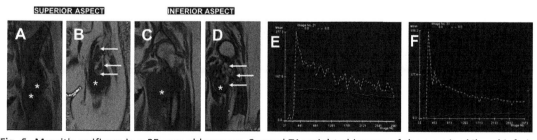

**Fig. 6.** Myositis ossificans in a 35-year-old woman. Coronal T1-weighted images of the superior (*A*) and inferior (*C*) aspects of a heterogeneous tumor in the left thigh. Note the soft tissue component of the lesion (*asterisks*), indicating the acute phase of myositis ossificans. Coronal T1 fat% images of the superior (*B*) and inferior (*D*) aspects of the lesion demonstrate areas of bone marrow (*white arrows*), suggesting a different stage (late phase of myositis ossificans). Note also the DCE-perfusion imaging of different components of the tumor demonstrating early enhancement of the soft tissue with type IV curve in the acute phase (*red line*) (*E*) and poor enhancement of the ossified component, with type II curve in the late phase (*F*).

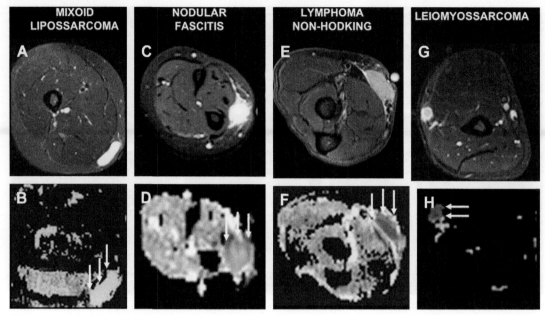

**Fig. 7.** Tissue characterization of superficial soft tissue masses. Myxoid liposarcoma of the thigh on postcontrast axial T1-weighted fat-suppressed (FS) image (*A*) with an ADC value of $2.6 \times 10^3$ mm²/s on axial ADC map (*B*) (*white arrows*). Nodular fasciitis of the forearm in a postcontrast axial T1-weighted FS image (*C*) with an ADC value of $1.4 \times 10^3$ mm²/s on axial ADC map (*D*) (*white arrows*). Lymphoma non-Hodgkin in the forearm on postcontrast axial T1-weighted FS image (*E*) with an ADC value of $0.65 \times 10^3$ mm²/s on axial ADC map (*F*) (*white arrows*). Leiomyosarcoma of the arm on postcontrast axial T1-weighted FS image (*G*) with an ADC value of $0.97 \times 10^3$ mm²/s on axial ADC map (*H*) (*white arrows*).

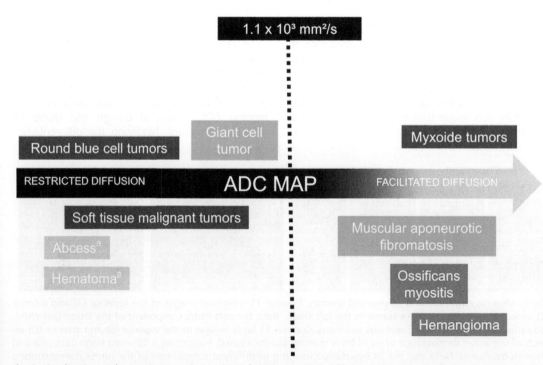

**Fig. 8.** Qualitative and quantitative relationship of ADC map with different histopathological types according to the WHO classification. [a] Pseudotumors.

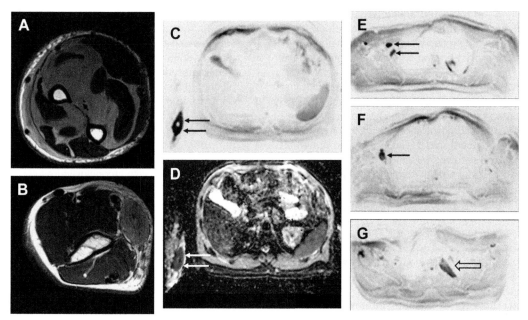

Fig. 9. Soft tissue lymphoma of the right arm in a 57-year-old man with a previous ultrasound diagnosis of sub-cutaneous lipoma. Proximal (A) and distal (B) axial T2-weighted images with infiltrative soft tissue lesion. Axial DWIBS image of an extended segment of the thorax with inverted grayscale (C) and ADC map (D) reveal a soft tissue lesion in the right arm with restricted diffusion (*white and black arrows*) and an ADC value of $0.58 \times 10^3$ mm$^2$/s, suggesting high cellularity. Axial DWIBS images of an extended segment of the arm and thorax with inverted grayscale in superior (F), middle (F), and inferior (G) levels allowing the detection of multicentric lesions with high cellularity in the arm and posterior thoracic wall (*open arrow*), as well as axillary lymphadenop-athy (*black arrows*).

between both. This overlapping is likely because ADC values can be affected by the tumor's collularity and extracellular matrix. Myxoid matrix is a component of interstitial spaces in many soft tissue tumors and can influence the ADC values. As a result, myxoid tumors have significantly higher ADC values than nonmyxoid tumors, regardless of being benign or malignant.[14]

DWI also can be used to monitor tumor response to treatment, most likely because effective anticancer therapy results in changes in the tumor's microenvironment, resulting in increased diffusion of water molecules and ADC value.[13]

**Diffusion-weighted imaging with background body signal suppression** Takahara and colleagues[15] have developed the concept of DWI with background body signal suppression (DWIBS) and proved the feasibility of DWI during free breathing, consequently facilitating the acquisition of images in the body segment and playing an important role in whole-body oncological imaging.

Once a malignant tumor is detected, it is important to determine the extent of the disease for appropriate treatment planning and prognosis determination. By covering a larger examination area beyond the tumor's location using DWIBS, it allows the evaluation of lesion multiplicity, providing an outstanding visualization of regional and distant lymph nodes and detecting simultaneous pathologies, improving diagnostic accuracy.

The assessment of an extended segment of the body could provide information that is unfeasible with localized conventional DWI, which is usually applied to detect and characterize soft tissue tumors. By covering a larger examination area beyond the tumor's location, DWIBS allows the evaluation of lesion multiplicity, providing an outstanding visualization of regional and distant lymph nodes and detecting simultaneous pathologies, improving diagnostic accuracy (**Fig. 9**).

During routine examinations at our institution, an extended segment of DWIBS is currently performed to assess soft tissue tumors, especially in the trunk and limbs, and is very useful in narrowing the differential diagnosis and staging the lesion. The finding of multifocal or extensive lesions limits the diagnostic considerations to angioma-tous lesions, neurofibromatosis, fibromatosis, lipomatosis, myxoma (Mazabraud syndrome), me-tastases, and lymphoma[16]

### Dynamic contrast-enhanced perfusion imaging

DCE-perfusion imaging provides physiologic information regarding tissue vascularization and perfusion, capillary permeability, and interstitial space volume.[17,18]

DCE-MR imaging is usually performed with fast volumetric gradient-echo T1 sequences that are repeated several times during approximately 5 minutes after administration of gadolinium-based intravenous contrast. It also can be performed as highly time-resolved MR angiographic sequences, allowing higher spatial resolution and the analysis of small vessels[7] (**Fig. 10**).

Subsequent to the acquisition of the images, qualitative, semiquantitative, and quantitative assessments may be obtained. The qualitative analysis is evaluated using time intensity curve (TIC) amplitude, which can be classified into 5 different patterns, and curve slope (% of increase of signal intensity per minute) (**Fig. 11**).[17]

Measurement of changes in tumor size based on the Response Evaluation Criteria in Solid Tumors (RECIST) guideline is commonly used to evaluate the response of solid tumors to treatment. However, previous studies[19] have suggested that tumor volume is not a reliable predictor of response to therapy in soft tissue sarcomas because variations in size are usually preceded by changes in tumor functions,[20,21] such as perfusion, cellularity, and metabolism. Consequently, assessing quantitative DCE-MR imaging could predict pathologic response to preoperative therapy (**Fig. 12**).

This technique could add important information including the following:

- *Tissue characterization*: Tissues with high vascularization and capillary permeability tend to have earlier and more intense contrast uptake compared with less vascularized tissues. Attempts have been made to use DCE-perfusion to differentiate benign (low slope) from malignant (high-slope) lesions, with sensitivity and specificity ranging from 72% to 83% and 77% to 89%, respectively. Verstraete and colleagues[22] observed a significant difference in slope values between benign and malignant lesions, but with some overlap (**Table 1**).

- *Identification of areas of viable tumor (high perfusion) to guide biopsy site*: Well-vascularized areas suggest viable tissue, preventing biopsies with inconclusive results.

- *Monitoring of preoperative chemotherapy*: A measurable outcome of preoperative chemotherapy, especially in patients with chemotherapy-sensitive soft tissue tumors is the percentage of tumor necrosis, which differentiates responders and nonresponders.[23] An increase, no change, or even a slight decrease in TIC amplitude and curve during follow-up indicates a poor response to treatment. Changes in TIC with a decrease of at least 60% in slope indicate a necrosis area larger than 90% and, consequently, a good response to treatment (see **Fig. 12**).[24]

- *Detection of residual or recurrent tumor distinguishing tumor from fibrosis*: Tumor tissue enhances early and fast during first-pass contrast, whereas post-therapeutic changes enhance later and more slowly.[23]

### Clinical Applications

#### Fibroblastic/myofibroblastic tumors and so-called fibrohistiocytic tumors

**Proliferative myositis (pseudosarcomatous)** Proliferative myositis is a rare benign inflammatory myopathy characterized by infiltration with basophilic giant cells and proliferative fibroblasts, which occurs most commonly in adults older than 40 and occasionally in children, and usually

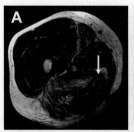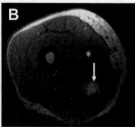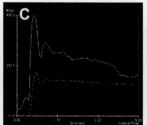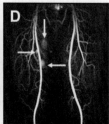

**Fig. 10.** Recurrence of undifferentiated sarcoma in a 64-year-old man. Axial proton density with fat saturation demonstrates a round heterogeneous lesion in the adductor compartment in the right thigh surrounded by edema (*white arrow*) (*A*). Axial DCE-perfusion imaging shows early enhancement of the lesion (*white arrow*) (*B*), with type IV curve (*dotted line*) in (*C*). Maximum intensity projection 3D reconstruction TWIST (time-resolved angiography with stochastic trajectories) perfusion imaging demonstrates the tumor and 2 other satellite lesions (*white arrows*) (*D*).

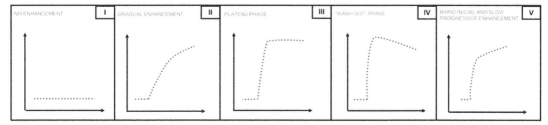

**Fig. 11.** Qualitative and quantitative relationship of ADC map with different histopathological types according to the WHO classification.

arises in the head and neck region or upper extremities.[25,26]

Patients usually present with a rapidly enlarging firm and painful mass that can double in size within a few days or weeks.[26] It shows no specific features on laboratory and imaging examinations. The usefulness of multiparametric approach in this setting is to differentiate proliferative myositis from other soft tissue masses, such as myositis ossificans, rhabdomyolysis, sarcomas, and lymphoma (**Fig. 13**).

**Myositis ossificans** Myositis ossificans is a pseudoinflammatory tumor of the muscle that may be mistaken clinically and even histologically for a malignant soft tissue tumor. A history of trauma is frequently elicited but is often absent (see **Fig. 7**). Myositis ossificans passes through 3 distinct phases, and MR appearance changes with the age of the lesion:

- Active phase (8–10 days): The immature lesion may show high perfusion areas and may mimic a malignant neoplasm (see **Fig. 6**).
- Subacute phase (2–3 weeks; "pseudosarcomatous appearance"): Characterized by an absence of restricted diffusion on DWI and a high-to-intermediate ADC.[17]
- Late phase (3–8 weeks): The maturation phase is characterized by bone production, observed at the periphery of the lesion ("zone phenomenon"), which can be identified on SWI.

**Extra-abdominal desmoid tumor** According to the WHO classification, extra-abdominal desmoid tumors (EADTs) are classified as intermediate tumors (locally aggressive) without metastasis. On conventional MR imaging, EADTs show a homogeneous isointense signal on T1-weighted images and a heterogeneous signal intensity on

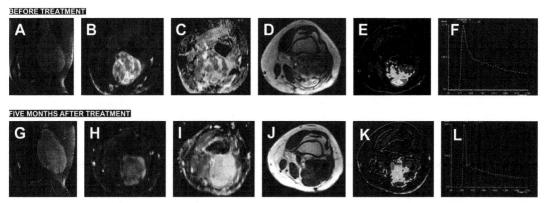

**Fig. 12.** High-grade sarcoma of the right knee in a 29-year-old man. Sagittal proton-density FS image before treatment (*A*) demonstrates heterogeneous tumor in the posterior compartment of the knee. Axial DWI (*B*) and ADC map (*C*) shows areas of restricted diffusion (ADC of $0.82 \times 10^3$ mm$^2$/s). Axial DCE-perfusion imaging (*D*) and color map (*E*) show posterior and superficial early enhancement of the lesion, with a type III curve (*red line*) in (*F*). After treatment, conventional MR image shows no substantial changes in sagittal proton density with fat saturation (*G*). However, axial DWI (*H*) and ADC map (*I*) show areas of facilitated diffusion (ADC of $2.1 \times 10^3$ mm$^2$/s). Axial DCE-perfusion (*J*) and color map (*K*) demonstrate changes with the TIC of early enhancement areas, with type V curve (*red line*) in (*L*), indicating a good response to treatment. The histologic analysis showed greater than 90% necrosis.

| Table 1 |  |
|---|---|
| Difference in slope values between benign and malignant lesions |  |
| **Highly Vascularized Benign Lesion** | **Poorly Vascularized Malignant Lesion** |
| Giant cell tumor | Highly necrotic tumors |
| Myositis ossificans (acute phase) | Late recurrences after chemotherapy or radiation therapy |
| Fibromatosis (occasionally) |  |

T2-weighted images with areas of low intensity ("collagen bands"), with an irregular margin owing to infiltrative growth pattern, and enhancement after gadolinium administration. Feld and colleagues[27] reported that low signal intensity on conventional MR imaging commonly seen in EADTs also could be observed in malignancies such as fibrosarcoma or undifferentiated pleomorphic sarcoma (**Fig. 14**).

Considering advanced techniques, DWI has the potential to differentiate EADTs from malignant soft tissue tumors, because the mean ADC of EADT tends to be higher than that of malignant soft tissue tumors.

Although surgery is the main therapeutic approach in EADTs, local recurrence rates with this treatment are high.[28] MR imaging after nonsurgical treatment can demonstrate decreased signal intensity on T2-weighted sequences, probably because of an increase in the collagen matrix content and a reduction on viable cellular tissue as responses to treatment.

**Giant cell tumors** Giant cell tumors of the tendon sheath are benign soft tissue tumors that arise from the synovium of the joint, bursae, and tendon sheath, and can be divided based on their site (intra-articular or extra-articular) and growth pattern (localized or diffuse), but featuring similar histologic features.[1,29] These lesions contain abundant collagen and hemosiderin, and appear isointense or hypointense to muscle on T1- and T2-weighted MR images, presenting with a "blooming" aspect on SWI and frequent enhancement (see **Fig. 4**).[30]

Nagata and colleagues[31] have described low ADC values in giant cell tumors of the tendon sheath and in diffuse-type. Giant cell tumors typically show high first-pass enhancement, followed by an early wash-out phase. DCE-MR imaging is useful for detecting recurrences or residual tumor tissue after surgery.[23]

### Myxoid tumors

Myxoid-containing soft tissue tumors are an uncommon, heterogeneous group of mesenchymal neoplasms characterized by the presence of abundant extracellular myxoid matrix with very high water content. This group of lesions includes myxomas, myxoid liposarcomas, and myxofibrosarcoma, and demonstrates substantial variability in their biological behavior and includes tumors that are entirely harmless, tumors with a tendency

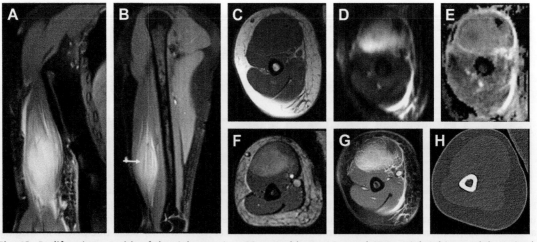

**Fig. 13.** Proliferative myositis of the right arm in a 38-year-old man. Coronal STIR-weighted image (*A*), sagittal STIR-weighted image (*B*), and axial T1-weighted image (*C*) demonstrating a fusiform lesion in the brachial muscle of the right arm with muscle fibers within the lesion (*arrow*). Axial DWI (*D*) and ADC map (*E*) reveal no areas of restricted diffusion, with an ADC of $1.6 \times 10^3$ mm$^2$/s. No blood product or calcification is suspected by axial SWI image (*F*). The lesion is greatly enhanced after gadolinium administration on axial T1-weighted FS image (*G*). Axial reconstruction with computed tomography (*H*) demonstrates no calcifications.

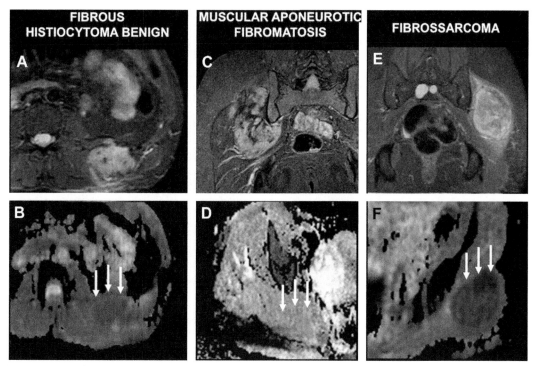

Fig. 14. Very similar morphologic characteristics on MR imaging in benign, intermediated, and malignant lesions of fibrous origin. Benign fibrous histiocytoma of the left paravertebral musculature on axial proton density–weighted image (A) with an ADC of $1.4 \times 10^3$ mm²/s on axial ADC map (B) (white arrows). Musculoaponeurotic fibromatosis (EADT) in the right gluteal musculature on coronal proton density–weighted image (C) with an ADC of $1.3 \times 10^3$ mm²/s on axial ADC map (D) (white arrows). Fibrosarcoma of the left gluteal musculature on coronal proton density–weighted image (E) with an ADC of $0.98 \times 10^3$ mm²/s on axial ADC map (F) (white arrows).

to recur locally but not metastasize, and malignant neoplasms. Differentiation of benign and malignant myxoid-containing soft tissue tumors based on imaging findings is often challenging due to an overlap of radiologic findings between both on conventional and functional MR sequences.

Conventional MR shows typical imaging features with low signal intensity on T1-weighted sequences and high signal intensity ("cystlike") on T2-weighted sequences.[32,33] Perfusion methods are useful for distinguishing cysts from myxoid tumors because myxoid tissue in sarcomas shows areas of intense and fast enhancement (Fig. 15).[23]

Myxoid tumors (benign or malignant) have higher diffusion coefficients than nonmyxoid tumors,[3,34] which reflects their contents of increased mucin, decreased collagen, and a large amount of water.

### Small round cell tumors

Small round cell tumors are a group of undifferentiated embryonal tumors with aggressive behavior that includes neuroblastoma, rhabdomyosarcoma, non-Hodgkin lymphoma, and the family of Ewing sarcomas (Fig. 16). Molecular techniques are required to diagnose these tumors, considering that they have similar histologic features and immunohistochemistry.[17] These are highly malignant tumors that feature dense, high cellularity and high nuclear/cytoplasmic ratio. Lymphomas have been shown to have significantly lower ADC values compared with other tumor types in different body regions (see Fig. 9).[35]

Pathologically, these tumors are more cellular, larger, and have more angulated nuclei and less extracellular space than other solid tumors.[31]

### Metastases

Metastases to soft tissue are rare and often present as a painless soft tissue mass that may be mistaken for a benign swelling or soft tissue sarcoma.[36]

The prevalence of muscle metastases is very low in both autopsy and radiological series. According to Haygood and colleagues,[37] the most common primary malignancies metastasizing to muscles are, in decreasing order of frequency,

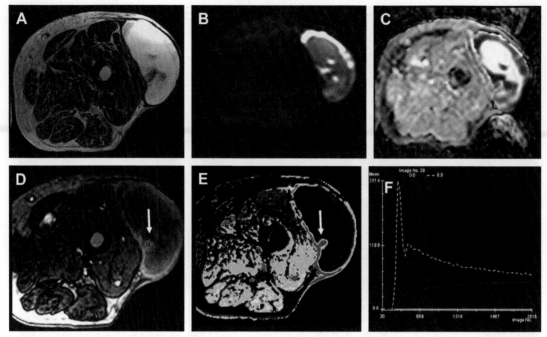

**Fig. 15.** Myxofibrosarcoma in an 84-year-old man. Axial T2-weighted image (*A*), demonstrating a well-defined, high signal intensity lesion in the lateral aspect of the left thigh. Axial DWI (*B*) and ADC map (*C*) reveal peripheral areas of restricted diffusion, suggesting a tissue with increased cellularity. Axial perfusion imaging (*D*) and color map (*E*) show nodular early enhancement in the lateral and inferior aspects of the lesion (*white arrows*), with type III curve (*red line*) in (*F*).

lung cancer, sarcomas, melanoma, renal cell carcinoma, and breast cancer.

Soft tissue metastases present with a broad spectrum of radiological features according to their histopathological content and primary site (**Fig. 17**).

## Pseudotumors (hematomas and abscesses)

Abscesses contain inflammatory cells, cellular debris, and bacteria in high-viscosity pus, with all of these factors restricting the motion of water. Signal intensity in the abscess cavity is increased on DWI and markedly reduced on ADC.[17]

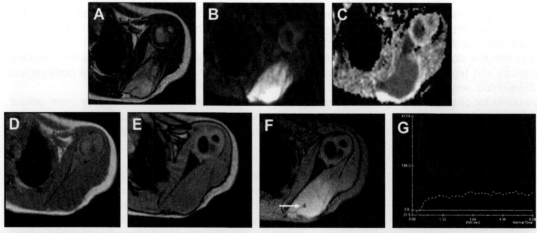

**Fig. 16.** Rhabdomyosarcoma of the left shoulder in a 3-year-old boy. Axial T2-weighted image (*A*) demonstrating an infiltrative lesion in the infraspinatus muscle. Axial DWI (*B*) and ADC map (*C*) reveal restricted diffusion of the lesion, with an ADC value of $0.69 \times 10^3$ mm$^2$/s, indicating high cellularity. In-phase (*D*) and out-phase images (*E*) demonstrate no fat tissue halo surrounding the lesion. Axial SWI (*F*) shows calcification (*arrow*) inside the lesion and (*G*) DCE-perfusion shows type II curve.

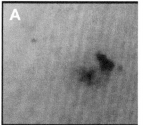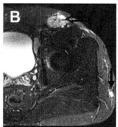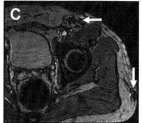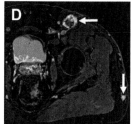

Fig. 17. Locoregional metastasis of melanoma in a 40-year-old man. Skin lesion in the lateral aspect of the left hip (*A*). Axial STIR-weighted image (*B*) shows subcutaneous soft tissue lesion in the left hip (*black arrow*) with locoregional dissemination to the ipsilateral inguinal region (*black open arrow*). Note the multiple hypointense foci within the lesions (*white arrows*) on SWI images (*C*) suggesting melanin. Axial DCE-perfusion imaging color map (*D*) shows early enhancement of both lesions and demonstrates locoregional dissemination (*white arrows*).

Abscesses may be highly vascularized with perfusion slopes similar to those seen in malignant tumors (**Fig. 18**).[38]

Necrotic neoplasms have facilitated diffusion in necrotic centers in comparison with abscess cavities, but tend to have more restricted diffusion on the ADC map in the solid wall of the tumor, which has higher cellularity.

Care must be taken during diagnostic imaging to differentiate hemorrhagic malignant tumors from hematomas. Some sarcomas tend to be misdiagnosed as chronic hematomas due to history of previous trauma. Hemosiderin causes local magnetic susceptibility effects that create accentuated markedly low signal intensity on SWI (see **Fig. 3**).[39] Acute and subacute hematomas have typical morphologic characteristics on conventional MR imaging and present with restricted diffusion on ADC maps of the central part of the lesion. Contrast enhancement in benign hematomas is rare.[40]

### Soft tissue sarcoma

Soft tissue sarcomas are a group of malignant neoplasms that includes a wide range of tumors associated with a high mortality rate. Considering many overlapping imaging appearances combined with their relative rarity in routine practice, contributing to a difficult diagnosis, the recognition of subtle suspicious signs with a potential of malignancy becomes crucial.

Zhao and colleagues[41] have demonstrated that morphologic parameters can be used to differentiate high-grade and low-grade soft tissue sarcomas. However, the numerous functional MR diagnostic techniques discussed previously have improved the knowledge for identification of different characteristics of sarcomas besides the morphologic criteria, and provided tools that enable a more accurate diagnosis,[42] prognosis, and therapeutic management.

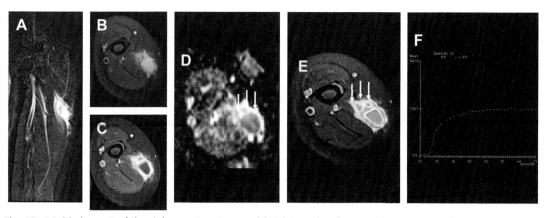

Fig. 18. "Cold abscess" of the right arm in a 2-year-old girl 4 weeks after vaccination. Coronal STIR-weighted image (*A*) and axial proton density–weighted image (*B*) demonstrating a soft tissue lesion in the right arm. Note an early peripheral enhancement after gadolinium administration on axial T1-weighted FS image (*C*). Axial ADC map (*D*) reveals restricted diffusion in the central portion of the lesion (*white arrows*). Axial DCE-perfusion imaging color map (*E*) shows an early peripheral enhancement (*white arrows*), with type III curve (*yellow line*) in (*F*).

Monitoring sarcoma treatment response Conventional MR imaging in the follow-up after treatment of soft tissue sarcomas is traditionally based on anatomic and morphologic approaches, such as tumor size and degree of contrast enhancement. However, this analysis has substantial limitations, including poor measurement reproducibility and persistence of (non-neoplastic) mass lesions after therapy.[43] Because cellular death and vascular changes in response to treatment precede changes in lesion measurement, multiparametric imaging may increase the sensitivity of MR imaging in determining the therapeutic response in soft tissue sarcomas.[17,44]

The DWI technique has been used to assess the viability of residual tumor tissue after treatment and detect early recurrence.[43] Differences in ADC are observed in post-therapeutic soft tissue changes and residual or recurrent tumor because solid tumors show high cellularity and intact cell membranes, whereas successful treatment results in decreased tumor cellularity and loss of cell membrane integrity.[45]

DCE-perfusion MR imaging is an essential method for monitoring preoperative response to chemotherapy and/or radiotherapy. Poor and good responders to chemotherapy can be detected on first-pass or subtraction images, or by evaluation of changes in slopes using the region of interest method.[23] The purpose of using this technology is to detect local tumor recurrence or residual tumor tissue and differentiate them from reactive tissue. Tumor tissue enhances fast during the first pass of contrast, whereas reactive tissue enhances later and slowly.[23] In soft tissue sarcomas, focal areas of early and rapidly progressive enhancement correspond to residual viable or recurrent tumor. In contrast, the absence of areas of early enhancement indicate a good response.

Radiation therapy can induce vascularization, resulting in increased perfusion in the irradiated area. Differentiation of a reactive mass with granulation tissue from residual tumors or recurrence tumor tissues may be difficult in the first 3 to 6 months after irradiation[23]; therefore, follow-up examinations are necessary because the perfusion of a reactive mass decreases but remains increased in residual tumor tissues because they grow and remain highly vascularized.[17]

## SUMMARY

Preventing an inadequate approach to soft masses is crucial for successful treatment of soft tissue sarcomas, minimizing oncological sequelae and extensively mutilating surgical procedures of these tumors, and increasing the survival and quality of life of the patients presenting with these tumors. Appropriate evaluation and treatment planning are required, along with an integrated and multidisciplinary approach by specialists using standard diagnostic methods and adequate techniques. The use of multiparametric MR imaging along with conventional and advanced MR sequences provides additional information on the detection, characterization, staging, and treatment follow-up of soft tissue tumors.

## ACKNOWLEDGMENTS

The authors thank Evandro Miguelote Vianna, MD, Walter Meohas, MD, Marcio Bernardes, and Ierecê Lins Aymoré for technical support.

## REFERENCES

1. Jo VY, Fletcher CD. WHO classification of soft tissue tumours: an update based on the 2013 (4th) edition. Pathology 2014;46(2):95–104.
2. van der Woude HJ, Verstraete KL, Hogendoorn PC, et al. Musculoskeletal tumors: does fast dynamic contrast-enhanced subtraction MR imaging contribute to the characterization? Radiology 1998; 208(3):821–8.
3. Costa FM, Ferreira EC, Vianna EM. Diffusion-weighted magnetic resonance imaging for the evaluation of musculoskeletal tumors. Magn Reson Imaging Clin N Am 2011;19(1):159–80.
4. Chung WJ, Chung HW, Shin MJ, et al. MRI to differentiate benign from malignant soft-tissue tumours of the extremities: a simplified systematic imaging approach using depth, size and heterogeneity of signal intensity. Br J Radiol 2012;85(1018):e831–6.
5. Rand SD, Prost R, Haughton V, et al. Accuracy of single-voxel proton MR spectroscopy in distinguishing neoplastic from nonneoplastic brain lesions. AJNR Am J Neuroradiol 1997;18(9):1695–704.
6. Fayad LM, Wang X, Salibi N, et al. A feasibility study of quantitative molecular characterization of musculoskeletal lesions by proton MR spectroscopy at 3 T. AJR Am J Roentgenol 2010;195(1):W69–75.
7. Vilanova JC, Baleato-Gonzalez S, Romero MJ, et al. Assessment of musculoskeletal malignancies with functional MR imaging. Magn Reson Imaging Clin N Am 2016;24(1):239–59.
8. Sah PL, Sharma R, Kandpal H, et al. In vivo proton spectroscopy of giant cell tumor of the bone. AJR Am J Roentgenol 2008;190(2):W133–9.
9. Fayad LM, Barker PB, Jacobs MA, et al. Characterization of musculoskeletal lesions on 3-T proton MR spectroscopy. AJR Am J Roentgenol 2007;188(6): 1513–20.
10. Gasparotti R, Pinelli L, Liserre R. New MR sequences in daily practice: susceptibility weighted

imaging. A pictorial essay. Insights Imaging 2011; 2(3):335–47.

11. Berglund J, Johansson L, Ahlstrom H, et al. Three-point Dixon method enables whole-body water and fat imaging of obese subjects. Magn Reson Med 2010;63(6):1659–68.

12. Hamstra DA, Rehemtulla A, Ross BD. Diffusion magnetic resonance imaging: a biomarker for treatment response in oncology. J Clin Oncol 2007;25(26): 4104–9.

13. Koh DM, Collins DJ. Diffusion-weighted MRI in the body: applications and challenges in oncology. AJR Am J Roentgenol 2007;188(6):1622–35.

14. Baur A, Reiser MF. Diffusion-weighted imaging of the musculoskeletal system in humans. Skeletal Radiol 2000;29(10):555–62.

15. Takahara T, Imai Y, Yamashita T, et al. Diffusion weighted whole body imaging with background body signal suppression (DWIBS): technical improvement using free breathing, STIR and high resolution 3D display. Radiat Med 2004;22:275–82.

16. Walker EA, Fenton ME, Salesky JS, et al. Magnetic resonance imaging of benign soft tissue neoplasms in adults. Radiol Clin North Am 2011;49(6): 1197–217, vi.

17. Costa FM, Canella C, Gasparetto E. Advanced magnetic resonance imaging techniques in the evaluation of musculoskeletal tumors. Radiol Clin North Am 2011;49(6):1325–58, vii–viii.

18. Schepper AM, Vanhoenacker FM, Parizel PM, et al. Imaging of soft tissue tumors. 3rd edition. Berlin: Springer; 2006.

19. van Rijswijk CS, Geirnaerdt MJ, Hogendoorn PC, et al. Dynamic contrast-enhanced MR imaging in monitoring response to isolated limb perfusion in high-grade soft tissue sarcoma: initial results. Eur Radiol 2003;13(8):1849–58.

20. Harry VN, Semple SI, Parkin DE, et al. Use of new imaging techniques to predict tumour response to therapy. Lancet Oncol 2010;11(1):92–102.

21. Padhani AR, Miles KA. Multiparametric imaging of tumor response to therapy. Radiology 2010;256(2): 348–64.

22. Verstraete KL, De Deene Y, Roels H, et al. Benign and malignant musculoskeletal lesions: dynamic contrast-enhanced MR imaging–parametric "first-pass" images depict tissue vascularization and perfusion. Radiology 1994;192(3):835–43.

23. Verstraete KL, Lang P. Bone and soft tissue tumors: the role of contrast agents for MR imaging. Eur J Radiol 2000;34(3):229–46.

24. Erlemann R, Vassallo P, Bongartz G, et al. Musculoskeletal neoplasms: fast low-angle shot MR imaging with and without Gd-DTPA. Radiology 1990;176(2): 489–95.

25. Enzinger FM, Dulcey F. Proliferative myositis. Report of thirty-three cases. Cancer 1967;20(12):2213–23.

26. Mulier S, Stas M, Delabie J, et al. Proliferative myositis in a child. Skeletal Radiol 1999;28(12): 703–9.

27. Feld R, Burk DL Jr, McCue P, et al. MRI of aggressive fibromatosis: frequent appearance of high signal intensity on T2-weighted images. Magn Reson Imaging 1990;8(5):583–8.

28. Micke O, Seegenschmiedt MH, German Cooperative Group on Radiotherapy for Benign Diseases. Radiation therapy for aggressive fibromatosis (desmoid tumors): results of a national Patterns of Care Study. Int J Radiat Oncol Biol Phys 2005;61(3): 882–91.

29. Murphey MD, Rhee JH, Lewis RB, et al. Pigmented villonodular synovitis: radiologic-pathologic correlation. Radiographics 2008;28(5):1493–518.

30. De Beuckeleer L, De Schepper A, De Belder F, et al. Magnetic resonance imaging of localized giant cell tumour of the tendon sheath (MRI of localized GCTTS). Eur Radiol 1997;7(2):198–201.

31. Nagata S, Nishimura H, Uchida M, et al. Diffusion-weighted imaging of soft tissue tumors: usefulness of the apparent diffusion coefficient for differential diagnosis. Radiat Med 2008;26(5):287–95.

32. Baheti AD, Tirumani SH, Rosenthal MH, et al. Myxoid soft-tissue neoplasms: comprehensive update of the taxonomy and MRI features. AJR Am J Roentgenol 2015;204(2):374–85.

33. Kim HS, Kim JH, Yoon YC, et al. Tumor spatial heterogeneity in myxoid-containing soft tissue using texture analysis of diffusion-weighted MRI. PLoS One 2017;12(7).e0181339.

34. Maeda M, Matsumine A, Kato H, et al. Soft-tissue tumors evaluated by line scan diffusion weighted imaging: influence of myxoid matrix on the apparent diffusion coefficient. J Magn Reson Imaging 2007; 25(6):1199–204.

35. Sumi M, Ichikawa Y, Nakamura T. Diagnostic ability of apparent diffusion coefficients for lymphomas and carcinomas in the pharynx. Eur Radiol 2007; 17(10):2631–7.

36. Plaza JA, Perez-Montiel D, Mayerson J, et al. Metastases to soft tissue: a review of 118 cases over a 30-year period. Cancer 2008;112(1):193–203.

37. Haygood TM, Wong J, Lin JC, et al. Skeletal muscle metastases: a three-part study of a not-so-rare entity. Skeletal Radiol 2012;41(8):899–909.

38. van Rijswijk CS, Geirnaerdt MJ, Hogendoorn PC, et al. Soft-tissue tumors: value of static and dynamic gadopentetate dimeglumine-enhanced MR imaging in prediction of malignancy. Radiology 2004;233(2): 493–502.

39. Wu JS, Hochman MG. Soft-tissue tumors and tumor-like lesions: a systematic imaging approach. Radiology 2009;253(2):297–316.

40. Oka K, Yakushiji T, Sato H, et al. Ability of diffusion-weighted imaging for the differential diagnosis

between chronic expanding hematomas and malignant soft tissue tumors. J Magn Reson Imaging 2008;28(5):1195–200.

41. Zhao F, Ahlawat S, Farahani SJ, et al. Can MR imaging be used to predict tumor grade in soft-tissue sarcoma? Radiology 2014;272(1):192–201.

42. Lauer S, Gardner JM. Soft tissue sarcomas–new approaches to diagnosis and classification. Curr Probl Cancer 2013;37(2):45–61.

43. Padhani AR, Khan AA. Diffusion-weighted (DW) and dynamic contrast-enhanced (DCE) magnetic resonance imaging (MRI) for monitoring anticancer therapy. Target Oncol 2010;5(1):39–52.

44. Soldatos T, Ahlawat S, Montgomery E, et al. Multiparametric assessment of treatment response in high-grade soft-tissue sarcomas with anatomic and functional MR imaging sequences. Radiology 2016;278(3):831–40.

45. Bley TA, Wieben O, Uhl M. Diffusion-weighted MR imaging in musculoskeletal radiology: applications in trauma, tumors, and inflammation. Magn Reson Imaging Clin N Am 2009;17(2):263–75.

# Multiparametric MR Imaging of Benign and Malignant Bone Lesions

Huasong Tang, MD, Shivani Ahlawat, MD,
Laura M. Fayad, MD*

## KEYWORDS

- MR imaging • Bone neoplasm • DWI • DCE-MR imaging • Chemical shift imaging

## KEY POINTS

- Multiple MR imaging sequences, both noncontrast and contrast-enhanced sequences, collectively provide valuable information for the characterization of bone lesions.
- For evaluating bone tumors, widely used MR imaging sequences include conventional T1, fluid-sensitive, and static postcontrast T1-weighted imaging. However, functional imaging with diffusion-weighted imaging, and dynamic contrast-enhanced MR imaging are fast sequences that are readily available for clinical use. In the musculoskeletal system, metabolic imaging with MR spectroscopy has been explored outside the realm of clinical usage.
- For the characterization of bone marrow signal abnormalities, chemical shift imaging is a fast non-contrast technique that helps distinguish a marrow-replacing lesion from dense red marrow or bone marrow edema.

## INTRODUCTION

Although radiography is the first test used in the evaluation of bone lesions (for detection as well as characterization), MR imaging is superior for defining the extent of a bone tumor, especially with conventional noncontrast spin-echo T1-weighted imaging. Such conventional sequences, along with fluid-sensitive sequences and contrast-enhancing static T1-weighted imaging, also provide information about the character of a bone lesion. With the emergence of functional sequences, including diffusion-weighted imaging (DWI) and dynamic contrast-enhanced (DCE) MR sequences, the role of MR imaging has further advanced with regard to lesion characterization, as more quantitative metrics have become available. Additionally, although conventional T1 and fluid-sensitive sequences depict marrow abnormalities exquisitely, areas of dense red marrow or marrow edema can be confused with a marrow tumor, necessitating the use of other sequences, such as chemical shift imaging with in-phase (IP) and opposed-phase (OP) sequences. In this review, the contribution of these varied MR imaging sequences for the assessment of benign and malignant bone lesions is discussed.

## BONE TUMOR MR IMAGING PROTOCOL
### Noncontrast MR Imaging Sequences

The foundation of a bone tumor MR imaging protocol is the spin-echo T1-weighted sequence, as this sequence superbly portrays a marrow-replacing lesion against normal fatty marrow (**Fig. 1A**).[1] In pediatric patients or patients with abundant red

Disclosures: Dr L.M. Fayad: GERRAF 2008 to 2010, Siemens Medical Systems 2011 to 2012, SCBT/MR 2004, William M.G. Gatewood Fellowship. Drs H. Tang and S. Ahlawat have nothing to disclose.
The Russell H. Morgan Department of Radiology and Radiological Science, The Johns Hopkins School of Medicine, 601 North Wolfe Street, Baltimore, MD 21287, USA
* Corresponding author.
*E-mail address:* lfayad1@jhmi.edu

mri.theclinics.com

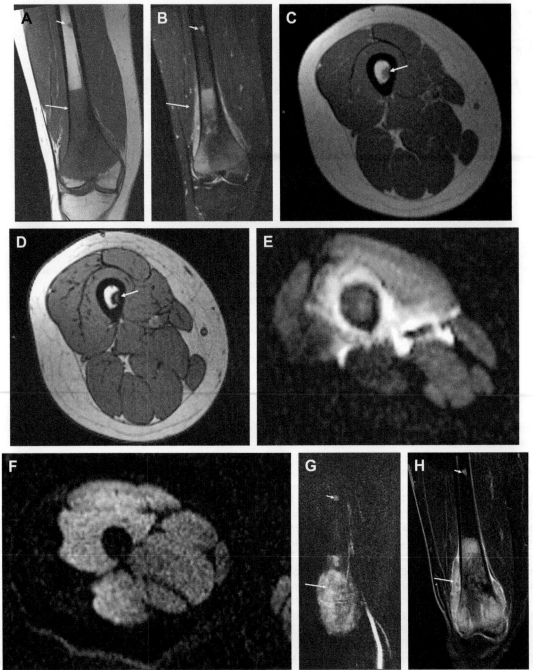

**Fig. 1.** A 14-year-old girl with right distal femoral osteoblastic osteosarcoma and a skip lesion in the mid-diaphysis. Coronal T1-weighted and T2–fat saturated (FS) image (*A, B*) through the distal right femur shows a large distal femoral osteosarcoma (*long arrow*) with a small signal abnormality in the mid-diaphysis (*short arrow*). Note how well defined the tumor is against the background of normal fatty marrow. On coronal fat-suppressed T2-weighted image (*B*), perilesional edema, soft tissue extension, and periosteal reaction are observed, consistent with the aggressive nature of this lesion. On axial IP (*C*) and OP (*D*) images through the mid-diaphysis of the right femur, the skip lesion (*arrow*) has an etching artifact along its margin visible on OP (*D*) due to fat-lesion interface and lacks signal dropout, consistent with a small focus of marrow replacement. Axial ADC map shows low signal within the marrow of the femur, with ADC values of 0.4 to 0.7 × 10$^{-3}$ mm$^2$/s, typical of malignancy (*E*). More superiorly, the normal marrow of the more proximal femur is dark, with ADC value of 0.1 × 10$^{-3}$ mm$^2$/s (*F*). The DCE sequence in the coronal plane through the right femur (*G*) shows early arterial enhancement of the large distal femoral osteosarcoma (*long arrow*), as well as the small skip lesion in the mid-diaphysis (*short arrow*). These findings are confirmed on the static postcontrast fat-suppressed T1-weighted coronal image through the femur, acquired with subtraction (precontrast subtracted from the postcontrast images) (*H*).

marrow (such as oncology patients), an additional T1-weighted imaging strategy, that of IP and OP chemical shift imaging, can provide "marrow-specific" imaging. With IP and OP sequences, the spin frequency difference between protons attached to water and those attached to lipid is exploited and used to identify whether a marrow signal abnormality contains lipid interspersed with water (as would be expected for red marrow or bone marrow edema), or whether the marrow signal abnormality is pure water (as would be expected with a marrow-replacing tumor).[2–4] Hence, if a signal abnormality in the marrow is shown to have a significant drop in signal on OP compared with IP imaging, there is presumed lipid interspersed with water, whereas if there is no significant drop in signal on the OP compared with the IP sequence, the area in question is presumed to be a true marrow-replacing lesion. Therefore, IP and OP imaging can be used for characterizing bone marrow signal abnormalities as marrow-replacing or non–marrow-replacing (such as red marrow or bone marrow edema) (**Fig. 1**B, C).

Fluid-sensitive sequences, with fat-suppressed T2-weighted imaging and short-tau inversion recovery, provide information on the aggressivity of the bone lesion by identifying perilesional edema, periosteal reaction, and extension to the soft tissues (**Fig. 1**D). Primary malignant bone tumors are often associated with perilesional signal abnormalities. However, not all malignant lesions are associated with perilesional edema (for example, see **Fig. 1**A showing a skip lesion without bone marrow edema in the proximal femur); metastatic disease and myeloma of bone may have no perilesional edema or periosteal reaction associated.

DWI is a noncontrast imaging technique that offers quantitative metrics for lesion assessment, including the apparent diffusion coefficient (ADC). DWI measures the Brownian motion of water, and the degree of restriction of that motion corresponds to the cellularity of a lesion, and, hence, its malignant potential.[5] For soft tissue tumor imaging, there is a higher likelihood of malignancy in lesions with lower ADC values.[6,7] In bone imaging, normal marrow has low ADC values because of the already reduced water content, and adipocytes that are densely packed, factors that result in the restriction of water diffusion (to a greater degree than a bone tumor). Hence, in bone tumor imaging, a bone tumor is expected to have greater ADC values than adjacent normal marrow; a bone tumor will also retain signal on a high b-value image compared with normal marrow, making it easy to identify against the background of normal marrow. Hence, DWI has been used as a whole-body technique for detecting metastatic bone disease by searching for bone lesions on high b-value imaging. Furthermore, once detected, the corresponding ADC map can be used for characterization of detected bone lesions, to differentiate benign and malignant skeletal lesions, as found by Ahlawat and colleagues[8] (see **Fig. 1**E, F).

### Contrast-Enhanced MR Imaging Sequences

A conventional musculoskeletal tumor protocol typically includes contrast-enhanced static T1-weighted imaging (**Fig. 2**). Fat suppression is used to improve the conspicuity of enhancing

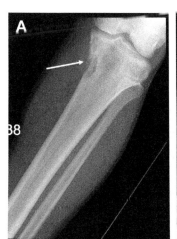
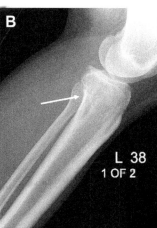
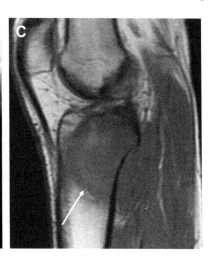

Fig. 2. A 21-year-old man with osteosarcoma. Anteroposterior (*A*) and lateral (*B*) radiographs of the proximal tibia show an aggressive skeletal lesion (*arrow*) within the proximal diametaphysis with mixed osteolysis and sclerosis. There is medial cortical destruction present. The radiographic features are compatible with osteosarcoma. Radiography is the first-line modality in the detection and characterization of a skeletal lesion. The T1-weighted image (*C*) is critical for showing the lesion extent (*arrow*) against the background of fatty marrow.

lesions against the suppressed background. Recently, 3-dimensional volumetric sequences with fat suppression and subtraction have been shown to offer fast, high-resolution imaging with high lesion conspicuity, important to identifying areas of enhancement within a bone tumor.[9] Additionally, when intravenous contrast is administered, the early enhancing phases can be acquired first (DCE-MR imaging); in a clinical setting, a time resolution of 7 seconds can be used (**Fig. 1**G), with dynamic acquisition for as long as desired, typically 2 to 5 minutes. The delayed static phase can be subsequently acquired (**Fig. 1**H). DCE-MR imaging has been shown to provide valuable information for differentiating malignant from benign tissue.[10]

## Magnetic Resonance Spectroscopy

MR spectroscopy (MRS) is a means of noninvasively identifying metabolic markers of malignancy. Although this test has been shown to be useful in detecting choline-containing metabolites in malignant bone and soft tissue tumors, MRS is not used routinely as a clinical tool. A review by Subhawong and colleagues[11] showed that quantitative MRS offers very high negative predictive value for the characterization of lesions, thus implying that MRS can be used to rule out malignancy.

## BONE TUMOR CHARACTERIZATION

Radiography remains an essential tool for the first-line assessment of a bone lesion. A patient with a bone lesion may experience pain or swelling that prompts the physician to obtain a radiograph that shows the bone lesion. This is particularly true in cases of malignancy of the extremities. MR imaging is then used when the visualized bone lesion is indeterminate (requiring MR imaging features for further characterization), or when information regarding the extent of disease is needed (malignant tumors) (see **Fig. 2**). However, for asymptomatic or nonaggressive benign bone lesions, the abnormality may be identified by MR imaging for the first time incidentally. In addition, radiographically occult lesions occur often in the axial skeleton (**Fig. 3**). As such, MR imaging must

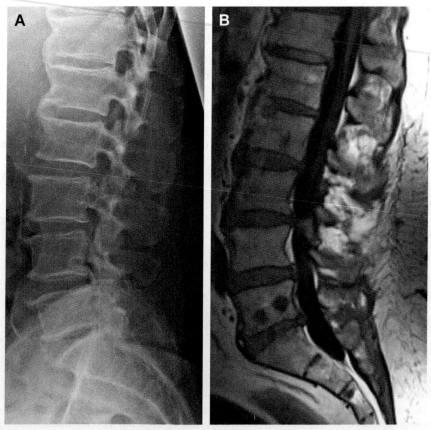

**Fig. 3.** A 66-year-old man with radiographically occult bone lesions in the spine, which were subsequently diagnosed as metastatic disease. Sagittal spine radiograph (*A*) shows no definite abnormality in the spine, while sagittal T1-weighted image (*B*) shows 2 lesions in L5.

play a role in the characterization of bone abnormalities. As sequences have emerged, normal marrow, benign lesions, and malignant tumors are more readily differentiated by MR imaging.

First, a well-circumscribed low–signal-intensity lesion distinguished against normal marrow on T1-weighted imaging may be benign or malignant. The strength of a spin-echo T1-weighted sequence is in providing detectability of bone marrow lesions, although it should be noted that in patients with extensive red marrow reconversion (as may be seen in children, oncology patients, obese individuals, or in those with a history of smoking or anemia), the T1-weighted sequence may provide insufficient contrast resolution for identifying the bone lesion against the adjacent normal red marrow.[12] In such cases, chemical shift imaging with IP and OP imaging details the location of the lesion in the bone marrow clearly (**Fig. 4**).[4] In addition, some bone marrow signal abnormalities that are detected by T1-weighted imaging may be indeterminate, in that it is unclear whether a marrow-replacing lesion is present or not. Chemical shift imaging can again be used to answer the latter question with confidence; if there is greater than 20% signal drop on the OP compared with IP sequence, then the signal abnormality can be deemed non–marrow-replacing (often red marrow or bone marrow edema), whereas if there is less than a 20% signal drop on the OP compared with IP sequence, the abnormality is considered marrow-replacing (see **Fig. 1C, D**). A potential caveat to the algorithm

described previously is that infiltrative disorders such as myeloma or leukemia may show significant signal drop on OP compared with IP,[3,13] although in the authors' experience, this is not a consistent feature.

Second, the absence of perilesional edema by fluid-sensitive sequences does not imply the lesion is benign. Similarly, the presence of perilesional edema, periosteal reaction, or soft tissue extension may not always herald malignancy, but rather, may be seen with an active benign lesion (such as Langerhans cell histiocytosis).[14] Other active benign lesions that may present with perilesional signal abnormalities include giant cell tumors (**Fig. 5**), aneurysmal bone cysts (**Fig. 6**), osteomyelitis, and any lesion that is associated with a pathologic fracture.[15]

Third, traditionally, cystic and solid masses in both skeletal and soft tissue can be readily distinguished by their contrast-enhancement characteristics (described further later in this article). If the lesion fails to enhance following contrast administration, it is regarded as a cyst. However, patients without intravenous access, adequate renal function, or who refuse contrast administration may be precluded from this approach. As previously mentioned, when performing DWI, high concentrations of cell membranes in cellular lesions will reduce the ADC, indicating a reduction in Brownian motion. Thus, in acellular environments such as a cystic lesion, the free diffusion of water will be marked by high ADC values (see **Fig. 6G**). In practice, DWI has proven to be accurate in

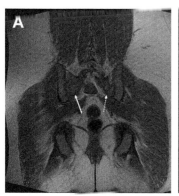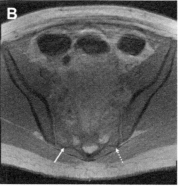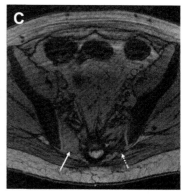

**Fig. 4.** A 40-year-old woman with left humerus Ewing sarcoma in the mid-diaphysis. The patient had low back pain and underwent MR imaging. Coronal T1-weighted image through the sacrum (*A*) reveals confluent T1 hypointense signal in the right sacrum (*solid arrow*). The dotted arrow describes an area of decreased T1 signal in the left sacrum and it is unclear whether this signal represents a marrow-replacing tumor or red marrow. The sacrum can be a challenging site to evaluate on T1-weighted images, particularly in patients with a history of malignancy or prior chemotherapy due to dense red marrow. CSI with IP (*B*) and OP (*C*) images confirm the presence of a metastatic lesion in the right sacrum (*solid arrow*) in this patient with both qualitative and quantitative lack of signal dropout between the 2 sequences. Note the signal dropout in the left hemisacrum on IP and OP (*dotted arrow*), indicating a lack of marrow replacement (in this case representing red marrow), although this region has similar signal characteristics to the right hemisacrum on the T1-weighted images.

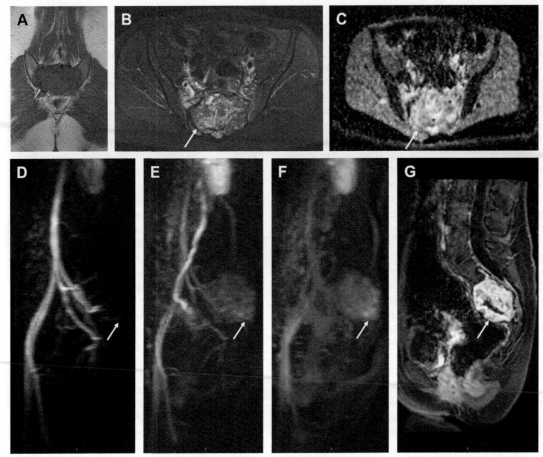

**Fig. 5.** A 32-year-old woman with sacral giant cell tumor of bone. Coronal T1-weighted image (*A*) and axial T2-FS image (*B*) through the pelvis show large skeletal lesion involving the entire sacrum (*arrow*). On the axial ADC map (*C*), the lesion (*arrow*) is heterogeneous but has intrinsically low ADC value (indicated by *asterisks* in the image) with a minimum ADC value of $0.6 \times 10^{-3}$ mm$^2$/s, suggestive of malignancy. On sequential sagittal DCE images through the pelvis (*D–F*), there is no enhancement on the early arterial phase (*D*) but late arterial and progressive enhancement on sequential images (*E*) and (*F*), a pattern associated with benign lesions. On sagittal static post-contrast T1-FS image through the pelvis (*G*), the lesion enhances with central nonenhancing regions (*arrow*).

separating cystic lesions from solid masses with very high specificity, and should be particularly considered in the aforementioned scenarios in which contrast administration is not an option.[16]

Fourth, when normal marrow and a cyst have been ruled out, another utility for DWI is in differentiating benign and malignant lesions. Through a qualitative approach to DWI, low and high b-value images can be compared, with the knowledge that malignant bone lesions retain signal on high b-value images, and are well outlined compared with normal surrounding marrow (which typically is fat-suppressed and has very low signal on high b-value images) (**Fig. 7**). As such, the addition of DWI to a whole-body MR imaging protocol for detecting metastatic disease has been proposed and shown to be similar to bone scan technique for detecting metastatic disease. A quantitative

metric associated with DWI is ADC mapping, a technique that quantitatively measures the Brownian movement of water.[17,18] In a study that measured ADC values of several benign and malignant entities, the analysis by Ahlawat and colleagues[8] showed that the minimum ADC value yielded the most accurate prediction of lesion histology (regarding malignant potential). Specifically, threshold values of $0.9 \times 10^{-3}$ mm$^2$/s corresponded to a sensitivity of 92% and specificity of 78%, and on average, minimum, mean, and maximum ADC values were higher in benign lesions compared with malignant tumors. Interestingly, it is worth noting that the biologically aggressive benign lesions (that often have perilesional aggressive characteristics), such as giant cell tumor, osteoblastoma, and Langerhans cell histiocytosis in this study, tended to have lower

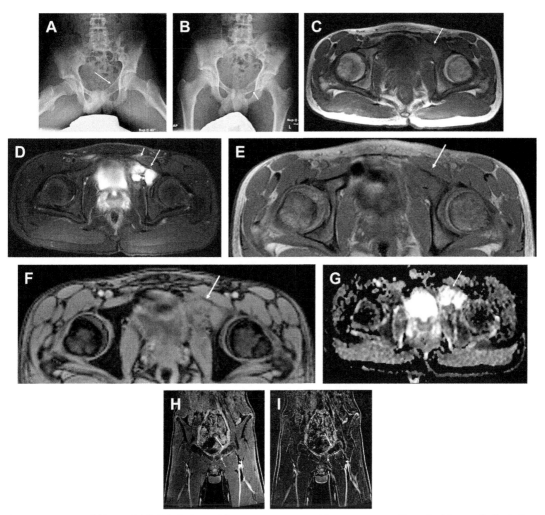

**Fig. 6.** A 15-year-old boy with left inferior pubic ramus aneurysmal bone cyst complicated with a pathologic fracture. Frog-leg lateral (*A*) and anteroposterior (AP) (*B*) images of the pelvis show an expansile, lytic lesion in the left pubic ramus (*long arrow*) with subtle pathologic fracture best seen on the AP image (*short arrow*). The lesion (*arrow*) is well visualized on the axial T1-weighted image (*C*) through the pelvis. The axial T2-FS image (*D*) shows the expansile, multilocular cystic appearance of the lesion (*arrow*). The short arrow demarcates the medial extent of the lesion. IP and OP images (*E* and *F*, respectively) qualitatively and quantitatively confirm the presence of a marrow-replacing lesion (*arrow*). The axial ADC map (*G*) shows markedly elevated ADC values within the lesion (*arrow*), with minimum ADC value of 2.5. Coronal T1-FS postcontrast images (*H*) and T1-weighted fat-suppressed postcontrast subtraction images (*I*) reveal perilesional enhancement (*dotted arrow*) due to the pathologic enhancement, as well as lack of internal enhancement. The solid arrow points to the lesion (*H*).

ADC values ($0.7 \times 10^{-3}$ mm$^2$/s) than their less aggressive benign peers ($1.3 \times 10^{-3}$ mm$^2$/s) (see **Fig. 5**C); this represents a palpable overlap with the corresponding ADC values of malignant lesions ($0.7 \times 10^{-3}$ mm$^2$/s), and is presumably secondary to the elevated underlying cellularity that is sometimes associated with these aggressive benign lesions. Low ADC values can also be present in lesions with blood products and fluid-fluid levels, as shown in **Fig. 8**.

Fifth, although the noncontrast imaging sequences discussed previously provide useful information, there are benefits to be retrieved from the administration of intravenous contrast material, including bone lesion characterization and assessment after treatment. With a contrast-enhanced study, the differentiation of a cyst from a solid lesion is possible; when uncomplicated, a unicameral bone cyst or primary aneurysmal bone cyst will show peripheral rim enhancement (see **Fig. 6**) and, perhaps, septal enhancement, without nodular internal contrast-enhancing areas. It should be understood, however, that in cases of pathologic fractures through a bone cyst, enhancing nodular granulation tissue may be present, along with enhancing periosteal reaction

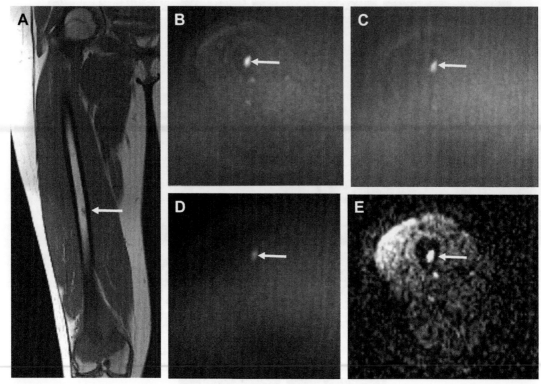

**Fig. 7.** A 14-year-old girl with right distal femoral osteoblastic osteosarcoma and a skip lesion in the mid-diaphysis (same patient as in **Fig. 1**) imaged after neoadjuvant therapy. The skip lesion is indicated by an arrow on the coronal T1-weighted image through the right femur (*A*). DWIs with b-value of 50 (*B*), 400 (*C*), and 800 (*D*) and ADC map (*E*) are shown. Note that the lesion remains visible on the high b-value image, underscoring the use of the high b-value image as a way to detect bone marrow malignant lesions.

and soft tissue enhancement that may confuse the appearance of the underlying benign bone cyst. In such cases, the radiographic appearance will provide additional valuable information for the characterization of the underlying cyst. Conversely, if the peripheral rim of enhancement of an uncomplicated presumed cystic lesion shows nodular thickening, an underlying bone tumor should be considered, as necrotic tumors will frequently have thick peripheral nodular enhancement and a nonenhancing central component.

For noncystic bone lesions, the perilesional enhancement characteristics following contrast medium administration can be useful. Similar to perilesional edema, perilesional enhancement on postcontrast imaging indicates an active lesion, either a benign aggressive lesion or a malignant tumor. The internal enhancement pattern of a bone lesion on postcontrast imaging also may be helpful for distinguishing benign and malignant status, especially with the use of DCE-MR imaging.

DCE-MR imaging differs from conventional static postcontrast sequences in its ability to provide temporal resolution. Because temporal resolution comes at the expense of spatial resolution,

DCE-MR imaging cannot be used as a stand-alone sequence; it should always be used in conjunction with static postcontrast sequences of high spatial resolution. The temporal enhancement characteristics of bone lesions have been successfully used to differentiate benign and malignant lesions in soft tissue and skeletal lesions.[19,20] The added temporal resolution provides information on the vascularity of lesions, whereby the rapid arterial enhancement of malignant lesions may be used to differentiate malignancy (see **Fig. 1**) from the gradual enhancing pattern of benign lesions (see **Fig. 5**). As previously mentioned, quantitative DWI may be limited in differentiating aggressive-appearing benign lesions such as Langerhans cell histiocytosis from malignant lesions due to the higher cellularity of Langerhans.[21] Adding temporal resolution with DCE-MR imaging potentially offers additional information for characterizing such lesions (see **Fig. 5**), although some aggressive benign entities have been shown to have rapid arterial enhancement.

Finally, MRS is a noncontrast technique that has been explored for identifying biomarkers of malignancy in bone and soft tissue tumors. As in other

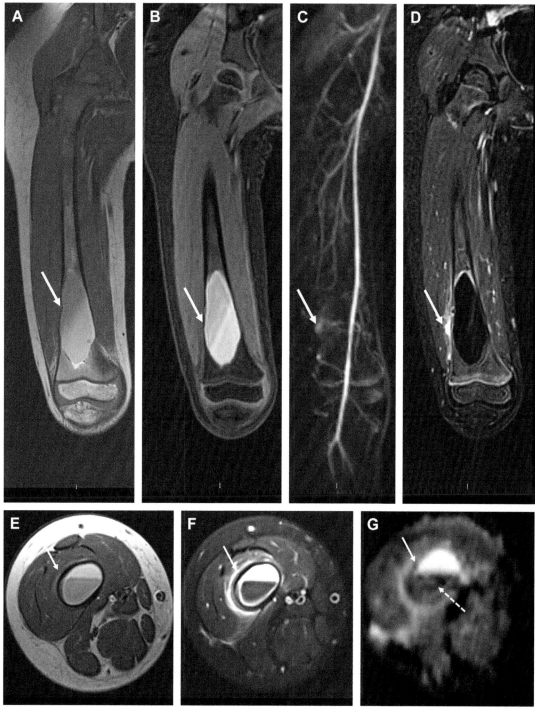

**Fig. 8.** A 4-year-old boy with right distal femoral unicameral bone cyst complicated with pathologic fracture. Coronal T1-weighted image (*A*) through the right femur shows a large skeletal lesion with internal T1 hyperintensity consistent with hemorrhagic products (*arrow*), also visible on coronal T1-weighted fat-suppressed image without contrast (*B*). DCE images (*C*) show minimal late arterial enhancement at the lateral cortex related to the pathologic fracture (*arrow*), also confirmed on static postcontrast T1-weighted fat-suppressed coronal image (*D*) through the lesion. On axial views, fluid-fluid level is evident by T1-weighted imaging (*E*), fat-suppressed T2-weighted image (*F*), and ADC map (*G*). The solid arrow points to the lesion and the dotted arrow to the fluid-fluid level within it (*G*).

parts of the body, choline-containing compounds are elevated in malignant lesions in the musculoskeletal system. This technique, while requiring additional scan time, has shown promise for the characterization of bone lesions. As shown by Fayad and colleagues[22] in a study that investigated the use of MRS in musculoskeletal lesions, giant cell tumors and bone cysts showed negligible concentrations of the choline-containing compounds compared with malignant sarcomas. Furthermore, in vitro, portions of bone specimens that contained benign lesional tissue (fibrous dysplasia, enchondroma) showed significantly different choline content than areas containing lesions with malignant degeneration (to malignant fibrous histiocytoma and chondrosarcoma), thereby making MRS a useful marker of malignancy and potentially a tool for guiding a biopsy.[23]

In conclusion, although radiography remains the first-line test for detecting and characterizing a bone lesion, MR imaging provides additional useful information for the evaluation of a bone lesion. Many sequences are available for the assessment of bone lesions, including conventional T1, fluid-sensitive sequences, chemical shift imaging (CSI), DWI, MRS, and postcontrast imaging with static and dynamic sequences. Differentiating normal components of bone marrow (red marrow and fatty marrow) from marrow-replacing bone lesions is done with noncontrast imaging, after which benign and malignant lesions can be differentiated by additional information obtained from DWI and postcontrast sequences. When the lesion remains indeterminate after evaluation by a full complement of MR imaging sequences (as often occurs in benign aggressive entities, such as Langerhans cell histiocytosis), a biopsy must be performed to establish the diagnosis. Malignancies are typically identified by radiographic features that are corroborated by MR imaging features, and also necessitate biopsy before initiating treatment.

## REFERENCES

1. Vogler JB 3rd, Murphy WA. Bone marrow imaging. Radiology 1988;168(3):679–93.
2. Zajick DC Jr, Morrison WB, Schweitzer ME, et al. Benign and malignant processes: normal values and differentiation with chemical shift MR imaging in vertebral marrow. Radiology 2005;237(2):590–6.
3. Dreizin D, Ahlawat S, Del Grande F, et al. Gradient-echo in-phase and opposed-phase chemical shift imaging: role in evaluating bone marrow. Clin Radiol 2014;69(6):648–57.
4. Del Grande F, Tatizawa-Shiga N, Jalali Farahani S, et al. Chemical shift imaging: preliminary experience as an alternative sequence for defining the extent of a bone tumor. Quant Imaging Med Surg 2014;4(3): 173–80.
5. Dudeck O, Zeile M, Pink D, et al. Diffusion-weighted magnetic resonance imaging allows monitoring of anticancer treatment effects in patients with soft-tissue sarcomas. J Magn Reson Imaging 2008; 27(5):1109–13.
6. Ahlawat S, Fayad LM. Diffusion weighted imaging demystified: the technique and potential clinical applications for soft tissue imaging. Skeletal Radiol 2018;47(3):313–28.
7. Del Grande F, Ahlawat S, Subhangwong T, et al. Characterization of indeterminate soft tissue masses referred for biopsy: what is the added value of contrast imaging at 3.0 tesla? J Magn Reson Imaging 2017;45(2):390–400.
8. Ahlawat S, Khandheria P, Subhawong TK, et al. Differentiation of benign and malignant skeletal lesions with quantitative diffusion weighted MRI at 3T. Eur J Radiol 2015;84(6):1091–7.
9. Ahlawat S, Morris C, Fayad LM. Three-dimensional volumetric MRI with isotropic resolution: improved speed of acquisition, spatial resolution and assessment of lesion conspicuity in patients with recurrent soft tissue sarcoma. Skeletal Radiol 2016;45(5): 645–52.
10. van Rijswijk CS, Geirnaerdt MJ, Hogendoorn PC, et al. Soft-tissue tumors: value of static and dynamic gadopentetate dimeglumine-enhanced MR imaging in prediction of malignancy. Radiology 2004;233(2): 493–502.
11. Subhawong TK, Wang X, Durand DJ, et al. Proton MR spectroscopy in metabolic assessment of musculoskeletal lesions. AJR Am J Roentgenol 2012;198(1):162–72.
12. Shiga NT, Del Grande F, Lardo O, et al. Imaging of primary bone tumors: determination of tumor extent by non-contrast sequences. Pediatr Radiol 2013; 43(8):1017–23.
13. Del Grande F, Subhawong T, Flammang A, et al. Chemical shift imaging at 3 Tesla: effect of echo time on assessing bone marrow abnormalities. Skeletal Radiol 2014;43(8):1139–47.
14. Samet J, Weinstein J, Fayad LM. MRI and clinical features of Langerhans cell histiocytosis (LCH) in the pelvis and extremities: can LCH really look like anything? Skeletal Radiol 2016;45(5):607–13.
15. Pettersson H, Gillespy T 3rd, Hamlin DJ, et al. Primary musculoskeletal tumors: examination with MR imaging compared with conventional modalities. Radiology 1987;164(1):237–41.
16. Subhawong TK, Durand DJ, Thawait GK, et al. Characterization of soft tissue masses: can quantitative diffusion weighted imaging reliably distinguish cysts from solid masses? Skeletal Radiol 2013;42(11): 1583–92.

17. Wilhelm T, Stieltjes B, Schlemmer HP. Whole-body-MR-diffusion weighted imaging in oncology. Rofo 2013;184(10):950–8.

18. Gutzeit A, Doert A, Froehlich JM, et al. Comparison of diffusion-weighted whole body MRI and skeletal scintigraphy for the detection of bone metastases in patients with prostate or breast carcinoma. Skeletal Radiol 2010;39(4):333–43.

19. Tuncbilek N, Karakas HM, Okten OO. Dynamic contrast enhanced MRI in the differential diagnosis of soft tissue tumors. Eur J Radiol 2005;53(3):500–5.

20. van der Woude HJ, Bloem JL, Verstraete KL, et al. Osteosarcoma and Ewing's sarcoma after neoadjuvant chemotherapy: value of dynamic MR imaging in detecting viable tumor before surgery. AJR Am J Roentgenol 1995;165(3):593–8.

21. Verstraete KL, Lang P. Bone and soft tissue tumors: the role of contrast agents for MR imaging. Eur J Radiol 2000;34(3):229–46.

22. Fayad LM, Wang X, Salibi N, et al. A feasibility study of quantitative molecular characterization of musculoskeletal lesions by proton MR spectroscopy at 3 T. AJR Am J Roentgenol 2010;195(1): W69–75.

23. Fayad LM, Bluemke DA, McCarthy EF, et al. Musculoskeletal tumors: use of proton MR spectroscopic imaging for characterization. J Magn Reson Imaging 2006;23(1):23–8.

# Advanced MR Imaging and Ultrasound Fusion in Musculoskeletal Procedures

Pedro Henrique Martins, MD[a],
Flávia Martins Costa, MD, PhD[a,b,*],
Flávia Paiva Proença Lobo Lopes, MD, PhD[a,b,c],
Clarissa Canella, MD, PhD[a,b,d]

## KEYWORDS

• MR imaging • Ultrasound • Imaging fusion • Guided biopsy • Musculoskeletal lesions

## KEY POINTS

• MR imaging–ultrasound (US) fusion is a new hybrid technique not yet established in the musculoskeletal field.
• Advanced MR imaging techniques are important tools for the characterization of soft tissue masses.
• The combination of MR imaging and US can improve procedures performed under US guidance.
• MR imaging–US fusion helps identify the best intralesional biopsy target within a heterogeneous soft tissue mass.
• To avoid radiation exposure, MR imaging–US fusion may emerge as an alternative method for procedures that are usually performed under computed tomography or fluoroscopy guidance.

## INTRODUCTION

Ultrasound (US)–MR imaging fusion is a new hybrid technique that allows a simultaneous display of images from previously acquired MR imaging and real-time US. This technique has been used in the last few years in a range of specialties and procedures, such as those involving the liver, prostate, and breast.[1] The fusion imaging utilization for detection of high-risk prostate cancer was shown to be superior to standard extended-sextant biopsy.[2]

Although this technique has yet to be established in the musculoskeletal field, the authors believe that it has a potential role in improving image-guided interventions, in particular, targeted tumor biopsies and therapeutic injections. This technique is especially useful in locating small lesions or enhancing soft tissue structures that are clearly visible on MR imaging but difficult to identify on US.

## TECHNICAL ASPECTS

Image fusion is obtained using a navigation and positioning system that allows accurate localization of the US transducer in space with the aid of an external magnetic field generator, which is usually located close to the patient.

Disclosures Statement: The authors have nothing to disclose.
[a] Radiology Department, Clínica de Diagnóstico por Imagem (CDPI)/DASA, Avenida das Américas, 4666, sala 301B, Centro Médico BarraShopping, CDPI, Barra da Tijuca, Rio de Janeiro, RJ CEP: 22640-102, Brazil; [b] Radiology Department, Alta Excelência Diagnóstica/DASA, Avenida das Américas, 4666, sala 301B, Centro Médico BarraShopping, CDPI, Barra da Tijuca, Rio de Janeiro, RJ CEP: 22640-102, Brazil; [c] Radiology Department, Federal University of Rio de Janeiro (UFRJ), Rua Rodolpho Paulo Rocco, 255, Cidade Universitária, Ilha do Fundão, Rio de Janeiro, RJ CEP: 21941-913, Brazil; [d] Radiology Department, Universidade Federal Fluminense, Av Marques do Paraná, 303, Centro, Niterói, RJ CEP: 24020-071, Brazil
* Corresponding author.
*E-mail address:* flavia26rio@hotmail.com

Magn Reson Imaging Clin N Am 26 (2018) 571–579
https://doi.org/10.1016/j.mric.2018.06.012

A small sensor receiver attached to the US probe communicates with the magnetic field generator, providing real-time positioning and orientation of the transducer to the workstation (**Fig. 1**). Subsequently, software-based fusion platforms incorporate complex algorithms to integrate the data from previously acquired MR imaging and real-time US. The US operator selects anatomic landmarks, often 3 or more, that are easily recognizable on both MR imaging and US images, and uses these landmarks as reference points, allowing the 2 images to be aligned. The correct matching of the landmarks selected on the US images with the equivalent points on MR imaging is crucial for spatial accuracy and synchronous movement of the images. The software fuses the images and may display them superimposed or side by side, showing the corresponding image from the MR imaging on the US.

The matching of MR imaging with US images can be difficult in body areas without easily identifiable fixed anatomic structures, such as in lesions located in the middle of the thigh or leg.

The MR imaging sequence used in the fusion is selected by the radiologist based on the most favorable anatomic depiction of the area of interest, such as isotropic 3D for perineural injection or postcontrast sequences for detection of viable tumor for biopsy in a heterogeneous soft tissue mass.

Another possible approach of this technology is cognitive fusion, which does not require additional equipment. In cognitive fusion, an experienced radiologist identifies suspicious areas on previous diagnostic MR imaging and attempts to locate the same suspicious areas while performing US based on anatomic landmarks and lesion morphology. To achieve good results, the operator must have good understanding of the position of the target by reviewing all available previous MR imaging.

## PROCEDURES

MR imaging–US fusion has already been tested in a few different procedures involving the musculoskeletal system, particularly in guided biopsies and sacroiliac injections[3–6]; however, the main applications of this method remain to be established.

### Biopsy

Soft tissue tumors are a heterogeneous group of benign, intermediate (locally aggressive), and malignant lesions arising from 9 different categories[7] for which diagnosis based on imaging and clinical features remains challenging in routine clinical practice. Sarcomas are a heterogeneous group of mesenchymal tumors that are usually underdiagnosed, with more than 50 different histologic subtypes that account for less than 1% of all malignancies and affect the extremities as the most common site (approximately 50% of the cases).[8]

Considering that sarcomas are rare and unsuspected on routine examinations, presumed misdiagnoses (eg, hematomas and lipomas) are usually

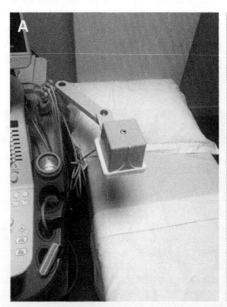
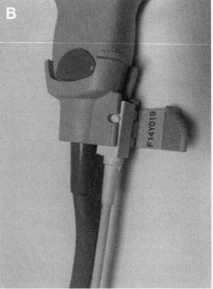

**Fig. 1.** The fusion imaging technique (Aplio 500 – Canon Medical Systems Tochigui – Japan) requires an external electromagnetic field generator (*A*) placed close to the patient and a position sensor attached to the US probe (PLT 1005 BT) (*B*) using a specific bracket. Both are connected to a position sensor unit embedded in the US machine.

made because of an inadequate imaging method and/or inaccurate interpretation. Consequently, unplanned excisions are often performed by surgeons not specialized in these tumors (eg, general, plastic, and orthopedic surgeons) in up to 50% of the cases, most frequently in young adults, which leads to higher local recurrence rates and a potential need for additional and more extensive mutilating surgery.[9]

Because excisional biopsy of a sarcoma is inappropriate and often may cause difficulties in further patient management, it is generally prudent to obtain a previous diagnostic biopsy for all soft tissue masses larger than 5 cm (unless it is a very obvious benign lesion; eg, subcutaneous lipoma) and for all subfascial or deep-seated tumors, almost independent of its size.[10] After that, the patient should be referred to a specialized tumor center before surgery for optimal treatment. Excisional biopsy should be avoided in those lesions because such an approach will make definitive reexcision more extensive due to the contamination of adjacent tissue planes.

Plain radiographs of such tumors are often normal unless the mass is large or contains calcification. In contrast, US is useful in determining whether a soft tissue mass is cystic or solid and assessing its vascularization using the Doppler mode, although this method has a limited role because it often reveals nonspecific imaging findings.

MR imaging is an important tool in the detection and characterization of soft tissue masses. Due to excellent tissue contrast, multiplanar capability, and lack of ionizing radiation, MR imaging has become the modality of choice in the assessment of soft-tissue masses. MR imaging also aids in planning surgery, staging of local extent, monitoring response to chemotherapy, and in the long-term follow-up for local recurrence. Conventional imaging is unable to define the extent of tumor necrosis and to detect the presence of viable cells, which are crucial information used to assess response to treatment and prognosis.

The combination of anatomic and functional sequences, including diffusion-weighted imaging (DWI) with apparent diffusion coefficient (ADC) mapping and dynamic contrast-enhanced (DCE) MR imaging sequences, can be helpful in distinguishing benign and malignant lesions and could help avoid biopsies of benign soft tissue lesions. For many patients, if MR imaging is unable to provide a specific histologic diagnosis and if it is unable to characterize a lesion as benign, the lesion should be considered indeterminate and undergo evaluation with biopsy to exclude malignancy.

According to the literature, the most common imaging findings predictive of malignancy on conventional MR imaging include a large lesion size

(mean diameter of more than 66 mm), heterogeneous sign intensity, necrosis, bone and neurovascular bundle involvement, perilesional edema, absence of calcification and fibrosis, and the lack of fat rim.[11–17]

Advanced techniques providing functional properties of tissue can add information to the conventional MR imaging, improving diagnostic accuracy and helping to determine the nature of the lesion.

However, despite the use of these advanced techniques, the differentiation between benign and malignant lesions is not always possible owing overlapping of imaging features between both; therefore, biopsy becomes necessary to diagnose those lesions that remain indeterminate after extensive imaging evaluation.

Open surgical biopsy offers the highest diagnostic accuracy to detect the lesion,[18] although image-guided percutaneous biopsy is also effective, less invasive, and associated with a lower complication rate.[19] Image-guided percutaneous biopsies also provide excellent spatial location of the lesion, which helps in avoiding contamination of the neurovascular bundle[20,21] and in selecting the best intralesional target for the biopsy.

Because percutaneous needle biopsy samples only a small part of the tumor, the selection of the biopsy target must be optimal within heterogeneous lesions to obtain sufficient and adequate material representing the tumor's aggressiveness and allow a correct diagnosis.[22] A biopsy that does not sample all the histologic features in a heterogeneous tumors could lead to a misdiagnosis and delay in appropriate treatment (Fig. 2).

Lesions associated with lower diagnostic accuracy rates on percutaneous biopsy include myxoid and round cell neoplasms, as well as infections.[18]

Myxoid tumors encompass a heterogeneous group of lesions characterized by abundant extracellular myxoid matrix with very high water content and are found on both benign (intramuscular myxoma) and malignant (myxoid sarcoma) tumors, whereas the differential diagnosis of small round cell neoplasms (undifferentiated embryonal tumors; eg, neuroblastoma, rhabdomyosarcoma, non-Hodgkin lymphoma, and the family of Ewing sarcomas) is particularly difficult due to their undifferentiated or primitive character, especially when the tumor is poorly differentiated.[23]

Heterogeneous sarcomas also can pose difficulties for successful biopsy because it may present intralesional necrosis, different grade areas within the tumor, and even benign and malignant components[20,24–26]; therefore, it is essential to avoid targeting areas of necrosis or myxoid changes within a heterogeneous lesion.

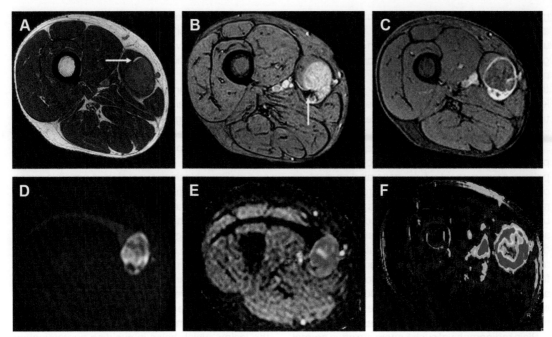

**Fig. 2.** Pleomorphic liposarcoma of the right thigh in a 62-year-old man. Axial T1-weighted image (*A*) demonstrates an oval, well-defined lesion in the medial muscular compartment of the thigh with an anterior peripheral area of high signal intensity, indicating a lipomatous origin (*white arrow*). Axial susceptibility-weighted imaging (SWI) shows areas of hemosiderin foci (*white arrow*) suggesting heterogeneity in the posterior part of the tumor (*B*). Axial T1-weighted image with fat saturation after gadolinium administration (*C*) demonstrates high peripheral enhancement, mostly in the posterior part of the tumor. However, axial DWI (*D*) and ADC maps (*E*) show areas of restricted diffusion and axial perfusion color map imaging (*F*) shows early enhancement of the lesion. A proper biopsy should contain adequate tissue that is representative of the whole lesion for a definitive diagnosis and accurate grading.

In lesions suspected to be malignant, biopsies must be carefully planned to respect the compartmental anatomy and reduce the risk of seeding malignant cells along the needle track[27,28] (**Table 1**). The radiologist and the orthopedic oncologic surgeon should discuss the choice of a biopsy entry site and pathway that will align with the plane of incision for potential surgery. Most limb masses are generally best sampled through a longitudinally oriented incision, so that the entire biopsy tract and immediate surrounding tissue can be completely removed en bloc with the tumor at the time of definitive resection.[29]

**Table 1**
**Compartmental anatomy to staging and biopsy of musculoskeletal tumors**

| Arm | Anterior (biceps, brachialis and coracobrachialis muscle) | Posterior (triceps) | |
|---|---|---|---|
| Forearm | Volar (flexor) | Dorsal (extensor) | |
| Thigh | Anterior (quadriceps, iliopsoas, sartorius and tensor fascia lata) | Medial (abductors and gracilis) | Posterior (hamstrings) |
| Leg | Anterior (tibialis anterior, extensor hallucis longus and extensor digitorum longus) | Lateral (peroneus longus and brevis) | Superficial posterior (flexor digitorum longus, tibialis posterior, flexor hallucis longus and popliteus) | Deep posterior (soleus and gastrocnemius) |

Identification of the local tumor extension and the neurovascular bundle status are essential for an accurate local staging of malignant soft tissue masses[30,31] and important parameters in the decision between limb conservation with reconstruction or amputation.[27] It is imperative to visualize the interface between the lesion and nearby major neurovascular bundles because contamination of major neurovascular structures can require their surgical removal and disqualify the patient from future limb sparing surgery. Because conventional MR imaging offers high-contrast and spatial resolution, MR imaging–US fusion biopsies allow a more accurate needle placement, restricting the biopsy track to the involved compartment and avoiding contamination of the neurovascular bundle or other compartments.

Advanced techniques are also important tools in guided biopsies. DCE is usually performed using a 3-dimensional fast spoiled gradient-echo with image sets obtained sequentially every few seconds for around 5 minutes after administration of gadolinium-based intravenous contrast. The dynamic images obtained during and after gadolinium bolus injection allows analysis of the initial distribution of the contrast from the capillaries to the interstitial space[32–34] and it helps to select highly vascularized intratumoral areas using the wash-in rate parameter, which indicates viable tissue regions within heterogeneous lesions to be targeted during biopsy because these regions are more likely to yield a diagnostic result on histology. A recent study reported a diagnostic yield of 100% with the targeting of areas with highest arterial enhancement on DCE, with a 100% correct prediction of a benign, indeterminate, or malignant status on histologic evaluation of the surgical specimen.[20]

DWI is also useful in the selection of viable tumor sites for biopsy, especially in patients in whom contrast agents are contraindicated.[20] This technique exploits the random motion of water molecules in the body (Brownian motion) and the microcirculation of the blood (perfusion),[35,36] which reflects tissue cellularity and cell membrane integrity.[37] Impeded diffusion of water molecules can be assessed quantitatively using ADC, with values tending to be lower in malignant tumors[15,38] owing to the high cellularity of these lesions, allowing targeted biopsy of representative areas within the lesion (**Fig. 3**).

Another advantage of DCE and DWI is their ability to distinguish posttreatment fibrosis and

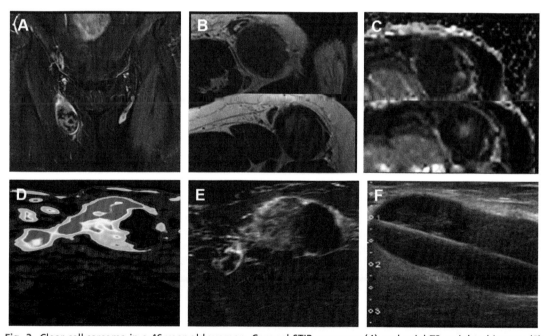

**Fig. 3.** Clear-cell sarcoma in a 46-year-old woman. Coronal STIR sequence (*A*) and axial T2-weighted images (*B*) reveal a large heterogeneous soft tissue mass at the thigh with a solid component at the upper portion of the lesion and a central necrosis area in the lower part. The corresponding ADC map (*C*) shows marked hypointensity of the upper part of the lesion, indicating restricted diffusion and suggesting high cellularity and, probably, the best biopsy target site within the lesion, whereas the lower portion has facilitated diffusion. DCE color-coded map (*D*) reflecting wash-in rates shows a hypervascularization zone, representing a site of viable tumor. Subtraction postcontrast volumetric T1-weighted image (*E*) was the selected sequence for the fusion technique. The US image (*F*) shows the needle passing through the cystic into the solid portion of the lesion.

granulation tissue from residual tumor, all of which appear similar on a conventional MR imaging protocol.[15,39] Reactive tissue or a pseudomass resulting from posttherapeutic changes enhances later and more slowly, at a rate equal to that of normal muscle, whereas tissue related to residual or recurrent tumor presents and early and rapidly progressive enhancement.[34] The placement of metallic clips under US guidance at the residual tumor detected on MR imaging can facilitate subsequent surgical excision and increase precision in postoperative radiation therapy (**Figs. 4** and **5**).[40]

## Other Procedures

Image fusion techniques are also feasible and effective in guiding sacroiliac joint injections, providing a rich anatomic definition of the injection target and expanding the field of view of the US. Computed tomography guidance is still the preferred method for sacroiliac joint injections, but US can be faster[4] while avoiding radiation exposure, which must be taken into consideration, especially in young patients or in those requiring repeated procedures.

MR imaging–US fusion has also been tested in muscle and tendon injuries associated with sports.[5] US provides an excellent evaluation of superficial lesions, whereas MR imaging is superior in assessing lower grade and deep muscle injuries.[41] The combination of both images may improve clinical decision-making and interventional US-guided procedures in deep muscle compartments.

With simultaneous visualization of images obtained with both MR imaging and US, fusion technology also has a potential educational purpose,[42] allowing residents and fellows to better understand and interpret the anatomy and the lesions seen on US with the visualization of the corresponding image on MR imaging.

Other previously tested uses for fusion application include piriformis and perineural injections, as well as barbotage of calcific tendinopathy.[1]

## LIMITATIONS

Limitations of MR imaging–US fusion include a difficult selection of landmark points in certain areas of the body, a process that is essential for this technique. The absence of fixed and easily recognizable anatomic structures close to the target in both sets of images may result in malalignment and a need to reset the system and repeat the process.

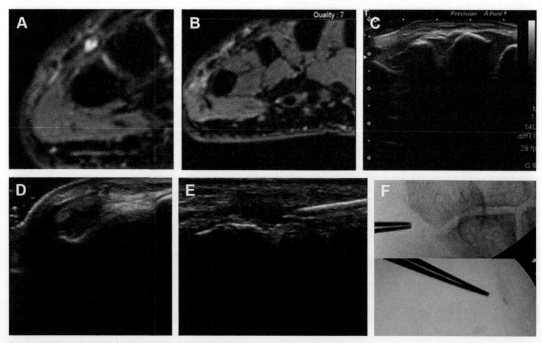

**Fig. 4.** MR imaging–US fusion guided wire marking in a residual myxofibrosarcoma in a 57-year-old woman. Axial postcontrast gradient-echo volumetric T1-weighted image (*A*) shows a small suspicious area of enhancement within the tumor bed. Because the lesion was very small, the fusion technique (*B*, *C*) was tested to localize the lesion during the US using the cortical of the metacarpal bones as anatomic landmarks to guide the placement of a marking wire (*D*, *E*) and facilitate the localization and removal of the lesion by the surgeon. The specimen radiograph (*F*) confirmed the successful excision of the marker (Clip C.R. Bard, Inc), and the residual tumor was confirmed by subsequent histopathological examination.

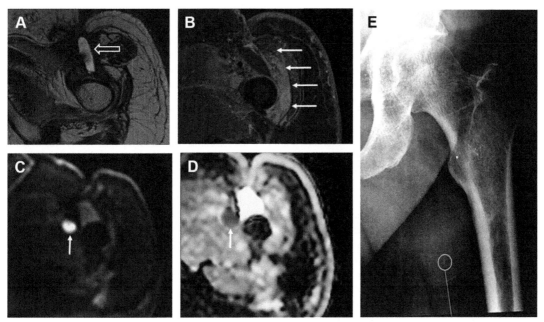

Fig. 5. Recurrent lesion of a synoviosarcoma in a 49-year-old man. Axial T2-weighted image (A) and T1-weighted image (B) with fat saturation after gadolinium administration demonstrating a postsurgery collection of the anterior aspect of the left thigh (*open arrow* on A) surrounded by posttherapeutic soft tissue changes (*white arrows* on B). There was no significant nodular area of enhancement identified after gadolinium administration. Axial DWI (C) and ADC mapping (D) revealed a nodular lesion presenting restricted diffusion in the medial aspect of the lesion (*white arrows*). The cognitive approach was used to guide a wire marking to help the surgeon to localize the lesion in the surgical bed (E). The MR imaging–US fusion guidance was not possible because the patient had an extensive area of subcutaneous fibrosis from the previous surgery, making the identification of anatomic landmarks difficult.

Another limitation is a need to maintain the external magnetic field transmitter close to the area of interest in the patient and, when the software processes the fusion, the transmitter must be maintained in a fixed position. Also, the distance between the transducer and the magnetic field generator should remain within 20 to 70 cm.

One possible disadvantage is the requirement of high-quality MR imaging, preferably 3 T, and volumetric sequences for optimal resolution and prevention of image distortion during rotation of the US probe.

## SUMMARY

MR imaging can be directly used to guide procedures; however, this method is complex, expensive, time-consuming, and uncomfortable for the patient. The combination of MR imaging and real-time US is effective and relatively easy to perform by an experienced musculoskeletal radiologist. The information provided by MR imaging can improve the navigation and the procedures performed under US guidance, although more research is needed to help define the actual usefulness of the MR imaging–US fusion technique.

In most cases, MR imaging–US fusion may not add a real benefit. It prolongs the duration of the procedure due to the process of importing data and selecting landmarks for correct alignment. However, MR imaging expands the limited field of view of the US and offers excellent spatial resolution and high contrast, providing additional anatomic details and facilitating deep biopsies and localization of small lesions. The use of MR imaging advanced techniques can aid the selection of the best targeting area in a heterogeneous soft tissue mass, decreasing the rate of inconclusive results.

The MR imaging–US fusion technique may also play an important role in the future as an alternative method for procedures that are usually performed under computed tomography or fluoroscopy guidance, avoiding unnecessary radiation exposure.

## ACKNOWLEDGMENTS

The authors thank Fernanda Philadelpho, PhD, for technical support.

## REFERENCES

1. Burke CJ, Bencardino J, Adler R. The potential use of ultrasound-magnetic resonance imaging fusion

applications in musculoskeletal intervention. J Ultrasound Med 2017;36(1):217–24.

2. Siddiqui MM, Rais-Bahrami S, Turkbey B, et al. Comparison of MR/ultrasound fusion-guided biopsy with ultrasound-guided biopsy for the diagnosis of prostate cancer. JAMA 2015;313(4):390–7.

3. Klauser AS, De Zordo T, Feuchtner GM, et al. Fusion of real-time US with CT images to guide sacroiliac joint injection in vitro and in vivo. Radiology 2010; 256(2):547–53.

4. Zacchino M, Almolla J, Canepari E, et al. Use of ultrasound-magnetic resonance image fusion to guide sacroiliac joint injections: a preliminary assessment. J Ultrasound 2013;16(3):111–8.

5. Wong-On M, Til-Perez L, Balius R. Evaluation of MRI-US fusion technology in sports-related musculoskeletal injuries. Adv Ther 2015;32(6):580–94.

6. Khalil JG, Mott MP, Parsons TW 3rd, et al. 2011 Mid-America Orthopaedic Association Dallas B. Phemister Physician in Training Award: can musculoskeletal tumors be diagnosed with ultrasound fusion-guided biopsy? Clin Orthop Relat Res 2012;470(8):2280–7.

7. Jo VY, Fletcher CD. WHO classification of soft tissue tumours: an update based on the 2013 (4th) edition. Pathology 2014;46(2):95–104.

8. Cormier JN, Pollock RE. Soft tissue sarcomas. CA Cancer J Clin 2004;54(2):94–109.

9. Pretell-Mazzini J, Barton MD Jr, Conway SA, et al. Unplanned excision of soft-tissue sarcomas: current concepts for management and prognosis. J Bone Joint Surg Am 2015;97(7):597–603.

10. Fletcher CDM, Unni KK, Mertens F, editors. World Health Organization Classification of Tumours. Pathology and genetics of tumours of soft tissue and bone. Lyon (France): IARC Press; 2002.

11. Del Grande F, Ahlawat S, Subhangwong T, et al. Characterization of indeterminate soft tissue masses referred for biopsy: what is the added value of contrast imaging at 3.0 tesla? J Magn Reson Imaging 2017;45(2):390–400.

12. Datir A, James SL, Ali K, et al. MRI of soft-tissue masses: the relationship between lesion size, depth, and diagnosis. Clin Radiol 2008;63(4):373–8 [discussion: 379–80].

13. Chen CK, Wu HT, Chiou HJ, et al. Differentiating benign and malignant soft tissue masses by magnetic resonance imaging: role of tissue component analysis. J Chin Med Assoc 2009;72(4): 194–201.

14. Costa FM, Canella C, Gasparetto E. Advanced magnetic resonance imaging techniques in the evaluation of musculoskeletal tumors. Radiol Clin North Am 2011;49(6):1325–58. vii-viii.

15. Jones BC, Fayad LM. Musculoskeletal tumor imaging: focus on emerging techniques. Semin Roentgenol 2017;52(4):269–81.

16. Kalayanarooj S. Benign and malignant soft tissue mass: magnetic resonance imaging criteria for discrimination. J Med Assoc Thai 2008;91(1): 74–81.

17. Pang KK, Hughes T. MR imaging of the musculoskeletal soft tissue mass: is heterogeneity a sign of malignancy? J Chin Med Assoc 2003;66(11): 655–61.

18. Rougraff BT, Aboulafia A, Biermann JS, et al. Biopsy of soft tissue masses: evidence-based medicine for the musculoskeletal tumor society. Clin Orthop Relat Res 2009;467(11):2783–91.

19. Daley NA, Reed WJ, Peterson JJ. Strategies for biopsy of musculoskeletal tumors. Semin Roentgenol 2017;52(4):282–90.

20. Noebauer-Huhmann IM, Amann G, Krssak M, et al. Use of diagnostic dynamic contrast-enhanced (DCE)-MRI for targeting of soft tissue tumour biopsies at 3T: preliminary results. Eur Radiol 2015; 25(7):2041–8.

21. Le HB, Lee ST, Munk PL. Image-guided musculoskeletal biopsies. Semin Intervent Radiol 2010; 27(2):191–8.

22. Guimaraes MD, Marchiori E, Odisio BC, et al. Functional imaging with diffusion-weighted MRI for lung biopsy planning: initial experience. World J Surg Oncol 2014;12:203.

23. Sharma S, Kamala R, Nair D, et al. Round cell tumors: classification and immunohistochemistry. Indian J Med Paediatr Oncol 2017;38(3):349–53.

24. Oliveira AM, Nascimento AG. Grading in soft tissue tumors: principles and problems. Skeletal Radiol 2001;30(10):543–59.

25. Sung KS, Seo SW, Shon MS. The diagnostic value of needle biopsy for musculoskeletal lesions. Int Orthop 2009;33(6):1701–6.

26. Carrino JA, Khurana B, Ready JE, et al. Magnetic resonance imaging-guided percutaneous biopsy of musculoskeletal lesions. J Bone Joint Surg Am 2007;89(10):2179–87.

27. Robinson E, Bleakney RR, Ferguson PC, et al. Oncodiagnosis panel: 2007: multidisciplinary management of soft-tissue sarcoma. Radiographics 2008; 28(7):2069–86.

28. Kim SY, Chung HW, Oh TS, et al. Practical guidelines for ultrasound-guided core needle biopsy of soft-tissue lesions: transformation from beginner to specialist. Korean J Radiol 2017;18(2):361–9.

29. Liu PT, Valadez SD, Chivers FS, et al. Anatomically based guidelines for core needle biopsy of bone tumors: implications for limb-sparing surgery. Radiographics 2007;27(1):189–205 [discussion: 206].

30. Anderson MW, Temple HT, Dussault RG, et al. Compartmental anatomy: relevance to staging and biopsy of musculoskeletal tumors. AJR Am J Roentgenol 1999;173(6):1663–71.

31. Rimner A, Brennan MF, Zhang Z, et al. Influence of compartmental involvement on the patterns of morbidity in soft tissue sarcoma of the thigh. Cancer 2009;115(1):149–57.

32. Erlemann R, Vassallo P, Bongartz G, et al. Musculoskeletal neoplasms: fast low-angle shot MR imaging with and without Gd-DTPA. Radiology 1990;176(2):489–95.

33. Erlemann R, Reiser MF, Peters PE, et al. Musculoskeletal neoplasms: static and dynamic Gd-DTPA–enhanced MR imaging. Radiology 1989;171(3):767–73.

34. Verstraete KL, Lang P. Bone and soft tissue tumors: the role of contrast agents for MR imaging. Eur J Radiol 2000;34(3):229–46.

35. Le Bihan D, Breton E, Lallemand D, et al. Separation of diffusion and perfusion in intravoxel incoherent motion MR imaging. Radiology 1988;168(2):497–505.

36. van Rijswijk CS, Kunz P, Hogendoorn PC, et al. Diffusion-weighted MRI in the characterization of soft-tissue tumors. J Magn Reson Imaging 2002;15(3):302–7.

37. Hamstra DA, Rehemtulla A, Ross BD. Diffusion magnetic resonance imaging: a biomarker for treatment response in oncology. J Clin Oncol 2007;25(26):4104–9.

38. Subhawong TK, Jacobs MA, Fayad LM. Diffusion-weighted MR imaging for characterizing musculoskeletal lesions. Radiographics 2014;34(5):1163–77.

39. Soldatos T, Ahlawat S, Montgomery E, et al. Multiparametric assessment of treatment response in high-grade soft-tissue sarcomas with anatomic and functional MR imaging sequences. Radiology 2016;278(3):831–40.

40. Nystrom LM, Reimer NB, Reith JD, et al. Multidisciplinary management of soft tissue sarcoma. ScientificWorldJournal 2013;2013:852462.

41. Woodhouse JB, McNally EG. Ultrasound of skeletal muscle injury: an update. Semin Ultrasound CT MR 2011;32(2):91–100.

42. Galiano K, Obwegeser AA, Bale R, et al. Ultrasound-guided and CT-navigation-assisted periradicular and facet joint injections in the lumbar and cervical spine: a new teaching tool to recognize the sonoanatomic pattern. Reg Anesth Pain Med 2007;32(3):254–7.

# Whole-Body Magnetic Resonance Imaging in Rheumatic and Systemic Diseases
## From Emerging to Validated Indications

Elie Barakat, MD[a], Thomas Kirchgesner, MD[a],
Perrine Triqueneaux, MSc[a], Christine Galant, MD[b],
Maria Stoenoiu, MD, PhD[c], Frederic E. Lecouvet, MD, PhD[d],*

## KEYWORDS

• MR imaging • Whole-body imaging • Diffusion-weighted MR imaging • Rheumatism • Arthritis
• Bone • Muscles • Joint

## KEY POINTS

- Whole-body (WB) magnetic resonance (MR) imaging plays an essential role in detecting and evaluating the extent of rheumatic disorders affecting the musculoskeletal system, as well as the activity of these diseases and their responses to treatment.
- Numerous multifocal skeletal and neuromuscular disorders benefit from the extended coverage and sensitivity of WB MR imaging to soft tissue alterations for disease diagnosis, quantification, and follow-up.
- The evolution and acceleration of sequences extend the indications of WB MR imaging as a noninvasive, nonirradiating tool in many musculoskeletal disorders, making older irradiating modalities obsolete in many settings.

## INTRODUCTION

Whole-body (WB) magnetic resonance (MR) imaging has been the focus of research of many studies during the last 2 decades. This imaging modality offers a large coverage of the skeleton and has a high sensitivity to bone alterations, proving to be effective for the detection of skeletal involvement by oncologic diseases, especially metastases from solid tumors, lymphoma, and multiple myeloma,[1–7] and evaluation of their responses to treatment.[8–10]

Advances in imaging techniques and hardware development have been continuously optimizing the coverage of the examinations and shortening their durations.[11] The sensitivity of MR imaging

Disclosure: The authors have nothing to disclose.
[a] Department of Radiology, Institut de Recherche Expérimentale et Clinique (IREC), Cliniques universitaires Saint-Luc, Université catholique de Louvain (UCL), Hippocrate Avenue, 10, Brussels B-1200, Belgium;
[b] Department of Pathology, Institut de Recherche Expérimentale et Clinique (IREC), Cliniques universitaires Saint-Luc, Université catholique de Louvain (UCL), Hippocrate Avenue, 10, Brussels B-1200, Belgium;
[c] Department of Rheumatology, Institut de Recherche Expérimentale et Clinique (IREC), Cliniques universitaires Saint-Luc, Université catholique de Louvain (UCL), Hippocrate Avenue, 10, Brussels B-1200, Belgium;
[d] Radiology Department, Institut de Recherche Expérimentale et Clinique, Université Catholique de Louvain, Cliniques Universitaires Saint-Luc, Hippocrate Avenue 10/2942, Brussels B-1200, Belgium
* Corresponding author.
E-mail address: frederic.lecouvet@uclouvain.be

Magn Reson Imaging Clin N Am 26 (2018) 581–597
https://doi.org/10.1016/j.mric.2018.06.005
1064-9689/18/© 2018 Elsevier Inc. All rights reserved.

to alterations in tissues such as bone marrow, joints, muscles, ligaments, and tendons, has led to a growing number of applications for this technique outside oncology, from spondyloarthropathies and peripheral seronegative arthritis to other systemic diseases and rheumatic conditions, and, lately, in numerous neuromuscular disorders.[12]

This article highlights the applications of WB MR imaging outside oncology, including rheumatologic disorders, muscle disorders, and bone disorders. Other emerging imaging applications outside these fields are overviewed. In addition, it illustrates the most appropriate MR imaging protocols for each disorder and the upcoming promising role of WB MR imaging in the near future.

## RHEUMATOLOGIC DISORDERS
### Inflammatory Rheumatisms

Rheumatologic disorders are the most established nononcologic indication of WB MR imaging, especially seronegative rheumatisms, including axial spondyloarthropathies; psoriatic arthritis (PsA); and, less frequently, reactive arthritis, enteropathic arthritis, and undifferentiated spondyloarthritis. WB MR imaging may be said to cover the body from eyes to thighs, which may be sufficient in the evaluation of patients with ankylosing spondyloarthritis (AS) or, more rarely, from head to toes, when the disorder affects distal extremities, as in PsA. Optimized protocols have been developed

to cover the upper extremities positioned behind the back or on the abdomen.[13]

### Ankylosing spondyloarthritis
AS (**Fig. 1**) typically affects the sacroiliac joints (SIJs) and the discovertebral junctions but may also involve peripheral joints and entheses. Established structural lesions include erosions and new bone formation and can evolve to ankylosis. These lesions are accessible to radiographic examination. MR imaging has extended the sensitivity of imaging tools to prestructural early inflammatory changes taking the form of bone marrow edema (BME) adjacent to joints and discs, enthesitis, and synovitis. In contrast, MR imaging also allows the detection of late chronic and structural changes such as erosions, new bone formation, and ankylosis.

MR imaging of the SIJ and lumbar spine is the modality of choice for early detection of AS and assessment of the response of the disease to treatment.[14–16] MR imaging is sufficient to establish the diagnosis of AS in most patients. Subchondral BME at the level of the SIJ reflects active inflammation and is a major diagnostic criterion for AS.[17] The diagnosis requires the presence of BME on 2 consecutive sections or 2 distinct BME areas in the same section.[18] At the chronic stage or after treatment, BME is replaced by fatty infiltration of the marrow, followed by the development of erosions, sclerosis, and, eventually, ankylosis.[19] At the spinal level, at least 3 typical lesions

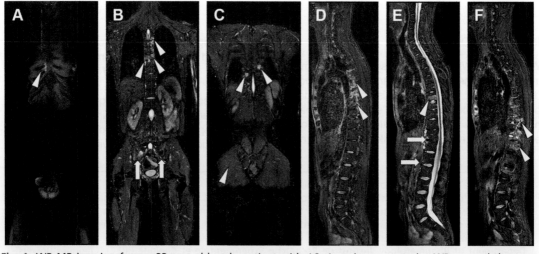

**Fig. 1.** WB MR imaging from a 33-year-old male patient with AS. Anterior to posterior WB coronal short-tau inversion-recovery (STIR) MR imaging (*A–C*) shows extensive sacroiliac joint (SIJ) inflammation (*arrows* in *B*), along with chondrosternal joint (*arrowhead* in *A*), midthoracic vertebral endplates (*arrowheads* in *B*), and costovertebral (*arrowheads* in *B* and *C*) involvement. Sagittal STIR MR imaging (*D–F*) shows vertebral angle involvement at the thoracolumbar junction (*arrows* in *E*), extensive endplate involvement at the midthoracic level (*arrowhead* in *E*), and severe involvement (*arrowheads* in *D* and *F*) of the lateral portion of the vertebral endplates and costovertebral joints (*arrowheads* in *D* and *F*).

of the anterior or posterior corners are required to establish the diagnosis of inflammatory disease and avoid confusion with degenerative disc disease, which is a frequent condition.[20]

WB MR imaging has the potential advantage of extending the screening of active and chronic lesions of bone margins, joints, tendons, and entheses to the entire axial and peripheral skeleton.[14] It allows the detection of potentially subclinical lesions within the entire spine, pelvis, shoulders, and extremities.[21] Extra-axial lesions are found in half of the patients, consisting most frequently in peripheral synovitis and enthesitis.[16] AS frequently involves the anterior thoracic wall, particularly the manubriosternal and sternoclavicular joint, and the chondrosternal and chondrocostal junctions (see **Fig. 1**).[22] WB MR imaging has driven the attention to specific spine lesions in AS, such as the involvement of costovertebral junctions, the most lateral endplates margins, and the posterior ligaments.[12] Hip involvement by synovitis, bursitis, or enthesitis is also frequent and parallels the disease activity.[23] In addition, the ability of WB MR imaging to detect AS lesions and be used to monitor them in active and chronic/nonactive stages makes it a valuable resource in staging and evaluating the therapeutic response of the disease.[24,25]

The major roles of WB MR imaging in AS are the improvement of diagnostic confidence in patients with negative or ambiguous SIJ observations and the evaluation of the disease activity in the peripheral skeleton in centrally ankylosed disease and the peripheral dominant or exclusive forms of the disease.[12]

### Juvenile spondyloarthritis

Juvenile spondyloarthritis (JSA) is a subtype of juvenile idiopathic arthritis associated with the human leukocyte antigen B27 antigen. JSA differs from adult spondyloarthritis by predominantly involving entheses and peripheral joints, mainly of the lower limbs, and its infrequent early involvement of the axial skeleton, which is later affected during the course of the disease.[26,27] WB MR imaging may demonstrate BME and perientheseal soft tissue involvement, synovitis, and joint or bursal fluid. Hips, knees, and ankles are most frequently affected, and tarsitis is a characteristic manifestation of the disease.[28] Synovitis, soft tissue edema, and perientheseal and joint/bursal fluid help distinguish JSA from edemalike findings of the bone marrow that may be seen as a normal variant in healthy children.[28] Arthritis affecting the hips, cervical spine, ankles, or wrists are well-known features of poor prognosis, irrespective of other factors.[29]

Early and accurate disease detection, and especially the detection of factors of poor prognosis in the disease, is essential for appropriate treatment selection. WB MR imaging is now available as a tool for early disease detection in AS and for monitoring activity and guiding therapy initiation and discontinuation.[28]

### Psoriatic arthritis

MR imaging is very effective in detecting synovitis and enthesitis in PsA.[30] In addition to the evaluation of the axial skeleton, WB MR imaging can detect and monitor alterations of tenosynovial sheaths and entheses, and may play an important role in therapeutic decisions and evaluation of treatment response.[31]

### Rheumatoid arthritis

Rheumatoid arthritis involves mainly the feet and hand joints, but, as a systemic inflammatory disease, it may also affect any joint, tendon, or enthesis in the body. Dedicated MR imaging is highly sensitive in assessing and monitoring disease activity, structural changes, and therapeutic response in rheumatoid arthritis.[32] Recent research has shown that WB MR imaging can be useful in the evaluation of total inflammatory disease load and monitoring of disease activity in axial and peripheral joints and entheses simultaneously.[33]

## Systemic Sclerosis

Systemic sclerosis (SSc) or scleroderma is a systemic rheumatic disease characterized by inflammation followed by fibrosis of the skin and subcutaneous tissue, with the potential to also affect other tissues, including muscles, joints, and tendons. Deep vital organs, such as the lungs, heart, esophagus, gut, and kidneys, are frequently involved and affect the prognosis of the disease. Joint and tendon involvement predicts disease progression and muscle involvement and has prognostic value, because it correlates with lesions in vital organs, especially lung fibrosis and myocarditis.[34,35] WB MR imaging can detect a wide variety of musculoskeletal involvement in SSc, including myositis, synovitis, tenosynovitis fasciitis, and enthesitis (**Fig. 2**).[36] This involvement is often generalized and mostly symmetric; it is present in more than 50% of the patients and correlates with the risk of organ damage.[37] WB MR imaging can also be used to monitor treatment response by detecting changes in fascial and subcutaneous thickening and fascial enhancement.[38]

## Polymyalgia Rheumatica

Polymyalgia rheumatica (PMR) is a clinically diagnosed rheumatologic disorder associated with a

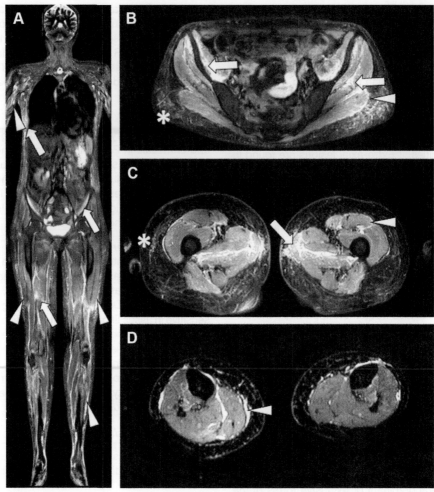

Fig. 2. WB MR imaging from a 53-year-old woman with a severe form of diffuse SSc with myocardial and pericardial involvement, presenting with tendon friction rubs, synovitis, tenosynovitis, and reduced range of motion in shoulders and ankles. Coronal (A) and transverse (B–D) STIR MR imaging reveals extensive musculoskeletal involvement with concurrent involvement of the muscles (arrows), fascias (arrowheads), and subcutaneous tissue at the level of the scapular and pelvic girdles (asterisks), thoracic and abdominal walls, and lower limbs.

moderate biological inflammatory syndrome and characterized by pain and stiffness affecting the shoulder and pelvic girdles. The symptoms typically show a rapid and impressive response to glucocorticoids. PMR has been regarded as a synovial disease but corresponds more with a periarticular and articular inflammatory process, whereas the presence of extrasynovial features such as bursitis and tendonitis has also been highlighted.[39] Facing uncertain clinical diagnosis, WB MR imaging may also be used to rule out other disorders. However, WB MR imaging might be a valuable tool for a positive diagnosis because extracapsular changes may be regarded as a distinctive feature of PMR, especially when observed around the greater trochanter and ischial tuberosity, in the periacetabular space, and below the symphysis pubis, with no BME.[40] The short-tau inversion recovery (STIR) sequence seems to be the most useful sequence to highlight these abnormalities (Fig. 3). The observation of these features identifies a subset of patients who are more responsive to glucocorticoid treatment. The diagnostic value of WB MR imaging in this indication must be compared with that of 18-fluorodeoxyglucose (18-FDG) PET/computed tomography, which shows similar findings (see Fig. 3).

## SKELETAL MUSCLE DISORDERS
### Idiopathic Inflammatory Myopathies

Idiopathic inflammatory myopathies (IIMs) are a heterogeneous group of autoimmune disorders characterized by nonsuppurative muscle inflammation,

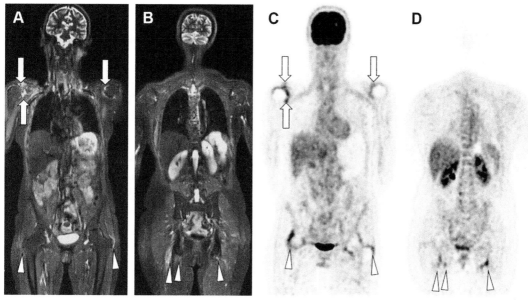

**Fig. 3.** WB MR imaging from a 52-year-old female patient with polymyalgia rheumatica. Coronal STIR MR imaging (*A, B*) shows bilateral shoulder involvement with inflammatory infiltration of the periarticular soft tissues and synovitis (*arrows* in *A*), hip involvement with peritrochanteric infiltration (*arrowheads* in *A*), and bilateral ischiatic tenosynovitis/bursitis (*arrowheads* in *B*). Corresponding reformatted coronal views of 18-fluorodeoxyglucose PET images (*C, D*) show the same lesions.

which sometimes affects extramuscular tissues. This group includes dermatomyositis (DM), polymyositis (PM), inclusion body myositis (IBM), necrotizing myopathy, and overlap myositis. In necrotizing myopathy, the muscular disorder is associated with a connective tissue disease.

DM, the most frequent type of IIM, affects the muscles and the skin. The onset of DM occurs in childhood, and the disease is more common in girls than in boys.[41] PM affects young adults and does not involve the skin. DM and PM present with muscular weakness, which is more pronounced proximally. IBM affects older male patients and typically involves the distal muscles of the upper limbs and proximal muscles of the lower limbs.[42] DM, PM, and IBM may be paraneoplastic observations associated with malignancy.[43]

MR imaging is very sensitive in detecting active muscle inflammation manifested by a high signal on STIR or water T2 Dixon images.[44] This method is more routinely used as an adjunct diagnostic test, along with clinical manifestations and biological tests such as measurement of muscle enzyme levels. Later in the disease course, MR imaging detects muscle atrophy and fatty involution, which correspond with less active advanced disease. This method also has an important role in guiding muscle biopsy, which is the gold standard for diagnosis of IIM, preventing false-negative results and repeated biopsies. Muscle biopsy should be

directed to a site of muscle edema and minimal fatty infiltration.[45] In early forms of the disease in which IIM is suspected despite normal muscle strength and minimal alterations in serum levels of muscle enzyme, MR imaging can be useful in detecting subclinical muscle changes and offers an opportunity for early treatment. In addition, this method allows noninvasive evaluation of treatment response (**Fig. 4**).

An advantage of WB MR imaging is its ability to detect distal and patchy lesions that sometimes are not assessed clinically and may be missed with focused conventional MR imaging.[46] This method also reveals disease activity in muscles that are difficult to examine clinically, detects subcutaneous edema suggestive of DM, and may detect occult malignancy in paraneoplastic forms.[47]

In addition, WB MR imaging may help differentiate between the types of IIM based mainly on the distribution of muscle involvement. DM presents with proximal symmetric involvement of the hip and shoulder girdles, frequently the quadriceps femoris, with edema of subcutaneous tissues and fascia. PM involves the thigh muscles globally or posteriorly, whereas IBM involves the thighs anteriorly.[48] Muscular involvement is patchy in DM and more diffuse in PM and IBM.[49] IBM characteristically affects the distal upper limb and proximal lower limb.[44]

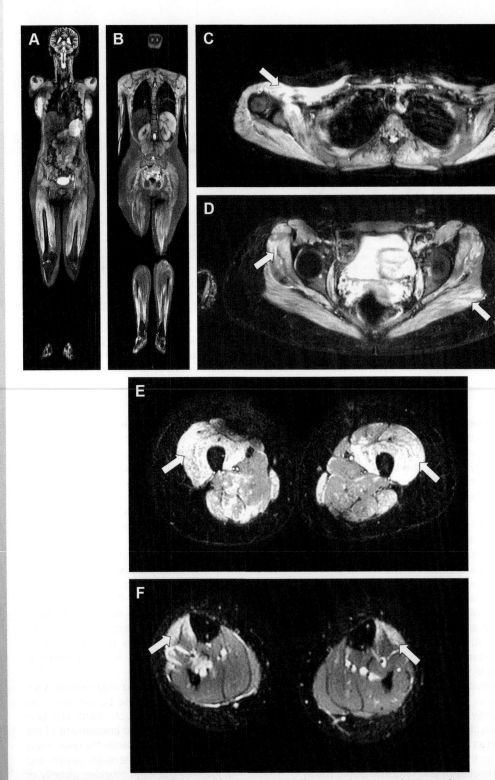

**Fig. 4.** WB MR imaging from a 26-year-old woman with diffuse muscle pain and increased serum creatine kinase level showing multifocal muscle abnormalities. Coronal (*A, B*) and transverse (*C–F*) STIR MR imaging shows severe multifocal (almost diffuse) abnormal signal intensity areas (*arrows*) involving the muscles in the upper and lower limbs. Dermatomyositis with autoantibodies was diagnosed after biopsy of an involved muscle (note the absence of evident subcutaneous tissue abnormalities on WB MR imaging). Corresponding coronal (*G, H*) and transverse (*I–L*) MR imaging after a 3-month treatment with high doses of glucocorticoids and methotrexate shows an almost complete disappearance of the muscle abnormalities.

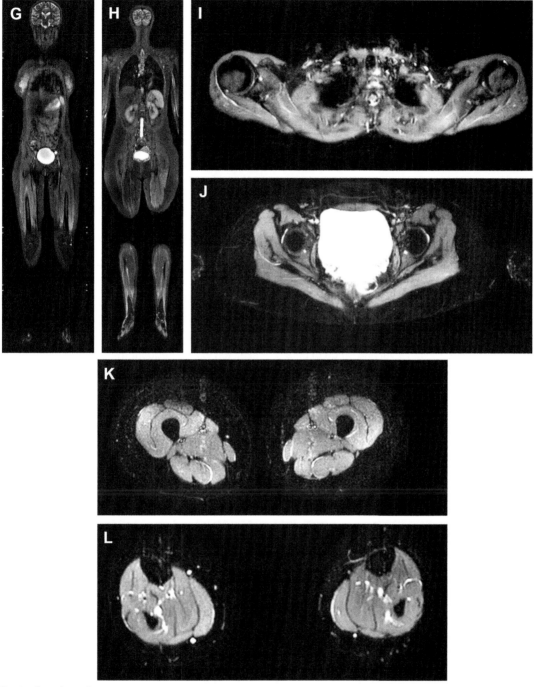

**Fig. 4.** (*continued*)

In addition to muscle inflammation and end-stage muscle atrophy and fatty transformation in IIM, WB MR imaging is also efficient in detecting steroid-induced myopathies manifested by fatty infiltration and muscle atrophy. In IIM, WB MR imaging detects side effects of steroid use, particularly early osteonecrosis.[50]

## Neuromuscular Diseases

WB MR imaging detects asymmetry of affected areas or disease-specific patterns of distribution within the body in neuromuscular disorders such as Duchenne and Becker disease, myotonic dystrophies, facioscapulohumeral muscular dystrophy, and glycogen storage diseases.[51–53] As in IIM, application of WB MR imaging in these inherited neuromuscular disorders offers valuable information about disease burden, distribution, and involvement of muscles difficult to assess clinically, such as the trunk and paraspinal muscles. WB MR imaging orients biopsy and targeted physiotherapy or functional exercises, depending on the affected muscles. It yields a baseline map of the affected sites, which can be used on follow-up examinations to estimate disease progression and treatment efficacy.

## MULTIFOCAL BONE DISORDERS
### Synovitis, Acne, Pustulosis, Hyperostosis, and Osteitis Syndrome and Chronic Recurrent Multifocal Osteomyelitis

Synovitis, acne, pustulosis, hyperostosis, and osteitis (SAPHO) and chronic recurrent multifocal osteomyelitis (CRMO) comprise a complex family of inflammatory disorders with a wide range of clinical presentations, of which multifocal aseptic osteitis is the main feature. In SAPHO, aseptic osteitis is associated with a varying range of cutaneous lesions, hyperostosis, and synovitis. CRMO usually consists of aseptic osteomyelitis, often multifocal, observed in a synchronous or metachronous fashion. CRMO is a pediatric condition, whereas SAPHO tends to affect adults between 30 and 50 years of age.[54,55] Many investigators consider CRMO as the pediatric form of SAPHO.[56] The cause of the disease is still unclear and most likely involves a genetic predisposition with an autoinflammatory process,[57] with infection by *Propionibacterium acnes* inconsistently proved in cases of SAPHO.[58]

Patients usually present with nonspecific focal or multifocal symptoms, including pain, swelling, and limited motion, associated with nonspecific serum biomarkers. Although it is possible to have a single affected site, in most cases multiple clinical or subclinical sites are affected at presentation or later in the disease course.

SAPHO and CRMO share as common features a multifocal skeletal involvement, and the observation of relapsing and remitting lesions typically coexisting at different stages. WB MR imaging may highlight several subclinical sites. These disorders also have distinct features, such as the predominant symmetric anterior chest wall involvement in SAPHO, which mainly affects the sternocostal joints, whereas chest wall involvement is less frequent in CRMO and can be limited to an isolated clavicular lesion. In CRMO, the most frequently affected locations are the distal femoral and tibial metaphyses; synovitis is not a characteristic feature, and the involvement of the axial skeleton is less frequent than in SAPHO.[59–63]

The appearance on MR imaging depends on the lesion's age and activity. BME and periosteal reactions are seen in early active stages, whereas fatty involution and sclerosis are characteristic of chronic lesions (**Fig. 5**). Hyperostosis and paravertebral enthesopathy may be observed in SAPHO.

The diagnoses of CRMO and SAPHO are made by exclusion, because both often mimic other diseases that must be ruled out, such as infectious

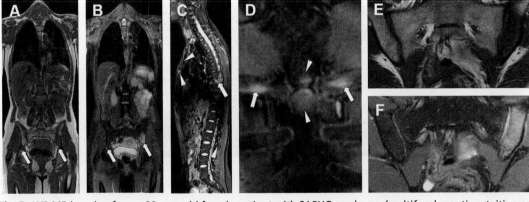

**Fig. 5.** WB MR imaging from a 38-year-old female patient with SAPHO syndrome (multifocal aseptic osteitis associated with palmoplantar pustulosis). Coronal T1 (*A*) and STIR (*B*) MR imaging of the WB and sagittal STIR images (*C*) of the spine show concurrent bone lesions at the level of the right and left iliac bone, and 1 thoracic vertebra (*arrows* in *A–C*) and suggest manubriosternal involvement (*arrowheads* in *C*). Zoomed coronal STIR image of the manubriosternal joint (*D*) confirms the involvement of this joint (*arrowheads* in *D*) and the adjacent second ribs (*arrows* in *D*). Oblique coronal T1 and STIR images (*E*, *F*) of the sacroiliac joints confirm an extensive lesion within the left iliac bone. The coexistence of bony lesions and anterior chest wall involvement, along with a clinical history of skin lesions, is pathognomonic of the disease.

osteomyelitis, Ewing sarcoma, Langerhans histiocytosis, osteosarcoma, and leukemia, which explains why, along with the observation of typical skin lesions, WB MR imaging has a major value by showing multifocal involvement by the disease, its characteristic distribution, and the concurrent observation of active and chronic lesions.

Another important role of WB MR imaging is the detection of asymptomatic or subclinical but active disease or lesions, allowing early treatment and preventing late complications such as vertebra plana and kyphosis in children. Standardized evaluation can be used for the assessment of progression, stability, and regression during the disease course and evaluation of therapeutic response.[64]

In addition, WB MR imaging has a major advantage compared with bone scintigraphy (the classic imaging technique in this setting), because it avoids the use of ionizing radiations, especially when considering the pediatric population. In this population, WB MR imaging can easily reveal the typical juxtaphyseal lesions that may be obscured on scintigraphy by normal physiologic uptake of the adjacent physis.[59]

## Multifocal Avascular Osteonecrosis

Avascular osteonecrosis (AVN) is a potentially disabling disorder that may lead to devastating secondary arthropathy if early diagnosis and treatment are missed, especially considering that early stages are often asymptomatic.[65] Its multifocal form affects mainly young adults and children treated with a high dose of corticosteroids for rheumatologic or hematologic diseases.

Corticosteroid use is the most common cause of multifocal osteonecrosis; other causes include alcohol abuse, coagulopathies, systemic lupus erythematosus, sickle cell disease, leukemia and lymphoma, renal failure, and Sjögren disease.

MR imaging is the best imaging technique to detect osteonecrosis, showing typical epiphyseal ischemic areas delineated by a geographic rim of low signal on T1-weighted MR imaging.[66] WB MR imaging allows, in a single examination, the evaluation of all possible sites of osteonecrosis in patients at risk and offers a diagnosis of preclinical disease. The risk of collapse may be evaluated in individual lesions to alert both clinician and patient for an early reaction on clinical signs of epiphyseal collapse and to allow early treatment and improvement of the prognosis of the affected joints.[50,67–69]

## Hereditary Multiple Exostoses

Hereditary osteochondromatosis or hereditary multiple exostoses is an autosomal dominant condition manifested by multiple benign osteochondromas growing from flat bones or metaphyses of long bones. Most cases are diagnosed in the early teens.[70] Patients may be asymptomatic or show bone deformities and muscular or neurovascular compression.

Malignant transformation is more common in hereditary osteochondromatosis than in sporadic osteochondromas, affecting 3% to 5% of the patients.[70] This complication should be suspected in patients with pain or tumor growth after puberty, cortical destruction, soft tissue mass, and thickened cartilage cap of more than 1.5 to 2 cm, as measured by ultrasonography or MR imaging studies.[71]

MR imaging can show so-called neobursitis or soft tissue edema around the lesion in cases of impingement or fracture of the stalk. Most importantly, this method is able to detect abnormal thickness of the cartilage cap and possible extension within surrounding tissues in cases of malignant transformation. Patients with multiple exostoses require long-term follow-up because of the higher risk of malignant transformation. WB MR imaging may assess multifocal lesions, especially lesions in which clinical examination is limited, such as those in the trunk, and may provide a baseline cartography and quantification of lesions for further systematic or clinically driven follow-up (**Fig. 6**).[72]

## Sarcoidosis

Sarcoidosis is a systemic disease that manifests with noncaseating granulomas affecting the bone, liver, spleen, lymph nodes, skin, muscles, and the central nervous system. WB MR imaging is a useful technique to assess these organs (**Fig. 7**). Extrathoracic organ involvement is found in 38% of the patients in WB MR imaging studies, with frequent lesions within the skeleton and muscles, which were probably underestimated before the advent of MR imaging.[73,74] WB MR imaging may show disease extension and activity; the concurrent observation of active and old fatty lesion, especially in the axial skeleton, helps in establishing the differential diagnosis.[75] WB MR imaging is also helpful in the choice of active lesions as biopsy targets.

## Langerhans Cell Histiocytosis

Langerhans cell histiocytosis ranges from single-organ involvement to a multisystemic disease affecting children and adolescents and mostly involving the skeleton. The radiographic appearance of the lesions is variable, and the MR imaging findings are nonspecific. Focal bone marrow

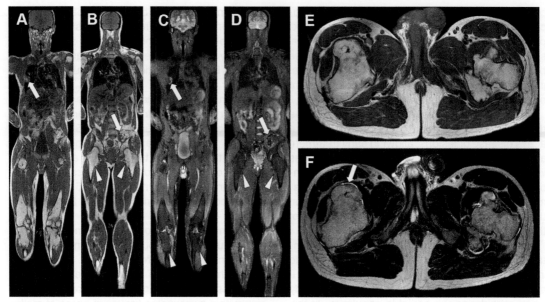

Fig. 6. WB MR imaging from a 22-year-old male patient with hereditary multiple exostoses. Coronal T1 (*A*, *B*) and STIR (*C*, *D*) MR imaging of the WB shows severe deformities predominantly at the level of the hip and knee joints (*arrowheads* in *B* and *D*) and involving the ribs (*arrows* in *A* and *C*) and the left iliac bone (*arrows* in *B* and *D*). Dedicated transverse T1-weighted (*E*) and T2-weighted (*F*) MR imaging shows lesions of the proximal femurs and allows delineation and measurement of the cartilage caps of the exostoses (*arrow* in *F*); these caps remain very thin, ruling out malignant degeneration.

replacement is the usual MR imaging finding, and perilesional edema may be seen in aggressive lesions. Skeletal histiocytosis is a great mimicker and should always be considered in the differential diagnosis of multifocal bone lesions in a child or adolescent. As in osseous sarcoidosis, the concurrent observation of active and quiescent lesions helps in the differential diagnosis with malignancies, although a biopsy may remain necessary. WB MR imaging helps to assess the extent of the disease, including asymptomatic lesions and extraskeletal lesions, and is more sensitive than radiography. Comparisons are ongoing with PET for lesion detection and monitoring.[76–78]

### Polyostotic Fibrous Dysplasia

Polyostotic fibrous dysplasia (PFD) is a nonneoplastic skeletal disorder that affects children and is characterized by multifocal proliferation of fibroosseous tissue in the medullary space. The lesions are usually asymptomatic unless pathologic fractures, deformities, or compression of adjacent structures occur. PFD can be associated with precocious puberty and café-au-lait spots (McCune-Albright syndrome), intramuscular myxomas (Mazabraud syndrome), and endocrinopathies.

The findings of PFD on MR imaging are nonspecific and must be confirmed by radiography once the diagnosis is established. WB MR imaging

may be used to evaluate the disease extension and as a baseline assessment for longitudinal monitoring, which may be triggered by the occurrence of symptoms, because the disease may present evolutive phases and complications, mainly pathologic fractures, which may be present insidiously.[79]

## OTHER APPLICATIONS AND PERSPECTIVES
### Peripheral Nerve Tumors

WB MR imaging has been used to assess tumor extent and to monitor extensive tumors involving peripheral nerves, such as those in neurofibromatosis (**Fig. 8**). Advances in imaging techniques and optimal application of anatomic and diffusion-weighted imaging sequences may offer a valuable approach for morphologic and volumetric analysis of the tumors and an effective tool for detection of malignant transformation.[80,81]

### Vascular Malformations

Hemangiomas and lymphangiomas can affect almost every organ, including the skeleton. WB MR imaging is a noninvasive tool for mapping, quantifying, and monitoring these malformations after treatment, regardless of their extension and the involved organs.[82,83] **Fig. 9** shows Parkes Weber syndrome.

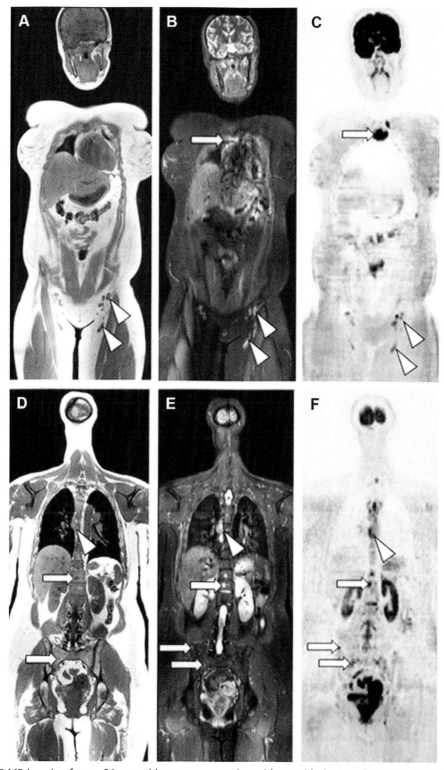

**Fig. 7.** WB MR imaging from a 34-year-old woman presenting with sarcoidosis. Anterior coronal T1 (*A*), STIR (*B*), and diffusion-weighted (*C*) MR imaging shows bone lesion (*arrows*) in the manubrium sterni, and inguinal lymphadenopathies (*arrowheads*). More posterior coronal slices (*D–F*) show bone lesion (*arrows*) in the spine and pelvis, and mediastinal lymphadenopathies (*arrowheads*). The coexistence of lymphadenopathies involving the mediastinum and inguinal areas is suggestive of sarcoidosis, although other malignant conditions, especially lymphoma, should be ruled out.

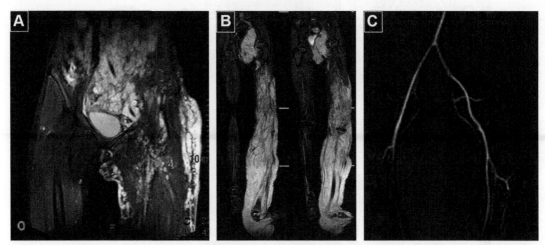

**Fig. 8.** Plexiform neurofibroma in a 16-year-old patient with neurofibromatosis type I. Coronal STIR-weighted image (*A*) and WB MR imaging (*B*) showing the involvement of the soft tissues, muscle groups, and skin of practically the entire left inferior limb, leading to hypertrophy and deformity. Note on angio-MR imaging (*C*) the tortuosity of the vessels.

## Body Fat Mapping

WB MR imaging using a T1 gradient recalled echo (GRE) Dixon sequence has been increasingly used for total body fat quantification and distribution assessment.[84] The main applications of WB MR imaging in this setting are monitoring and treatment of

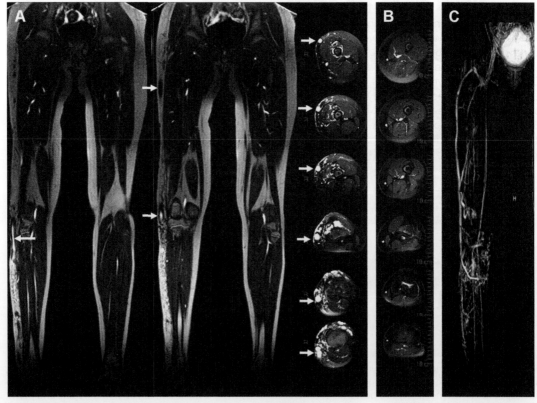

**Fig. 9.** Parkes Weber syndrome. WB MR imaging coronal T1-weighted images (*A*) and axial STIR images (*B*) showing the enlargement of the right inferior limb caused principally by arteriovenous malformation (*white arrows*). Note on angio-MR imaging (*C*) the arteriovenous malformation without an important fistula component.

patients with obesity and metabolic syndrome, but this method may also be used in training programs of athletes or in syndromes with lipodystrophy, such as neonatal progeroid syndrome, in which generalized loss of subcutaneous fat is a cardinal feature.[85]

## Specific Pediatric Applications

In pediatrics, continuous development of the WB MR imaging technique and improvement of this method's sensitivity allow newer applications, including evaluation of fractures/BME and organ injury in nonaccidental trauma,[85] pathologic fractures in susceptible children (such as those with rickets or osteogenesis imperfecta), and hidden focus of inflammation/infection in children with fever of unknown origin.[86] In addition, WB MR imaging has a promising role in virtual autopsy in children and adults.[87]

## TECHNICAL NOTE: WHOLE-BODY MAGNETIC RESONANCE IMAGING PROTOCOLS IN NONONCOLOGIC DISORDERS

WB MR imaging protocols are tailored to cover the body and provide exhaustive multiparametric (multisequence) information about the disease, varying with the suspected disorder (Table 1).

In axial spondyloarthropathies and rheumatisms, most protocols include coronal T1-weighted and STIR (or fat-saturated T2-weighted) WB images, sagittal T1 and STIR images of the whole spine, and high-resolution oblique coronal T1-weighted and STIR images of the SIJ. Additional dedicated sequences may be added: high-resolution coronal study of the wrists, hands, and feet in PsA and rheumatoid arthritis; axial images of the hindfoot to detect frequent involvement of the Achilles tendon, ankle tendons, and plantar aponeurosis in seronegative rheumatisms.

**Table 1**
Summary of current and potential indications of whole-body MR imaging beyond oncology and suggested whole-body MR imaging protocols

| Disorder | Proposed Protocols | | |
| | WB | Whole Spine | Additional Areas |
| --- | --- | --- | --- |
| Spondyloarthropathies | Coronal (T1 and) STIR DWI (investigational) | Sagittal T1 and STIR | SIJ: oblique coronal T1 and STIR/FST2/T2 Dixon |
| PsA | Coronal (T1 and) STIR | Sagittal T1 and STIR | Feet/hands: high-resolution STIR/FST2/T2 Dixon |
| Systemic sclerosis | Coronal STIR | — | Transverse STIR/FST2/Dixon T2 scapular and pelvic girdles or on affected areas detected on coronal views |
| Polymyalgia rheumatica | Coronal STIR or FST1 postgadolinium | — | Transverse STIR/FST2/ Dixon T2/ |
| Multifocal nononcologic bone diseases (CRMO, SAPHO, AVN, sarcoidosis, Langerhans cell histiocytosis) | Coronal T1 and STIR | Sagittal T1 and STIR | Transverse T1 or STIR to choose a site for biopsy |
| Multiple exostoses | Coronal T1 and STIR | — | Adapted plane, high-resolution T2 (T1) of suspect lesions (clinics, coronal study) |
| Inflammatory myopathies and related disorders | Whole-body (coronal and) transverse T1 and STIR or T2 Dixon DWI (investigational) | — | — |
| Peripheral nerve tumors, vascular malformations | Whole-body (coronal and) transverse T1 and STIR or Dixon T2 | — | Whole-body T1 after gadolinium injection in some studies |
| Fat mapping | Whole-body T1 Dixon | — | — |

Abbreviations: DWI, diffusion-weighted imaging; FST1, fat-saturated T1; FST2, fat-saturated T2.

This coronal T1-STIR approach is also valuable for most WB MR imaging studies targeting muscles, bones, and nerves, providing a global view of the disease in an acceptable time frame. Transverse sections are also obtained for confident identification of anatomic structures, evaluation of trophicity, and side-by-side comparison of the involvement in muscle disease. These axial slices cover (either systematically or guided by the clinical findings or the findings on global coronal MR imaging views) the scapular and pelvic girdles; lower limbs; and, if the explored field of view allows, the upper limbs as well. These axial slices or tailored planes may also be planned on demand to complement the study of focal bone lesions detected on coronal images, such as exostoses.

The combination of T1 and STIR or fat-saturated T2 images may become obsolete because T2 Dixon images provide in one single sequence combined information on the inflammatory activity through water images and on the fatty degeneration through fat images: this can be transposed to inflammatory and tumoral conditions involving joints, bones, and muscles.[88] Along with anatomic T1, T2, and STIR sequences, the role of diffusion-weighted MR imaging, widely used in WB MR imaging studies performed in oncology and providing functional information on tissues, is also promising in rheumatology, providing sensitivity and high signal to background for subtle lesion screening, as, for example, in spondyloarthropathies.[12]

## SUMMARY

WB MR imaging has been proved feasible and useful in numerous nononcologic disorders, of which rheumatologic disorders are the most established, including the study of spondyloarthropathies, PsA, and SSc. WB MR imaging should be used to confirm suspected CRMO and SAPHO syndrome and for an exhaustive evaluation of benign multifocal disorders, such as eosinophilic granuloma and sarcoidosis. It is a noninvasive tool for the diagnosis of inflammatory conditions involving muscles, fascia, and subcutaneous tissue, and its roles range from diagnosis to evaluation of disease burden, choice of lesions for biopsy, and evaluation of treatment response. Tailored protocols have been proposed to address these different indications.

## ACKNOWLEDGMENTS

Heartfelt thanks are expressed to Flávia Costa, MD, and Roberto Domingues, MD, for stimulating discussions and for iconographic support.

## REFERENCES

1. Antoch G, Vogt FM, Freudenberg LS, et al. Whole-body dual-modality PET/CT and whole-body MRI for tumor staging in oncology. JAMA 2003;290(24): 3199–206.
2. Baur-Melnyk A, Buhmann S, Becker C, et al. Whole-body MRI versus whole-body MDCT for staging of multiple myeloma. AJR Am J Roentgenol 2008; 190(4):1097–104.
3. Eustace S, Tello R, DeCarvalho V, et al. A comparison of whole-body turboSTIR MR imaging and planar 99mTc-methylene diphosphonate scintigraphy in the examination of patients with suspected skeletal metastases. AJR Am J Roentgenol 1997;169(6):1655–61.
4. Horvath LJ, Burtness BA, McCarthy S, et al. Total-body echo-planar MR imaging in the staging of breast cancer: comparison with conventional methods–early experience. Radiology 1999;211(1): 119–28.
5. Lauenstein TC, Freudenberg LS, Goehde SC, et al. Whole-body MRI using a rolling table platform for the detection of bone metastases. Eur Radiol 2002; 12(8):2091–9.
6. Lauenstein TC, Goehde SC, Herborn CU, et al. Whole-body MR imaging: evaluation of patients for metastases. Radiology 2004;233(1):139–48.
7. Pasoglou V, Michoux N, Peeters F, et al. Whole-body 3D T1-weighted MR imaging in patients with prostate cancer: feasibility and evaluation in screening for metastatic disease. Radiology 2015;275(1):155–66.
8. Lecouvet FE, Larbi A, Pasoglou V, et al. MRI for response assessment in metastatic bone disease. Eur Radiol 2013;23(7):1986–97.
9. Lecouvet FE, Talbot JN, Messiou C, et al. Monitoring the response of bone metastases to treatment with magnetic resonance imaging and nuclear medicine techniques: a review and position statement by the European Organisation for Research and Treatment of Cancer imaging group. Eur J Cancer 2014;50(15): 2519–31.
10. Padhani AR, Makris A, Gall P, et al. Therapy monitoring of skeletal metastases with whole-body diffusion MRI. J Magn Reson Imaging 2014;39(5):1049–78.
11. Lecouvet FE. Whole-body MR imaging: musculoskeletal applications. Radiology 2016;279(2):345–65.
12. Lecouvet FE, Michoux N, Nzeusseu Toukap A, et al. The increasing spectrum of indications of whole-body MRI beyond oncology: imaging answers to clinical needs. Semin Musculoskelet Radiol 2015; 19(4):348–62.
13. Poggenborg RP, Eshed I, Ostergaard M, et al. Enthesitis in patients with psoriatic arthritis, axial spondyloarthritis and healthy subjects assessed by 'head-to-toe' whole-body MRI and clinical examination. Ann Rheum Dis 2015;74(5):823–9.

14. Althoff CE, Sieper J, Song IH, et al. Active inflammation and structural change in early active axial spondyloarthritis as detected by whole-body MRI. Ann Rheum Dis 2013;72(6):967–73.

15. Barkham N, Keen HI, Coates LC, et al. Clinical and imaging efficacy of infliximab in HLA-B27-positive patients with magnetic resonance imaging-determined early sacroiliitis. Arthritis Rheum 2009; 60(4):946–54.

16. Rudwaleit M, Schwarzlose S, Hilgert ES, et al. MRI in predicting a major clinical response to anti-tumour necrosis factor treatment in ankylosing spondylitis. Ann Rheum Dis 2008;67(9):1276–81.

17. Rudwaleit M, van der Heijde D, Landewe R, et al. The development of Assessment of SpondyloArthritis international Society classification criteria for axial spondyloarthritis (part II): validation and final selection. Ann Rheum Dis 2009;68(6):777–83.

18. Aydin SZ, Maksymowych WP, Bennett AN, et al. Validation of the ASAS criteria and definition of a positive MRI of the sacroiliac joint in an inception cohort of axial spondyloarthritis followed up for 8 years. Ann Rheum Dis 2012;71(1):56–60.

19. van Onna M, van Tubergen A, van der Heijde DM, et al. Bone marrow edema on magnetic resonance imaging (MRI) of the sacroiliac joints is associated with development of fatty lesions on MRI over a 1-year interval in patients with early inflammatory low back pain: a 2-year followup study. J Rheumatol 2014;41(6):1088–94.

20. Hermann KG, Baraliakos X, van der Heijde DM, et al. Descriptions of spinal MRI lesions and definition of a positive MRI of the spine in axial spondyloarthritis: a consensual approach by the ASAS/OMERACT MRI study group. Ann Rheum Dis 2012;71(8):1278–88.

21. Althoff CE, Appel H, Rudwaleit M, et al. Whole-body MRI as a new screening tool for detecting axial and peripheral manifestations of spondyloarthritis. Ann Rheum Dis 2007;66(7):983–5.

22. Weber U, Lambert RG, Rufibach K, et al. Anterior chest wall inflammation by whole-body magnetic resonance imaging in patients with spondyloarthritis: lack of association between clinical and imaging findings in a cross-sectional study. Arthritis Res Ther 2012;14(1):R3.

23. Jans L, van Langenhove C, Van Praet L, et al. Diagnostic value of pelvic enthesitis on MRI of the sacroiliac joints in spondyloarthritis. Eur Radiol 2014; 24(4):866–71.

24. Appel H, Hermann KG, Althoff CE, et al. Whole-body magnetic resonance imaging evaluation of widespread inflammatory lesions in a patient with ankylosing spondylitis before and after 1 year of treatment with infliximab. J Rheumatol 2007;34(12): 2497–8.

25. Karpitschka M, Godau-Kellner P, Kellner H, et al. Assessment of therapeutic response in ankylosing spondylitis patients undergoing anti-tumour necrosis factor therapy by whole-body magnetic resonance imaging. Eur Radiol 2013;23(7):1773–84.

26. Burgos-Vargas R, Pacheco-Tena C, Vazquez-Mellado J. A short-term follow-up of enthesitis and arthritis in the active phase of juvenile onset spondyloarthropathies. Clin Exp Rheumatol 2002;20(5): 727–31.

27. Tse SM, Laxer RM. New advances in juvenile spondyloarthritis. Nat Rev Rheumatol 2012;8(5):269–79.

28. Aquino MR, Tse SM, Gupta S, et al. Whole-body MRI of juvenile spondyloarthritis: protocols and pictorial review of characteristic patterns. Pediatr Radiol 2015;45(5):754–62.

29. Beukelman T, Patkar NM, Saag KG, et al. 2011 American College of Rheumatology recommendations for the treatment of juvenile idiopathic arthritis: initiation and safety monitoring of therapeutic agents for the treatment of arthritis and systemic features. Arthritis Care Res 2011;63(4):465–82.

30. Coates LC, Hodgson R, Conaghan PG, et al. MRI and ultrasonography for diagnosis and monitoring of psoriatic arthritis. Best Pract Res Clin Rheumatol 2012;26(6):805–22.

31. Weckbach S, Schewe S, Michaely HJ, et al. Whole-body MR imaging in psoriatic arthritis: additional value for therapeutic decision making. Eur J Radiol 2011;77(1):149–55.

32. Ostergaard M, Emery P, Conaghan PG, et al. Significant improvement in synovitis, osteitis, and bone erosion following golimumab and methotrexate combination therapy as compared with methotrexate alone: a magnetic resonance imaging study of 318 methotrexate-naive rheumatoid arthritis patients. Arthritis Rheum 2011;63(12):3712–22.

33. Axelsen MB, Eshed I, Ostergaard M, et al. Monitoring total-body inflammation and damage in joints and entheses: the first follow-up study of whole-body magnetic resonance imaging in rheumatoid arthritis. Scand J Rheumatol 2017;46(4):253–62.

34. Avouac J, Walker UA, Hachulla E, et al. Joint and tendon involvement predict disease progression in systemic sclerosis: a EUSTAR prospective study. Ann Rheum Dis 2016;75(1):103–9.

35. West SG, Killian PJ, Lawless OJ. Association of myositis and myocarditis in progressive systemic sclerosis. Arthritis Rheum 1981;24(5):662–8.

36. Stoenoiu MS, Houssiau FA, Lecouvet FE. Tendon friction rubs in systemic sclerosis: a possible explanation–an ultrasound and magnetic resonance imaging study. Rheumatology 2013;52(3):529–33.

37. Schanz S, Henes J, Ulmer A, et al. Magnetic resonance imaging findings in patients with systemic scleroderma and musculoskeletal symptoms. Eur Radiol 2013;23(1):212–21.

38. Schanz S, Henes J, Ulmer A, et al. Response evaluation of musculoskeletal involvement in patients with

deep morphea treated with methotrexate and prednisolone: a combined MRI and clinical approach. AJR Am J Roentgenol 2013;200(4):W376–82.

39. Salvarani C, Cantini F, Olivieri I, et al. Proximal bursitis in active polymyalgia rheumatica. Ann Intern Med 1997;127(1):27–31.

40. Mackie SL, Pease CT, Fukuba E, et al. Whole-body MRI of patients with polymyalgia rheumatica identifies a distinct subset with complete patient-reported response to glucocorticoids. Ann Rheum Dis 2015;74(12):2188–92.

41. Wedderburn LR, Rider LG. Juvenile dermatomyositis: new developments in pathogenesis, assessment and treatment. Best Pract Res Clin Rheumatol 2009; 23(5):665–78.

42. Badrising UA, Maat-Schieman ML, van Houwelingen JC, et al. Inclusion body myositis. Clinical features and clinical course of the disease in 64 patients. J Neurol 2005;252(12):1448–54.

43. Tiniakou E, Mammen AL. Idiopathic inflammatory myopathies and malignancy: a comprehensive review. Clin Rev Allergy Immunol 2017;52(1):20–33.

44. Badrising UA, Kan HE, Verschuuren JJ. MRI in inflammatory myopathies and autoimmune-mediated myositis. In: Weber MA, editor. Magnetic resonance imaging of the skeletal musculature. Berlin: Springer; 2013.

45. Kumar Y, Wadhwa V, Phillips L, et al. MR imaging of skeletal muscle signal alterations: systematic approach to evaluation. Eur J Radiol 2016;85(5): 922–35.

46. Malattia C, Damasio MB, Madeo A, et al. Whole-body MRI in the assessment of disease activity in juvenile dermatomyositis. Ann Rheum Dis 2014;73(6): 1083–90.

47. Day J, Patel S, Limaye V. The role of magnetic resonance imaging techniques in evaluation and management of the idiopathic inflammatory myopathies. Semin Arthritis Rheum 2017;46(5):642–9.

48. Dion E, Cherin P, Payan C, et al. Magnetic resonance imaging criteria for distinguishing between inclusion body myositis and polymyositis. J Rheumatol 2002;29(9):1897–906.

49. Cantwell C, Ryan M, O'Connell M, et al. A comparison of inflammatory myopathies at whole-body turbo STIR MRI. Clin Radiol 2005; 60(2):261–7.

50. Zhen-Guo H, Min-Xing Y, Xiao-Liang C, et al. Value of whole-body magnetic resonance imaging for screening multifocal osteonecrosis in patients with polymyositis/dermatomyositis. Br J Radiol 2017; 90(1073):20160780.

51. Regula JU, Jestaedt L, Jende F, et al. Clinical muscle testing compared with whole-body magnetic resonance imaging in facio-scapulo-humeral muscular dystrophy. Clin Neuroradiol 2016;26(4): 445–55.

52. Shelly MJ, Bolster F, Foran P, et al. Whole-body magnetic resonance imaging in skeletal muscle disease. Semin Musculoskelet Radiol 2010;14(1):47–56.

53. Javan R, Horvath JJ, Case LE, et al. Generating color-coded anatomic muscle maps for correlation of quantitative magnetic resonance imaging analysis with clinical examination in neuromuscular disorders. Muscle Nerve 2013;48(2):293–5.

54. Iyer RS, Thapa MM, Chew FS. Chronic recurrent multifocal osteomyelitis: review. AJR Am J Roentgenol 2011;196(6 Suppl):S87–91.

55. Li C, Zuo Y, Wu N, et al. Synovitis, acne, pustulosis, hyperostosis and osteitis syndrome: a single centre study of a cohort of 164 patients. Rheumatology 2016;55(6):1023–30.

56. Earwaker JW, Cotten A. SAPHO: syndrome or concept? Imaging findings. Skeletal Radiol 2003; 32(6):311–27.

57. Hofmann SR, Roesen-Wolff A, Hahn G, et al. Update: cytokine dysregulation in chronic nonbacterial osteomyelitis (CNO). Int J Rheumatol 2012;2012: 310206.

58. Crouzet J, Claudepierre P, Aribi EH, et al. Two cases of discitis due to *Propionibacterium acnes*. Rev Rhum Engl Ed 1998;65(1):68–71.

59. Falip C, Alison M, Boutry N, et al. Chronic recurrent multifocal osteomyelitis (CRMO): a longitudinal case series review. Pediatr Radiol 2013;43(3):355–75.

60. Greenwood S, Leone A, Cassar-Pullicino VN. SAPHO and recurrent multifocal osteomyelitis. Radiol Clin North Am 2017;55(5):1035–53.

61. Magrey M, Khan MA. New insights into synovitis, acne, pustulosis, hyperostosis, and osteitis (SAPHO) syndrome. Curr Rheumatol Rep 2009;11(5): 329–33.

62. Walsh P, Manners PJ, Vercoe J, et al. Chronic recurrent multifocal osteomyelitis in children: nine years' experience at a statewide tertiary paediatric rheumatology referral centre. Rheumatology 2015; 54(9):1688–91.

63. Colina M, Govoni M, Orzincolo C, et al. Clinical and radiologic evolution of synovitis, acne, pustulosis, hyperostosis, and osteitis syndrome: a single center study of a cohort of 71 subjects. Arthritis Rheum 2009;61(6):813–21.

64. Arnoldi AP, Schlett CL, Douis H, et al. Whole-body MRI in patients with non-bacterial osteitis: radiological findings and correlation with clinical data. Eur Radiol 2017;27(6):2391–9.

65. Kaste SC, Pei D, Cheng C, et al. Utility of early screening magnetic resonance imaging for extensive hip osteonecrosis in pediatric patients treated with glucocorticoids. J Clin Oncol 2015;33(6):610–5.

66. Zibis AH, Varitimidis SE, Dailiana ZH, et al. Fast sequences MR imaging at the investigation of painful skeletal sites in patients with hip osteonecrosis. Springerplus 2015;4:3.

67. Albano D, Patti C, La Grutta L, et al. Osteonecrosis detected by whole body magnetic resonance in patients with Hodgkin lymphoma treated by BEACOPP. Eur Radiol 2017;27(5):2129–36.

68. Castro TC, Lederman H, Terreri MT, et al. The use of joint-specific and whole-body MRI in osteonecrosis: a study in patients with juvenile systemic lupus erythematosus. Br J Radiol 2011;84(1003):621–8.

69. Miettunen PM, Lafay-Cousin L, Guilcher GM, et al. Widespread osteonecrosis in children with leukemia revealed by whole-body MRI. Clin Orthop Relat Res 2012;470(12):3587–95.

70. Murphey MD, Choi JJ, Kransdorf MJ, et al. Imaging of osteochondroma: variants and complications with radiologic-pathologic correlation. Radiographics 2000;20(5):1407–34.

71. de Souza AMG, Bispo Júnior RZ. Osteochondroma: ignore or investigate? Rev Bras Ortop 2014;49(6): 555–64.

72. Herget GW, Kontny U, Saueressig U, et al. Osteochondroma and multiple osteochondromas: recommendations on the diagnostics and follow-up with special consideration to the occurrence of secondary chondrosarcoma. Radiologe 2013;53(12):1125–36 [in German].

73. Hostettler KE, Bratu VA, Fischmann A, et al. Whole-body magnetic resonance imaging in extrathoracic sarcoidosis. Eur Respir J 2014;43(6):1812–5.

74. Wieers G, Lhommel R, Lecouvet F, et al. A tiger man. Lancet 2012;380(9856):1859.

75. Kuzyshyn H, Feinstein D, Kolasinski SL, et al. Osseous sarcoidosis: a case series. Rheumatol Int 2015;35(5):925–33.

76. Goo HW, Yang DH, Ra YS, et al. Whole-body MRI of Langerhans cell histiocytosis: comparison with radiography and bone scintigraphy. Pediatr Radiol 2006;36(10):1019–31.

77. Mueller WP, Melzer HI, Schmid I, et al. The diagnostic value of 18F-FDG PET and MRI in paediatric histiocytosis. Eur J Nucl Med Mol Imaging 2013; 40(3):356–63.

78. Dallaudiere B, Kerger J, Malghem J, et al. Adult onset asynchronous multifocal eosinophilic granuloma of bone: an 11-year follow-up. Acta Radiol Open 2015; 4(2). 2047981614552217.

79. Ferreira EC, Brito CC, Domingues RC, et al. Whole-body MR imaging for the evaluation of McCune-Albright syndrome. J Magn Reson Imaging 2010; 31(3):706–10.

80. Ahlawat S, Fayad LM, Khan MS, et al. Current whole-body MRI applications in the neurofibromatoses: NF1, NF2, and schwannomatosis. Neurology 2016; 87(7 Suppl 1):S31–9.

81. Van Meerbeeck SFL, Verstraete KL, Janssens S, et al. Whole body MR imaging in neurofibromatosis type 1. Eur J Radiol 2009;69(2):236–42.

82. Darge K, Jaramillo D, Siegel MJ. Whole-body MRI in children: current status and future applications. Eur J Radiol 2008;68(2):289–98.

83. Kellenberger CJ, Epelman M, Miller SF, et al. Fast STIR whole-body MR imaging in children. Radiographics 2004;24(5):1317–30.

84. Brennan DD, Whelan PF, Robinson K, et al. Rapid automated measurement of body fat distribution from whole-body MRI. AJR Am J Roentgenol 2005; 185(2):418–23.

85. O'Neill B, Simha V, Kotha V, et al. Body fat distribution and metabolic variables in patients with neonatal progeroid syndrome. Am J Med Genet A 2007;143A(13):1421–30.

86. Damasio MB, Magnaguagno F, Stagnaro G. Whole-body MRI: non-oncological applications in paediatrics. Radiol Med 2016;121(5):454–61.

87. Griffiths PD, Paley MN, Whitby EH. Post-mortem MRI as an adjunct to fetal or neonatal autopsy. Lancet 2005;365(9466):1271–3.

88. Ozgen A. The value of the T2-weighted multipoint Dixon sequence in MRI of sacroiliac joints for the diagnosis of active and chronic sacroiliitis. AJR Am J Roentgenol 2017;208(3):603–8.

# Magnetic Resonance Imaging in Rheumatology

Robert G.W. Lambert, MB BCh, FRCR, FRCPC[a],*, Mikkel Østergaard, MD, PhD, DMSc[b,c],
Jacob L. Jaremko, MD, PhD, FRCPC[d]

## KEYWORDS

- MR imaging • Rheumatology • Techniques • Spondyloarthritis • Rheumatoid arthritis
- Juvenile idiopathic arthritis • Indications

## KEY POINTS

- Magnetic resonance (MR) imaging is an excellent tool for detection of inflammation and cartilage damage in arthritis, providing information that may not be available by any other means.
- MR imaging is essential for early diagnosis of axial spondyloarthritis and cartilage degeneration in areas for which physical examination provides limited information.
- New MR imaging techniques for clinical assessment and research in rheumatology are rapidly advancing, including faster acquisition, new sequences, and new methods of quantification.
- MR imaging may be useful as a problem-solving tool in all arthropathies but is not routinely necessary for management of peripheral inflammatory or crystalline arthritis.

## INTRODUCTION

Since the first radiograph was published, imaging in rheumatology has been synonymous with conventional radiography. However, in the last 30 years, new imaging modalities, especially magnetic resonance (MR) imaging, have dramatically changed the information available to clinicians and researchers imaging bones, joints, and soft tissues.

Diagnosis of a rheumatic disorder synthesizes information from history, physical examination, laboratory testing, medical imaging, and disease course, including response to therapy. MR imaging may be only a small part of this puzzle but has become increasingly important. With modern highly effective therapeutic strategies and new agents, it is often imperative to diagnose accurately an inflammatory arthropathy as early as possible, which is challenging because the diagnosis or prognosis is often unclear at first presentation before the condition manifests classic features. In addition to assisting in determining the diagnosis, disease extent, and suitability for specific therapies at baseline, serial MR imaging is useful to monitor change in disease activity, structural damage, and complications.

This article reviews recent advances in MR imaging that are relevant to rheumatology, and the use of MR imaging in common arthropathies and research applications.

Disclosure: Dr R.G.W. Lambert has received consulting fees from Abbvie, BioClinica, Parexel, and UCB. Dr M. Østergaard has received research support and/or consultancy/speaker fees from Abbvie, BMS, Boehringer Ingelheim, Celgene, Eli-Lilly, Centocor, GSK, Hospira, Janssen, Merck, Mundipharma, Novartis, Novo, Orion, Pfizer, Regeneron, Roche, Takeda, UCB, and Wyeth. Dr J.L. Jaremko is the Capital Health Chair in Diagnostic Radiology. Drs J.L. Jaremko and R.G.W. Lambert's research is supported by Medical Imaging Consultants.
[a] Department of Radiology and Diagnostic Imaging, University of Alberta, WMC 2A2.41, 8440 – 112 Street, Edmonton, Alberta T6G 2B7, Canada; [b] Center for Rheumatology and Spine Diseases, Copenhagen Center for Arthritis Research, Center for Rheumatology and Spine Diseases, Rigshospitalet, Valdemar Hansens Vej 1-23, Glostrup 2600, Denmark; [c] Department of Clinical Medicine, Faculty of Health and Medical Sciences, University of Copenhagen, Blegdamsvej 3B, Copenhagen 2200, Denmark; [d] Department of Radiology and Diagnostic Imaging, University of Alberta, 8440 – 112 Street, Edmonton, Alberta T6G 2B7, Canada
* Corresponding author.
*E-mail address:* rlambert@ualberta.ca

## TECHNIQUES AND TECHNICAL INNOVATION

MR imaging technology has improved dramatically over the last 20 years, primarily through advances in coil technology, gradient hardware, and rapid evolution of software (**Fig. 1**). MR imaging is customized to answer specific questions and target specific joints, tissues, and pathologic processes. Small joints usually require small coils and a focused approach tailored for the patient. Prolonged overhead positioning of the hands is impractical for patients with polyarticular inflammatory arthropathy, so hand/wrist MR imaging usually focuses only on the most symptomatic side. For diagnostic purposes, most MR imaging features should be viewed in 2 planes to limit the effect of artifacts and misinterpretation. However, once the diagnosis is established, imaging of an individual feature in a single plane may be sufficient for prognostication, monitoring, or quantification. Wholebody MR imaging is a promising technique in development (see Elie Barakat and colleague's article, "Whole-Body Magnetic Resonance Imaging in Rheumatic and Systemic Diseases: From Emerging to Validated Indications," in this issue).

## INFLAMMATION
### Detection

For detection and quantification of most inflammatory signal changes, such as bone marrow edema

(BME) or bone marrow lesions (BMLs), joint or tendon sheath effusion, or soft tissue inflammation, any water-sensitive sequence usually suffices as long as there is adequate suppression of fat signal (**Fig. 2**). The literature comparing water-sensitive sequences is inconsistent, with an apparent superiority of one technique over another often caused by lack of optimization of the other sequence. A new sequence may not be available on all platforms, or may only be superior in specific circumstances. Most centers continue to use either inversion recovery (IR) sequences, such as short-tau IR (STIR), or a spin-echo (SE) sequence with spectral selective fat saturation (FS), typically T2 weighted (T2w). Water excitation or Dixon techniques are also based on spectral selection. Hybrid sequences that use elements of both IR and spectral selection include spectral-attenuated IR and spectral presaturation with IR.[1] For all these sequences, the distinction between fluid (effusion) and intensely inflamed tissue (synovitis) is difficult and inconsistent. T1 SE with FS and gadolinium-contrast enhancement (T1-FS + Gd) sequences visualize pathologic tissues with high perfusion and permeability, especially inflamed synovium (**Fig. 3**). Contrast enhancement increases sensitivity for synovitis in peripheral joints,[2] whereas BME is detected equally well on T2w sequences, in children and adults.[3,4] Dynamic acquisition can quantify speed and intensity of

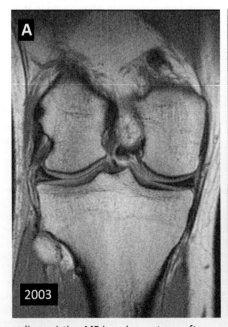
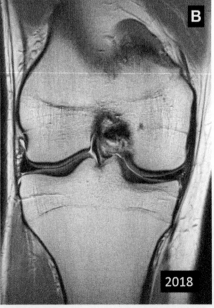

**Fig. 1.** Upgrading existing MR imaging systems often results in considerably improved image quality. Coronal MR imaging of two 25-year-old male athletes scanned on the same 1.5-T MR imaging scanner (installed in 1999). The 2003 image (*A*) proton density, time echo (TE) 14 ms, extremity coil; 2018 image (*B*) intermediate weighted, TE effective 28 ms, 15-channel array knee coil; both images 3 mm thick, 512 × 256 resolution. Improved surface coil and software technology allow markedly improved image quality on the same MR imaging unit with the same gradient coils 15 y later.

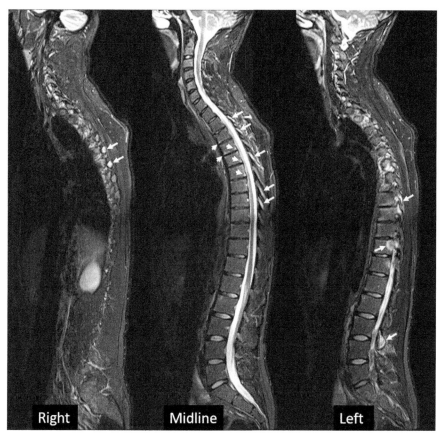

Fig. 2. Good fat suppression is essential for detection of inflammation, and high resolution is required to interpret small lesions. Full-spine sagittal short-tau IR (STIR) MR imaging in 2 acquisitions takes a total of 5 min and 40 s. STIR provides consistent fat suppression over large fields of view. In this 32-year-old man with early spondyloarthritis, multiple foci of BME are scattered through the spine in a typical distribution: right, upper thoracic transverse processes (*arrows*); midline, spondylitis with anterior and posterior corner inflammatory lesions (CILs) (*arrowheads*) and spinous processes (*arrows*); left, facet and costovertebral joints (*arrows*).

contrast enhancement but is seldom used in rheumatology practice.

## Quantification

Formal diagnosis and monitoring of rheumatologic inflammation, especially in clinical trials, requires objective validated MR imaging criteria for disease presence and extent. Because inflammation is a frequent target of therapy, methods for quantification of inflammatory signal change have been intensely investigated. Some features can be scored in a binary fashion (eg, present/absent), whereas others, such as BME, are often scored by grading the feature (eg, mild, moderate, severe) or by visually estimating the proportion of involvement of the structure.[5] Recent work has shown that reliability can be increased by semiquantitative binary BME scoring (present/absent) in each sector of a grid overlay at the articular bone.

With technological advances, this scoring can be quickly performed on consecutive images in a Web-based environment using a touchscreen (**Fig. 4**). The Hip Inflammation MRI Scoring System (HIMRISS) is one example of semiquantitative scoring in rheumatology, using modern technology to assess imaging more objectively and faster than previous spreadsheet-based methods.[6] Fully automated quantification and artificial intelligence image processing will further refine these techniques in the future. Current objective methods for quantifying abnormal inflammatory signal include diffusion-weighted imaging (DWI), which might increase specificity for clinically significant BME. However, the few available publications applying DWI to articular disease have understated the importance of conventional sequence interpretation for selection of a region of interest for DWI analysis. The apparent superiority of DWI results seems to rely on conventional sequences

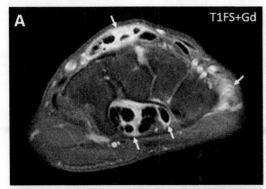

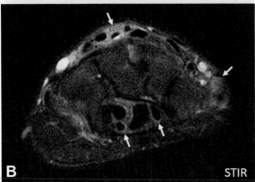

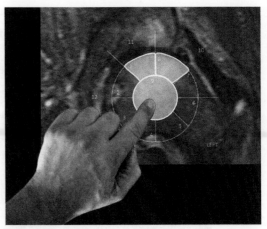

**Fig. 4.** Scoring BME in the left femoral head using a grid overlay and a touchscreen. Within a Web browser environment, coronal STIR images of the hip are displayed with a grid overlay fitted to the femoral head. The user touches each region judged to contain BME, which changes color for visual confirmation, and scoring is updated in an online database. Scrolling through the images as normal, the user touches all regions containing BME on each slice with the grid staying in place. The HIMRISS (Hip Inflammation MRI Scoring System) BME score is supplied per slice, per region, and in total, for analysis.

**Fig. 3.** Postcontrast enhanced images (T1-FS + Gd) (*A*) are more sensitive and specific for detection of synovitis than T2-FS or STIR (*B*). Axial wrist MR imaging in a 44-year-old man presenting with pain and mild swelling in several joints, suspicious for rheumatoid arthritis but with atypical right wrist symptoms suggestive of carpal tunnel syndrome. Prominent tenosynovitis in dorsal compartments, carpal tunnel, and thumb (*arrows*) is more easily seen on T1-FS + Gd. Wrist synovitis is minimal.

as a crucial step in the analysis, and therefore cannot be considered to be fully automated or truly objective.

## STRUCTURAL CHANGE
### Detection

T1-weighted (T1w) sequences provide excellent anatomic detail, strong signal, few artifacts, and consistency across MR imaging platforms. T1w images are best for the depiction of postinflammatory fat metaplasia/fatty lesions and are important for detection of erosion and new bone formation/ankylosis. However, no single sequence has yet been shown to reliably detect the earliest stage of mineralization within fibrous tissue, such as small syndesmophytes in ankylosing spondylitis, which remains an obstacle to the universal application of MR imaging for assessment of spinal structural damage in spondyloarthritis (SpA). Ultrashort time echo or zero-time echo sequences may assist in using MR imaging as a substitute for computed

tomography (CT) and radiography but are still experimental.[7] T1w or proton density (PD)–weighted sequences with FS may improve evaluation of erosion. For a detailed assessment of the bone/cartilage interface, high-resolution three-dimensional (3D) gradient-echo sequences, which exaggerate the paramagnetic effect of calcium in bone (or the loss of calcium in eroded bone), seem to optimize erosion detection. Recent unpublished data (courtesy of Drs Diekhoff and Hermann) from the SIMACT (Sacrolliac MAgnetic resonance Computed Tomography) trial show that, compared with low-dose CT (ldCT), high-resolution 3D MR imaging is clearly superior to T1 for erosion detection (sensitivity/specificity: T1, 0.79/0.93; 3D MR imaging, 0.95/0.93), with similar reader reliability to ldCT (Cohen's kappa: ldCT, 0.77; T1, 0.54; 3D MR imaging, 0.71) (**Fig. 5**).[8] The combination of accuracy of high-resolution 3D MR imaging for erosion detection and its ability to detect inflammation makes MR imaging the clear test of choice for evaluation of sacroiliitis.

### Quantification

The potential for molecular imaging quantification with MR imaging is exciting, but this remains experimental. Numerous sequences have been developed to evaluate the chemical and biophysical structure of musculoskeletal tissues, especially

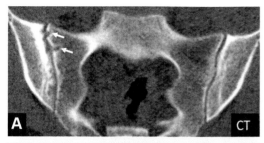

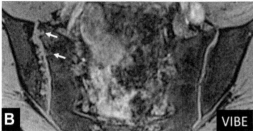

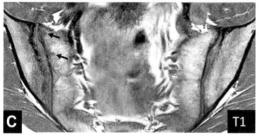

**Fig. 5.** High-resolution MR imaging allows detection of small lesions. ldCT (*A*) and MR imaging were performed in the SIMACT study,[8] which showed that high-resolution 3D MR imaging with a VIBE (volumetric interpolated breath-hold examination) (*B*) sequence detected articular erosion in the sacroiliac (SI) joints with excellent accuracy and reliability. In the subchondral bone of the left sacrum, ldCT and VIBE show erosions equally well (*arrows*), whereas, on the T1-weighted image (*C*), no definite sacral erosion is seen. All 3 images show iliac erosion equally well. (*Courtesy of* Drs Diekhoff, MD and Hermann, MD, PhD, Berlin, Germany.)

articular cartilage: T2 or T2* relaxation-time mapping, delayed gadolinium-enhanced MR imaging of cartilage, T1ρ imaging (T1 properties in the rotating frame of reference), glycosaminoglycan chemical exchange saturation transfer, diffusion-tensor imaging (DTI), and sodium MR imaging. All of these require dedicated software and/or hardware and are challenging to perform consistently. Of these developments, DTI has particularly interesting potential (**Fig. 6**).[9] The signal produced depends on water movement, with one component primarily related to its speed (apparent diffusion coefficient [ADC]) and another primarily related to its direction (fractional anisotropy [FA]). In hyaline cartilage, the ADC is affected mostly by glycosaminoglycan

concentration and distribution, whereas the FA is heavily dependent on the orientation and degree of organization of collagen fibers. Thus, in cartilage, DTI has potential to provide most of the molecular information available from all the other technologies combined. This potential remains to be translated to validated clinically useful sequences.

## AXIAL SPONDYLOARTHRITIS
### Detection

SpA is a group of inflammatory arthropathies characterized by its propensity for bone proliferation, with ankylosing spondylitis (AS) being the most common form of SpA to affect the axial skeleton; that is, the spine and sacroiliac (SI) joints. The usual presentation of AS is inflammatory-type back pain, but symptoms do not discriminate well between various causes; additionally, the spine is much harder to physically examine for inflammation compared with the peripheral joints. Radiography of the SI joints is the traditional method of confirming AS. However, detection of radiographic abnormality depends on visualization of structural damage changes of bone erosion, sclerosis, or ankylosis indicating the presence of chronic sacroiliitis; this frequently delays the diagnosis by 7 to 10 years. The structural damage changes are preceded by inflammation, and MR imaging is now established as the preeminent method for detecting early SpA[10] because of its ability to sensitively detect inflammatory processes long before radiographic changes are evident.

The earliest manifestation of axial SpA is an inflammatory process that starts most often in the subchondral bone of the SI joints. Structural damage changes on MR imaging include bone erosion, backfill, sclerosis, periarticular fat metaplasia (fatty lesions), bone spurs, and ankylosis (**Fig. 7**). Typical signs of activity in the spine include corner inflammatory lesions (CILs) in the vertebral bodies (spondylitis) and at vertebral endplates (spondylodiscitis), and arthritis of the facet, costovertebral, and costotransverse joints (see **Fig. 2; Fig. 8**).[11] Bone erosion occurs less often in the spine, but corner fat lesions, bone spurs (syndesmophytes), and ankylosis are common (see **Fig. 8**).[12] Enthesitis also commonly affects the interspinous and supraspinous ligaments and the SI interosseous ligaments.

### Role of Magnetic Resonance Imaging

MR imaging has essential roles in the diagnosis and management of axial SpA (**Table 1**). Detection of inflammatory sacroiliitis by MR imaging is key to an early diagnosis. Recently updated ASAS (Assessment of Spondyloarthritis International

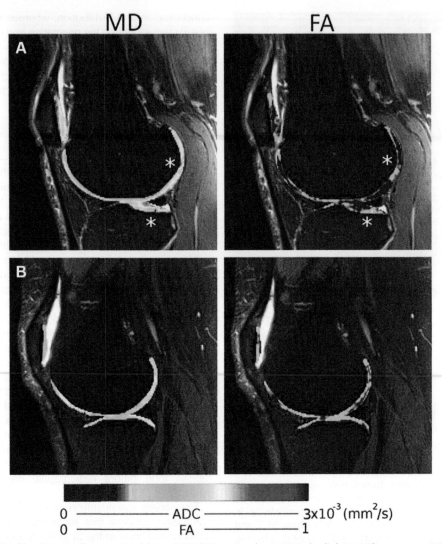

**Fig. 6.** DTI of hyaline cartilage: sagittal knee 3-T MR imaging by RAISED (radial SE DTI) sequence. DTI displays voxel intensity to represent specific properties of microscopic movement of tissue water. Mean diffusivity (MD) is the mean of the apparent diffusion coefficients (ADCs) and represents the speed of water movement (more red = faster). Fractional anisotropy (FA) records to what extent the direction of water movement is constrained by the tissue microarchitecture (lighter blue = more directionally dependent and less random). (*A*) This patient has Kellgren-Lawrence grade 2 osteoarthritis (OA). The cartilage MD appears more red (*asterisks*) in comparison with the subject in (*B*), a healthy volunteer, because damage to cartilage in early OA results in proteoglycan loss allowing water in cartilage to be less tightly bound and to move faster. The structure of the collagen network may also be damaged in early OA, and the FA map in (*A*) shows that some of the cartilage has less FA and appears as a darker blue (*asterisks*) compared with the healthy volunteer (*B*). As the highly organized collagen network starts to break down, water motion becomes more random and less directionally dependent. By using these measurements, DTI has the unique capacity to separately detect damage in hyaline cartilage to both collagen and proteoglycan. (*Courtesy of* Dr José Raya, PhD, New York, New York.)

Society) classification criteria emphasize the critical need for the presence of active inflammation in subchondral bone of sufficient size and intensity to be considered highly suggestive of SpA.[13] In most cases, structural damage changes are also seen. The contextual interpretation of all findings together is critical to an accurate interpretation,

because solitary BME lesions less than 1 cm in size are frequently seen in healthy controls and degeneration is common at the perimeter of the joint.[14] The presence of 2 or more erosions in the SI joint is highly specific for SpA.[15] In contrast, detecting SI joint fat lesions and/or spine lesions has not been documented to improve the

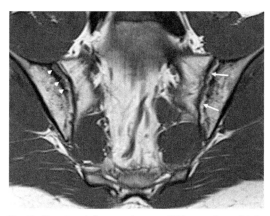

Fig. 7. Structural damage in sacroiliitis may have highly variable MR imaging appearances, especially after treatment. On this T1-weighted image in a young male patient, the right ilium shows subchondral sclerosis with erosion (*arrowheads*). On the left side, a well-defined serpiginous line of bright signal (*arrows*) parallels the distorted joint space on the articular side of iliac subchondral sclerosis. This appearance is typical of backfill, which represents tissue metaplasia, containing lipid-laden macrophages, filling the space created by erosion of subchondral bone and occurring as a repair process when inflammation subsides. Backfill may occur spontaneously or after biologic therapy.

diagnostic utility of MR imaging,[16] and MR imaging of the spine is not necessary for the diagnosis of SpA in most cases. If spine MR imaging is performed for a specific indication, it is essential to include the lower thoracic spine.

The number, location, distribution, and morphology of SpA lesions are all important to distinguish from spondylosis. The significance of spinal lesions varies with age, and the presence of concomitant disc degeneration as Modic-type degenerative changes in vertebral corners may appear similar to SpA lesions. Early SpA spine involvement most often occurs in the thoracic spine or thoracolumbar junction. Multiple symmetric lesions are more likely inflammatory in origin, and the shape of the CIL is important too because the classic inflammatory lesion is taller in vertical height than its horizontal dimension (see **Fig. 8**). Inflammation of the costovertebral joints is highly specific for SpA. Complete spine fusion does not preclude the presence of active inflammation, and patients with complete discovertebral ankylosis may have active facet joint arthropathy and vice versa. MR imaging is useful as a problem-solving tool in established SpA for evaluation of unexplained deterioration or failure to respond to treatment and may detect occult fracture or infection in immunosuppressed patients.

MR imaging can provide objective evidence of currently active inflammation in patients with SpA. Several validated scoring methods, mainly for use in trials, are available for assessment of disease activity in the SI joints and spine,[17] and extensive inflammation on pretreatment MR imaging is related to a good response to biologic therapy. MR imaging is established for quantification of structural changes in the SI joints but not in the spine, because MR imaging has poor sensitivity for detection of syndesmophytes. The use of MR imaging for prognostic purposes in clinical practice is limited, although intense SI subchondral BME together with human leukocyte antigen (HLA)-B27 positivity is a strong predictor of future AS.

## RHEUMATOID ARTHRITIS
### Detection

MR imaging is used for the diagnosis of rheumatoid arthritis (RA) much less often than in axial SpA because, in the peripheral skeleton, the symptomatic joint is much easier to identify and examine. In most cases of RA, the diagnosis is established clinically and confirmed with widely available laboratory tests, radiographs, and/or ultrasonography (US). MR imaging is still useful in problematic cases (**Fig. 9**). MR imaging has advantages compared with US because it can assess all the structures involved in RA, including synovium, effusion, cartilage, bone, ligaments, tendons, and tendon sheath, and can aid in investigating patients with atypical presentation or early disease (**Fig. 10**). MR imaging signs of synovial disease closely correlate with histopathologic and miniarthroscopic findings.[18] BME represents inflammatory infiltrates in the bone marrow (osteitis). Although erosion of bone reflects structural damage, BME seems to represent the link between joint inflammation and bone destruction.[19] CT documents that MR imaging erosion represents true bone damage with a high level of agreement.[20]

### Role of Magnetic Resonance Imaging

In undifferentiated arthritis, follow-up studies have documented an independent predictive value of MR imaging in the diagnosis of RA. In classification criteria for RA, MR imaging or US can be used to determine joint involvement. Several published systems use MR imaging for quantitative, semiquantitative, or qualitative evaluation. The OMERACT (Outcome Measures in Rheumatology) RA MR imaging scoring system (RAMRIS) is the most frequently used system: it involves semiquantitative assessment of synovitis, bone erosion, and

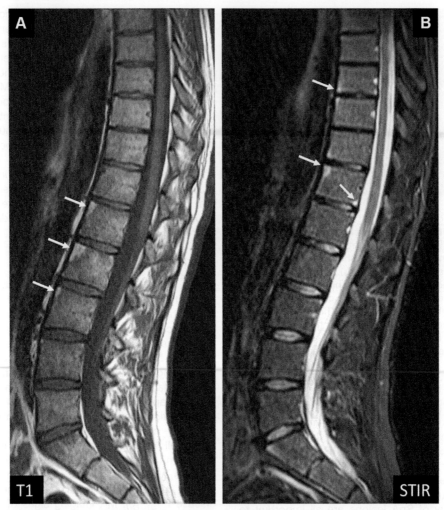

**Fig. 8.** Vertebral body corner lesions in spondylitis may have characteristic features. The corner fat lesions seen anteriorly in the lumbar spine (*A, arrows*) are longer in height than horizontal width. This finding is characteristic of SpA, and this shape is rarely seen with degeneration. Multiple CILs are seen on STIR (*B, arrows*). These CILs are small with nonspecific shape but, combined with the fat lesions and minimal evidence of disc degeneration, the appearances are typical of persistent active inflammation caused by SpA. This 34-year-old man with recurrent symptoms but normal C-reactive protein level was seen in follow-up after biologic treatment (same patient as **Fig. 2**, 2 years later).

BME in RA hands and wrists, based on consensus MR imaging definitions of these findings on a core set of basic MR imaging sequences. Scoring systems of joint space narrowing to assess cartilage damage, and of tenosynovitis, as adjuncts to RAM-RIS have been developed and validated.[21] MR imaging allows more sensitive monitoring of inflammation and bone erosion than clinical and radiographic assessments. Trials have documented the superior ability of MR imaging to discriminate the ability of different therapies to inhibit progressive damage of bone and cartilage.[22] MR imaging findings, particularly BME in wrist and/or metacarpophalangeal joints, independently predict radiographic progression in early RA.[23]

Synovitis on MR imaging and US is found frequently in patients despite clinical remission, and several reports indicate that baseline MR imaging and/or US inflammation is significantly related to subsequent progressive structural damage.[24] These studies encourage further exploration of MR imaging and US for predicting disease course and defining remission.

## JUVENILE IDIOPATHIC ARTHRITIS
### Detection

Juvenile idiopathic arthritis (JIA) is an umbrella term referring to arthritis presenting before the age of 16 years, lasting more than 6 weeks, and

**Table 1**
**Indications for MR imaging in suspected/present axial spondyloarthritis**

| Patients | SpA Status Before MR Imaging | MR Imaging Scan | Comment |
|---|---|---|---|
| Suspected early axSpA | No or normal or equivocal radiograph of SI joints | SI joints. To ascertain presence/absence of sacroiliitis | MR imaging spine not routinely necessary |
| Patients with nonspecific back pain in a higher-risk population | Predisposing factors such as uveitis, Crohn disease, or family history of SpA | SI joints. To exclude presence of unsuspected sacroiliitis | MR imaging spine not indicated for axSpA but possibly for other reasons |
| Atypical presentation with neck, dorsal, or chest wall pain | Not yet diagnosed | Possibly indicated. Spine and SI joints | More common in psoriatic arthritis |
| Known axSpA Before first biologic therapy (Bio Rx) No recent MR imaging | Active disease known or suspected, but objective evidence lacking or incomplete | Indicated and recommended. SI joints and spine | May be required for prescription of therapy Baseline data can only be collected once |
| Known axSpA Failure to respond or maintain response to Bio Rx | Symptoms may have more than 1 cause, especially in middle-aged patients | Possibly indicated. SI joints and/or spine | Must be compared with baseline MR imaging Seeking objective evidence of response/failure to respond |
| Known axSpA New symptoms in patient with established disease | Unexplained clinical deterioration | Possibly indicated. Symptomatic area | Fracture, degeneration, active SpA, or complication of therapy may be present |

*Abbreviations:* axSpA, axial spondyloarthritis; Bio Rx, biologic therapy.

of unknown cause.[25] JIA includes a heterogeneous collection of subtypes and clinical presentations, categorized by the International League of Associations for Rheumatology (ILAR)[25] as oligoarthritis (about half of the cases), polyarthritis, systemic disease, psoriatic arthritis (PsA), enthesitis-related arthritis (ERA), or undifferentiated arthritis. ERA can include enthesitis and/or involvement of SI joints, the HLA-B27 gene type, and/or family history of ERA or SpA. As with adult SpA, radiographs mainly detect late findings of structural damage or indirect consequences of chronic arthritis (eg, bony overgrowth caused by hyperemia). US can be helpful in detecting and differentiating between synovitis, enthesitis, and tenosynovitis but is not helpful to assess deep structures; even in well-visualized joints, US is subjective, with little standardization or validation of diagnostic criteria.[26] MR imaging in children faces unique challenges. Because awake children must be cooperative enough to lie completely still for 20 to 30 minutes, general anesthesia is necessary in most children less than 6 years of age and in many school-aged children, involving major

logistical difficulties, high cost, and increased risk. Intravenous contrast injection is often emotionally traumatic, and tiny veins may be difficult to cannulate. Furthermore, pediatric joints are difficult to image because of their small size. Thinner, higher-resolution slices may show anatomy and disorder more clearly but require longer scan times, and the child is more likely to wiggle during the scan. Imagers must also be aware of wide ranges of normal variation in children, such as the normal periarticular "flare" at SI joints (**Fig. 11**), which can mimic arthritis.

### Role of Magnetic Resonance Imaging

Given these challenges, MR imaging is used sparingly in JIA to assess regions difficult to examine clinically or by US. It is a useful problem-solving modality to evaluate complex disease or anatomy. MR imaging increasingly functions as the primary imaging modality for assessment of axial disease involving the spine and SI joints, but a keen awareness of its limitations is necessary. For example, although MR imaging is more sensitive than

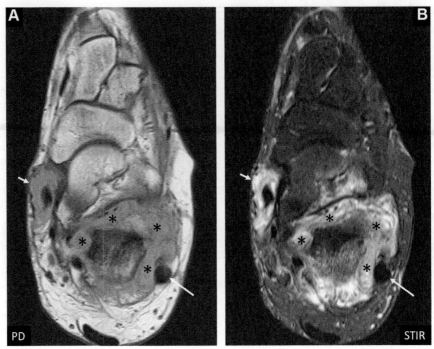

Fig. 9. MR imaging may be helpful in challenging clinical cases. Axial PD (*A*) and STIR (*B*) images of the right foot in a 45-year-old woman with known RA. Severe symptoms were thought to be due primarily to talocrural synovitis and bilateral tenosynovitis with possible tendon tear. Tibialis posterior tenosynovitis (*short arrows*) was expected, but all tendons were intact and the peroneal tendon sheath was normal (*long arrows*). Severe subtalar synovitis (*asterisks*) was unsuspected.

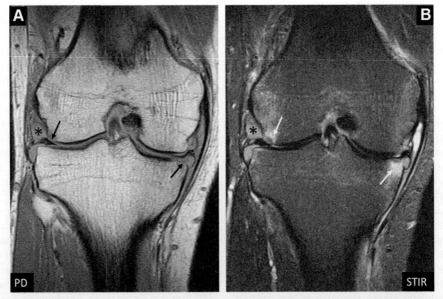

Fig. 10. MR imaging may confirm early erosive arthropathy when radiographs are normal. Coronal knee MR imaging in a 28-year-old man with unexplained joint effusion shows subtle erosion of subchondral bone in the lateral femoral condyle and medial tibial plateau on PD (*A, arrows*) with surrounding BME on STIR (*B, arrows*). Synovial thickening (*asterisks*) is nonspecific, but the combination of synovial thickening with subtle erosion and surrounding BME is typical of early RA in any joint.

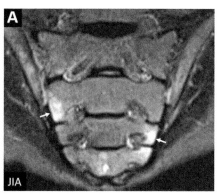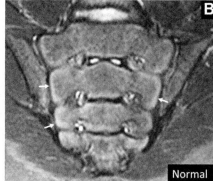

**Fig. 11.** Age-related normal variation should not be misinterpreted as BME on coronal STIR MR imaging of the SI joints. Patchy sacral BME (*A, arrows*) is typical for active inflammation in a 12-year-old boy with known ERA subtype JIA. Normal periphyseal flaring (*B, arrows*) is present in a 7-year-old boy with a thin high signal rim in sacral subchondral bone, somewhat asymmetrical in intensity because of scan inhomogeneity.

radiographs for sacroiliitis, only half of the patients eventually diagnosed with axial involvement of JIA have any abnormality visible on SI joint MR imaging at the time of the first presentation.[27] The formal integration of MR imaging into pediatric rheumatology clinical practice in general lags far behind that in adults and the ILAR diagnostic criteria for sacroiliitis do not include MR imaging.[25] OMERACT is currently working to determine to what extent adult ILAR criteria can be adapted to pediatric sacroiliitis[28] and, eventually, JIA. Particularly the confusing ERA and undifferentiated subtypes may be more clearly defined by MR imaging criteria, leading to more effective evidence-based therapy.

## OSTEOARTHRITIS
### Detection

MR imaging is ideally suited for assessment of inflammation, compositional change in cartilage, and other structural lesions in osteoarthritis (OA). A comprehensive discussion of the vast literature on MR imaging for OA is beyond the scope of this article. MR imaging allows direct assessment of thickness, surface contour, and internal architecture of articular cartilage in OA, and is far superior to radiography for detection of cartilage damage (**Fig. 12**). Central and marginal osteophytes are well visualized. Subchondral changes include sclerosis, cysts, and BMLs; areas with inhomogeneous,

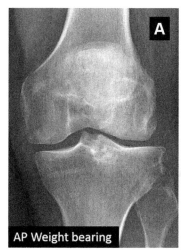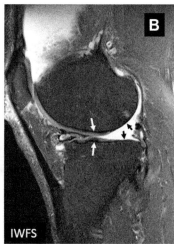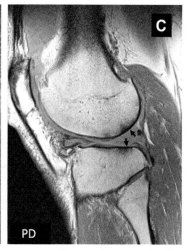

**Fig. 12.** MR imaging is far superior to radiography for detection of cartilage damage. On an anteroposterior (AP) weight-bearing radiograph, mild joint space narrowing is present (*A*). Sagittal MR imaging shows that, in full extension, intact hyaline cartilage anteriorly in the lateral compartment (*B, white arrows*) is responsible for the radiographic appearance, whereas large areas of severe cartilage loss elsewhere in the compartment (*black arrows*) are associated with sclerosis and attrition of subchondral bone (*C*). IWFS, intermediate-weighted fat saturated. PD, proton density.

intermediate-low signal on T1w and high signal on water-sensitive techniques. On histologic samples obtained by surgery in advanced OA, BMLs show trabecular microfracture and bone marrow fibrosis and/or necrosis but limited interstitial edema,[29] and BML is the preferred term for T2 high-signal lesions in bone in OA rather than BME. Synovitis is seen frequently by MR imaging in OA but to a lesser degree than in RA.

### Role of Magnetic Resonance Imaging

Classification criteria for OA are based on clinical and conventional radiographic findings. However, in the diagnosis of articular degeneration, MR imaging can sensitively depict most of the pathologic changes, and the role of MR imaging in OA is rapidly expanding. Several quantitative and semi-quantitative methods have been developed for use in the hip, knee, and hand. These measures have high reliability and better sensitivity to change than radiograph methods.[30] In a systematic literature review,[31] quantitative cartilage volume change and presence of cartilage defects or BML were significantly related to subsequent total knee replacement. Enlargement of BML correlates to increased pain and improvement in BML to decreased pain.[32] In contrast, inconsistent and generally weak relations between cartilage loss and symptom change, and a weak relation between change in synovitis and change in pain, have been reported. The presence of meniscal

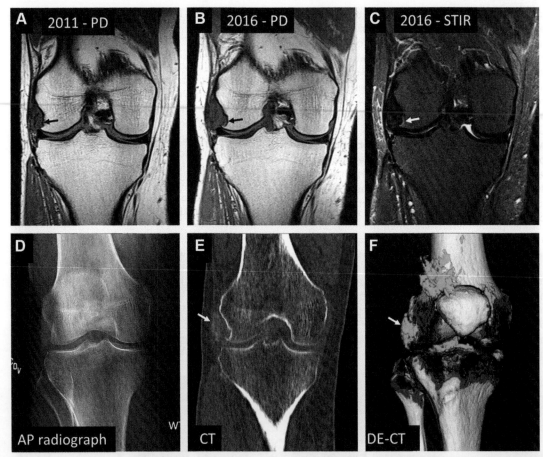

**Fig. 13.** Periarticular changes caused by gout can be challenging to interpret on MR imaging. A 67-year-old man with chronic knee pain had MR imaging done in 2011 (*A*) for possible meniscal tear. The scan shows a small soft tissue mass on the lateral side causing subtle erosion of the lateral condyle (*arrow*). Still undiagnosed, MR imaging was repeated 5 years later (*B* and *C*) for suspected meniscal tear. Periarticular/intra-articular soft tissue swelling is now present in multiple locations, most pronounced on the lateral side (*arrows*), with condylar erosion, and peripatellar changes (not shown). Soft tissue swelling is low signal on all sequences with only a whisker of BME (*C, arrow*). AP radiograph, after the 2016 MR imaging, shows only subtle soft tissue swelling with faint increased density (*D*). Subsequent dual-energy CT (DE-CT) (*E* and *F*) confirms gout with extensive deposition of periarticular/intra-articular urate crystals (*arrows*) (urate deposits are green in *F*).

damage, cartilage defects, and/or BML predicts subsequent MR imaging progression.[31]

## PSORIATIC ARTHRITIS

The clinical presentation of PsA is diverse, with potential involvement of the spine, SI joints, peripheral joints, and/or entheses, and bears resemblance with both RA and SpA; this also applies to its MR imaging features.[33] The locations to be imaged are individualized based on the presentation pattern. Whole-body MR imaging may be a future solution to this problem, but its utility requires validation. MR imaging findings include synovitis, tenosynovitis, periarticular inflammation, enthesitis, BME, bone erosion, and bone proliferation. Dactylitis has been shown on MR imaging to be caused by tenosynovitis with effusion, sometimes associated with diffuse soft tissue edema and/or synovitis in nearby finger or toe joints. There are few MR imaging studies in axial PsA, but findings are similar to AS findings, although more frequently asymmetric. PsA can be clinically silent and, in patients with psoriasis without arthritic signs or symptoms, pathologic findings on MR imaging have been reported much more frequently than in healthy controls,[34] although the clinical importance of these findings is unclear. Scoring systems of inflammation and damage have been developed and validated.[35] However, their clinical utility needs further testing, and only a few longitudinal studies of the prognostic value of MR imaging findings in PsA are available.[36]

## GOUT

MR imaging can directly visualize inflammation and bone erosion in gout. MR imaging can also visualize tophi, with the signal on MR imaging being typically low on T1w images; variable postcontrast enhancement; and low, medium, or high signal on T2w images. The T2 signal depends on the degree of cellular tissue surrounding or infiltrating the crystalline mass, the extent of inflammatory reaction, and the degree of microscopic calcification, which can lead to low signal on T2w imaging (Fig. 13). Gouty lesions can be hard to identify on MR imaging if the inflammatory reaction is minimal and the calcification is subtle. Deeper tophi are hard to detect clinically and may be unsuspected at the time of the MR imaging. The diagnostic accuracy of MR imaging for gout is unclear, so, although MR imaging can detect synovial changes and tophi, the diagnosis of gout is best confirmed with joint aspirate of monosodium urate crystals or dual-energy CT, which specifically highlights urate crystal deposition. US is more useful than MR imaging for diagnostic ascertainment. MR imaging can be used to quantify tophus volume but scoring systems have not been developed, and use of MR imaging for gout in clinical follow-up or clinical trials is minimal.

## SUMMARY

Imaging is integral to the management of patients with rheumatic diseases. For early diagnosis of bone marrow inflammation in SpA and articular cartilage degeneration in OA, MR imaging may be essential for patient care. For most other arthropathies, MR imaging plays a subsidiary role and is usually reserved for problem solving in specific clinical situations. Advances in MR imaging progress at a rapid pace and future important developments will likely include rapid image acquisition, new MR imaging sequences, and quantitative assessment systems that incorporate artificial intelligence techniques.

## REFERENCES

1. Del Grande F, Santini F, Herzka DA, et al. Fat-suppression techniques for 3-T MR imaging of the musculoskeletal system. Radiographics 2014; 34(1):217–33.
2. Ostergaard M, Conaghan PG, O'Connor P, et al. Reducing invasiveness, duration, and cost of magnetic resonance imaging in rheumatoid arthritis by omitting intravenous contrast injection – Does it change the assessment of inflammatory and destructive joint changes by the OMERACT RAMRIS? J Rheumatol 2009;36(8):1806–10.
3. Baraliakos X, Hermann KG, Landewé R, et al. Assessment of acute spinal inflammation in patients with ankylosing spondylitis by magnetic resonance imaging: a comparison between contrast enhanced T1 and short tau inversion recovery (STIR) sequences. Ann Rheum Dis 2005;64(8): 1141–4.
4. Madsen KB, Egund N, Jurik AG. Grading of inflammatory disease activity in the sacroiliac joints with magnetic resonance imaging: comparison between short-tau inversion recovery and gadolinium contrast-enhanced sequences. J Rheumatol 2010; 37(2):393–400.
5. Roemer FW, Hunter DJ, Winterstein A, et al. Hip Osteoarthritis MRI Scoring System (HOAMS): reliability and associations with radiographic and clinical findings. Osteoarthritis Cartilage 2011;19(8): 946–62.
6. Jaremko JL, Azmat O, Lambert RGW, et al. Validation of a knowledge transfer tool according to the OMERACT filter: does web-based real-time iterative calibration enhance the evaluation of bone marrow

lesions in hip osteoarthritis? J Rheumatol 2017; 44(11):1713–7.

7. Siriwanarangsun P, Statum S, Biswas R, et al. Ultra-short time to echo magnetic resonance techniques for the musculoskeletal system. Quant Imaging Med Surg 2016;6(6):731–43.

8. Diekhoff T, Hermann KG, Greese J, et al. Comparison of MRI with radiography for detecting structural lesions of the sacroiliac joint using CT as standard of reference: results from the SIMACT study. Ann Rheum Dis 2017;76(9):1502–8.

9. Raya JG, Dettmann E, Notohamiprodjo M, et al. Feasibility of in vivo diffusion tensor imaging of articular cartilage with coverage of all cartilage regions. Eur Radiol 2014;24(7):1700–6.

10. Mandl P, Navarro-Compan V, Terslev L, et al. EULAR recommendations for the use of imaging in the diagnosis and management of spondyloarthritis in clinical practice. Ann Rheum Dis 2015;74(7):1327–39.

11. Lambert RGW, Pedersen SJ, Maksymowych WP, et al. Active inflammatory lesions detected by magnetic resonance imaging in the spine of patients with spondyloarthritis: definitions, assessment system and reference image set. J Rheumatol 2009; 36(Suppl 84):3–17.

12. Østergaard M, Maksymowych WP, Pedersen SJ, et al. Structural lesions detected by magnetic resonance imaging in the spine of patients with spondyloarthritis: definitions, assessment system and reference image set. J Rheumatol 2009;36(Suppl 84):18–34.

13. Lambert RG, Bakker PA, van der Heijde D, et al. Defining active sacroiliitis on MRI for classification of axial spondyloarthritis: update by the ASAS MRI working group. Ann Rheum Dis 2016;75(11):1958–63.

14. Weber U, Lambert RG, Ostergaard M, et al. The diagnostic utility of magnetic resonance imaging in spondylarthritis: an international multicenter evaluation of one hundred eighty-seven subjects. Arthritis Rheum 2010;62(10):3048–58.

15. Weber U, Ostergaard M, Lambert RG, et al. Candidate lesion-based criteria for defining a positive sacroiliac joint MRI in two cohorts of patients with axial spondyloarthritis. Ann Rheum Dis 2015; 74(11):1976–82.

16. Weber U, Zubler V, Zhao Z, et al. Does spinal MRI add incremental diagnostic value to MRI of the sacroiliac joints alone in patients with non-radiographic axial spondyloarthritis? Ann Rheum Dis 2015;74(6):985–92.

17. Ostergaard M, Poggenborg RP, Axelsen MB, et al. Magnetic resonance imaging in spondyloarthritis– how to quantify findings and measure response. Best Pract Res Clin Rheumatol 2010;24(5):637–57.

18. Ostendorf B, Peters R, Dann P, et al. Magnetic resonance imaging and miniarthroscopy of metacarpophalangeal joints: sensitive detection of morphologic changes in rheumatoid arthritis. Arthritis Rheum 2001;44(11):2492–502.

19. McQueen FM, Gao A, Østergaard M, et al. High grade MRI bone oedema is common within the surgical field in rheumatoid arthritis patients undergoing joint replacement and is associated with osteitis in subchondral bone. Ann Rheum Dis 2007;66:1581–7.

20. Dohn UM, Ejbjerg BJ, Court-Payen M, et al. Are bone erosions detected by magnetic resonance imaging and ultrasonography true erosions? A comparison with computed tomography in rheumatoid arthritis metacarpophalangeal joints. Arthritis Res Ther 2006;8(4):R110.

21. Glinatsi D, Bird P, Gandjbakhch F, et al. Development and validation of the OMERACT Rheumatoid Arthritis Magnetic Resonance Tenosynovitis Scoring System in a multireader exercise. J Rheumatol 2017; 44(11):1688–93.

22. Peterfy C, Emery P, Tak PP, et al. MRI assessment of suppression of structural damage in patients with rheumatoid arthritis receiving rituximab: results from the randomised, placebo-controlled, double-blind RA-SCORE study. Ann Rheum Dis 2016; 75(1):170–7.

23. Hetland ML, Ejbjerg B, Horslev-Petersen K, et al. MRI bone oedema is the strongest predictor of subsequent radiographic progression in early rheumatoid arthritis. Results from a 2-year randomised controlled trial (CIMESTRA). Ann Rheum Dis 2009; 68(3):384–90.

24. Gandjbakhch F, Haavardsholm EA, Conaghan PG, et al. Determining a magnetic resonance imaging inflammatory activity acceptable state without subsequent radiographic progression in rheumatoid arthritis: results from a followup MRI study of 254 patients in clinical remission or low disease activity. J Rheumatol 2014;41(2):398–406.

25. Petty RE, Southwood TR, Manners P, et al. International League of Associations for Rheumatology classification of juvenile idiopathic arthritis: second revision, Edmonton, 2001. J Rheumatol 2004;31(2): 390–2.

26. Chauvin NA, Doria AS. Ultrasound imaging of synovial inflammation in juvenile idiopathic arthritis. Pediatr Radiol 2017;47(9):1160–70.

27. Jaremko JL, Liu L, Winn NJ, et al. Diagnostic utility of magnetic resonance imaging and radiography in juvenile spondyloarthritis: evaluation of the sacroiliac joints in controls and affected subjects. J Rheumatol 2014;41(5):963–70.

28. Herregods N, Dehoorne J, Van den Bosch F, et al. ASAS definition for sacroiliitis on MRI in SpA: applicable to children? Pediatr Rheumatol Online J 2017;15(1):24.

29. Taljanovic MS, Graham AR, Benjamin JB, et al. Bone marrow edema pattern in advanced hip

osteoarthritis: quantitative assessment with magnetic resonance imaging and correlation with clinical examination, radiographic findings, and histopathology. Skeletal Radiol 2008;37(5):423–31.

30. Hunter DJ, Zhang W, Conaghan PG, et al. Responsiveness and reliability of MRI in knee osteoarthritis: a meta-analysis of published evidence. Osteoarthritis Cartilage 2011;19(5):589–605.

31. Hunter DJ, Zhang W, Conaghan PG, et al. Systematic review of the concurrent and predictive validity of MRI biomarkers in OA. Osteoarthritis Cartilage 2011;19(5):557–88.

32. Zhang Y, Nevitt M, Niu J, et al. Fluctuation of knee pain and changes in bone marrow lesions, effusions, and synovitis on magnetic resonance imaging. Arthritis Rheum 2011;63(3):691–9.

33. Poggenborg RP, Sorensen IJ, Pedersen SJ, et al. Magnetic resonance imaging for diagnosing,

monitoring and prognostication in psoriatic arthritis. Clin Exp Rheumatol 2015;33(5 Suppl 93):S66–9.

34. Emad Y, Ragab Y, Bassyouni I, et al. Enthesitis and related changes in the knees in seronegative spondyloarthropathies and skin psoriasis: magnetic resonance imaging case-control study. J Rheumatol 2010;37(8):1709–17.

35. Glinatsi D, Bird P, Gandjbakhch F, et al. Validation of the OMERACT Psoriatic Arthritis Magnetic Resonance Imaging Score (PsAMRIS) for the hand and foot in a randomized placebo-controlled Trial. J Rheumatol 2015;42(12):2473–9.

36. Poggenborg RP, Wiell C, Boyesen P, et al. No overall damage progression despite persistent inflammation in adalimumab-treated psoriatic arthritis patients: results from an investigator-initiated 48-week comparative magnetic resonance imaging, computed tomography and radiography trial. Rheumatology (Oxford) 2014;53(4):746–56.

# Magnetic Resonance Neurography in Musculoskeletal Disorders

Marcelo Bordalo-Rodrigues, MD, PhD[a,b,c],*

## KEYWORDS

• MR imaging • Neurography • Nerves • Musculoskeletal system

## KEY POINTS

• Magnetic resonance (MR) neurography enables direct visualization of peripheral nerves.
• A dedicated protocol with high-resolution technique is important to obtain reliable diagnostic images.
• Knowledge of peripheral nerve anatomy and clinical syndromes are crucial to interpretation of MR neurography studies.
• Fascicular alteration, thickening, and increased T2-signal are MR signs of neuropathy.

## INTRODUCTION

Magnetic resonance (MR) neurography is a specific imaging technique optimized for the study of peripheral nerves that was introduced in 1992.[1] The development of dedicated hardware and imaging techniques has allowed the visualization of small nerves and their disorders and established the increasing role of MR neurography in the management of conditions affecting the peripheral nerves.[2]

This article intends to discuss current imaging techniques in MR neurography and review the main applications of this method in the musculoskeletal system, especially in disorders of the brachial and lumbosacral plexuses, as well as those affecting nerves in the upper and lower extremities, demystifying the clinical applications of this technique in daily practice.

### Imaging Techniques

MR neurography enables the visualization of the peripheral nerve anatomy, contours, fascicular arrangement, signal, and caliber alterations.[3,4] The surrounding anatomic and pathologic conditions leading to nerve compression are also depicted by this method. Several techniques have been described to highlight and isolate peripheral nerves, especially fat suppression, and 3-dimensional (3D) volumetric and diffusion-weighted (DW) sequences.

T1-weighted sequences are excellent in demonstrating nerve anatomy, allowing excellent contrast with the surrounding fat. However, this method is limited in terms of intraneural characterization (Fig. 1). T2-weighted sequences, in turn, demonstrate variations in fluid content in the endoneurial tissue. In order to better demonstrate T2 signal characteristics, long echo times (TEs) of 30 to 90 milliseconds are obtained. Nerve morphology, caliber, and fascicle configuration are well demonstrated in T2-weighted sequences (Fig. 2).

3D volumetric sequences are essential for examination of peripheral nerves. The small size and

Disclosure Statement: The author has nothing to disclose.
[a] Institute of Orthopedics and Traumatology, Diagnostic Center, Clinics Hospital, University of São Paulo Medical School, Rua Ovídio Pires de Campos, 333, Térreo, São Paulo, São Paulo 05403-010, Brazil; [b] Radiology Institute, Clinics Hospital, University of São Paulo Medical School, R. Dr. Ovídio Pires de Campos, 75, São Paulo, SP 05403-010, Brazil; [c] Sirio-Libanese Hospital, R. Adma Jafet, 115, São Paulo, SP 01307-000, Brazil
* Corresponding author. Instituto de Ortopedia, HC/FMUSP, Centro Diagnóstico, Rua Ovídio Pires de Campos, 333, Térreo, São Paulo, São Paulo 05403-010, Brazil.
E-mail address: marcelo.bordalo@hc.fm.usp.br

Magn Reson Imaging Clin N Am 26 (2018) 615–630
https://doi.org/10.1016/j.mric.2018.06.007

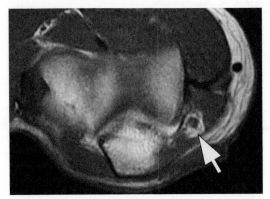

Fig. 1. Normal nerve anatomy. Axial T1-weighted image of the elbow demonstrates normal ulnar nerve (*arrow*) and enhanced contrast with the surrounding fat tissue.

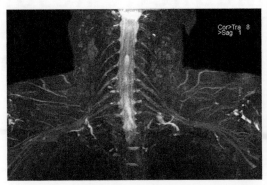

Fig. 3. MIP reconstruction of volumetric STIR SPACE images of a normal brachial plexus.

tortuous course of these structures allow 3D imaging to better demonstrate their anatomy and signal changes when compared with routine transaxial images. High-contrast volumetric sequences are available from major vendors with the commercial names of Cube (GE Healthcare, Waukesha, WI, USA), SPACE (Siemens Healthcare, Erlangen, Germany), and VISTA (Philips, Best, The Netherlands). These sequences offer an isotropic resolution of 1 mm in acceptable imaging times (5–7 minutes). Multiplanar and maximal intensity projection (MIP) reconstructions allow excellent nerve anatomy visualization with optimal signal-to-noise and contrast-to-noise ratios (**Fig. 3**). Fat suppression can be obtained with SPAIR (spectral attenuated inversion recovery) or short TI inversion recovery (STIR) techniques. Gradient echo volumetric

sequences are reserved to evaluate postcontrast enhancement.[3]

Because of the restricted diffusion of peripheral nerves compared with the surrounding tissues, they are better evaluated with DW sequences, appearing with high-signal intensity on DW images. In order to maximize the signal-to-noise ratio, b values in the range of 100 to 300 $mm^2$ are preferred (**Fig. 4**).[4]

## Imaging Evaluation

The initial approach to MR neurography includes evaluation of high field-of-view images for global recognition of the anatomic area and assessment of conditions related to a specific nerve pathologic condition, such as the presence of tumors, fractures, and muscle denervation changes (atrophy and edema). Routine axial spin-echo and 3D volumetric images are used to differentiate nerves from adjacent blood vessels and depict nerve morphology, caliber, signal, and fascicle configuration.[5,6]

In neuropathies, the nerve remains isointense on T1-weighted images but is hyperintense to muscle on fluid-sensitive sequences due to increased endoneurial free water. The nerve may appear

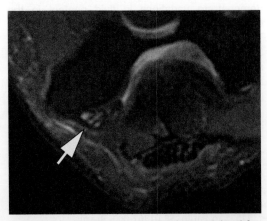

Fig. 2. Normal nerve anatomy. Axial T2-weighted fat-suppressed image of the elbow shows a normal ulnar nerve with normal size, morphology, and characteristic high signal. Note the normal fascicular pattern (*arrow*).

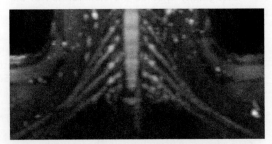

Fig. 4. MIP reconstruction of DW sequence of a normal brachial plexus (b value of 150 s/$mm^2$).

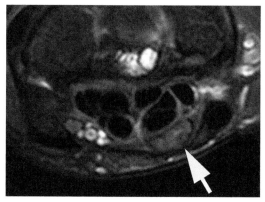

Fig. 5. Neuropathy of the median nerve. Axial T2-weighted fat-suppressed image of the wrist depicts thickening of the median nerve, slightly increased signal, and loss of the normal fascicular pattern (*arrow*).

fusiform or present focal thickening that is usually proximal or at the level of the compression, although nerve compression may not necessarily demonstrate morphologic or signal changes, despite clinical evidence of neuropathy. The injured nerve may also present distortion of the normal fascicular architecture (**Fig. 5**).

Signal abnormalities in denervated muscles may be demonstrated. In acute denervation, prolongation of T2 relaxation times can occur as early as 4 days after nerve injury and present as high-signal intensity on fluid-sensitive sequences (**Fig. 6**). Chronic denervation may lead to atrophy and fat replacement of the muscles, optimally seen on T1 weighted images (**Fig. 7**).[7,8]

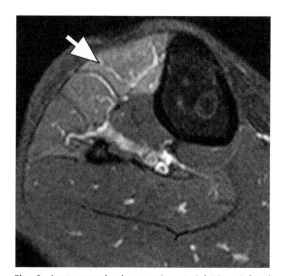

Fig. 6. Acute muscle denervation. Axial T2-weighted fat-suppressed image of the leg shows edema of the extensor muscles (*arrow*), related to a fibular nerve compression.

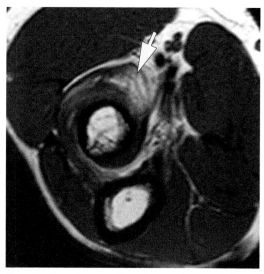

Fig. 7. Chronic muscle denervation. Axial T1-weighted image of the elbow shows fatty atrophy of the supinator muscle (*arrow*), related to PIN compression.

## Musculoskeletal Disorders

### Brachial plexopathy

Traumatic brachial plexus injuries may occur in high-energy trauma, usually involving motor vehicles, or in neonatal injuries, due to the position of the newborn's arm during delivery.[9–11] In adults, traumatic injuries are divided into preganglionic and postganglionic. MR neurography using steady-state acquisition (fast imaging employing steady state acquisition [FIESTA]), 3D volumetric images with multiplanar/MIP reconstructions, and DW images has comparable accuracy with computed tomographic (CT) myelography, with the advantage of allowing postganglionic evaluation by MR. High-contrast volumetric images, based on sampling perfection with application-optimized contrasts using different flip-angle evolutions (SPACE), enables evaluation of the trunks and cords. However, the definition of the brachial plexus may not be clear due to overlap with vessels. The T1 relaxation time of blood is known to be as reduced after gadolinium contrast administration as that of fat tissue in STIR sequences. Consequently, the performance of 3D-STIR sequences with paramagnetic contrast provides a better definition of the brachial plexus outline (**Fig. 8**).[12,13]

Traumatic injuries of the brachial plexus may be classified as preganglionic avulsion, postganglionic rupture, and postganglionic lesion-in-continuity. Steady-state sequences are used to diagnose preganglionic avulsions and are comparable to CT myelography (**Fig. 9**).

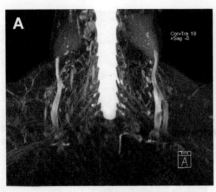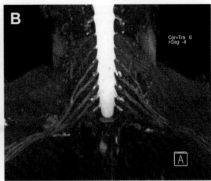

**Fig. 8.** Value of postcontrast on 3D STIR images of the brachial plexus. MIP reconstruction of a volumetric SPACE STIR acquisition before (*A*) and after (*B*) intravenous paramagnetic contrast administration. Note the almost complete disappearance of vascular structures surrounding the brachial plexus.

Pseudomeningoceles are associated with nerve root avulsions in approximately 90% of the cases and are an important red flag for the presence of avulsion (**Fig. 10**).[14] Postganglionic evaluation is performed on sagittal and coronal fluid-sensitive images. In general, nerve thickening and enhancement are seen in all types of postganglionic lesions (**Fig. 11**).

Neonatal traumatic injuries occur in up to 0.5% of the live births. The superior plexus is the most commonly involved (C5 and C6, and eventually, C7), although the inferior plexus (C8 and T1) may be affected as well. In addition, MR is useful in diagnosing preganglionic avulsions (**Fig. 12**).[15]

In thoracic outlet syndrome (TOS), the brachial plexus can be compressed in 3 areas along its course, namely, the interscalene triangle, costoclavicular space, and retropectoral space, which may also involve vessels. The main causes of compression are the presence of congenital fibrous bands along the first thoracic rib, a cervical rib, or muscle hypertrophy. In the setting of TOS, 3D volumetric images with postural maneuvers (elevation of the arm) can be performed in order to better evaluate nerve compression and the relationship of the compression with other anatomic landmarks (**Fig. 13**).[16]

In regards to tumoral involvement, the brachial plexus is more commonly affected by metastatic tumors than primary tumors. Breast and lung neoplasms are the most common primary tumors associated with brachial plexus metastasis. MR is useful in differentiating tumors that are adjacent to the brachial plexus and which compress or invade the nerves from tumors that originate within the nerve (**Fig. 14**). The most common primary tumors are schwannomas, neurofibromas, and malignant peripheral nerve sheath tumors (**Fig. 15**). Other tumors in the vicinity of the brachial plexus can invade or compress the

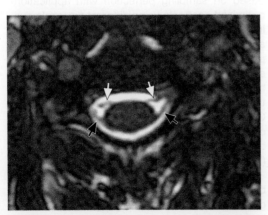

**Fig. 9.** Axial 3D FIESTA image of the cervical spine shows the ventral (*white arrows*) and dorsal (*black arrows*) nerve roots emerging from the spinal cord.

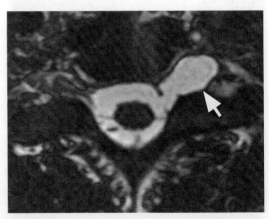

**Fig. 10.** Pseudomeningocele. Axial 3D FIESTA image of the cervical spine demonstrates a pseudomeningocele extending to the left extraforaminal region (*arrow*).

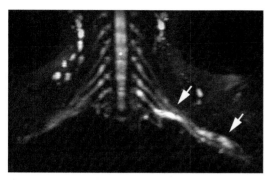

Fig. 11. Postganglionar rupture. MIP coronal reconstruction of a DW acquisition of the brachial plexus (b value, 150 s/mm²). There is thickening and increased signal of the left brachial plexus at the level of the cords (*arrows*). A postganglionar rupture was confirmed at surgery.

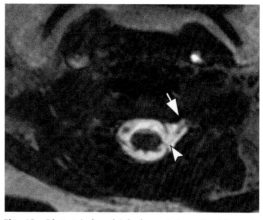

Fig. 12. Obstetric brachial plexus injury. An 11-week-old neonate with a left brachial plexus injury. Axial 3D FIESTA image of the cervical spine demonstrates a left pseudomeningocele (*arrow*) associated with a complete avulsion of the left ventral and dorsal roots (*arrowhead*).

plexus, such as Pancoast tumor, lymphomas, fibromatosis, lipomas, hemangiomas, and lymphangiomas (**Fig. 16**).

Actinic injury to the brachial plexus occurs in less than 1% of the patients irradiated, especially after breast irradiation, and may occur from 6 months to more than 10 years after radiation therapy. The MR findings in actinic injury are difficult to differentiate from tumoral involvement; however, diffuse homogeneous thickening and increased signal, with or without contrast enhancement, are more indicative of radiation plexopathy (**Fig. 17**).

## Suprascapular neuropathy

The most common cause of suprascapular nerve injury is nerve entrapment at the suprascapular

and/or spinoglenoid notches. In athletes, dynamic nerve entrapment has been shown to be more common at the spinoglenoid notch, whereas in the general population, it occurs more frequently at the suprascapular notch.[17]

The suprascapular nerve runs across the superior border of the scapula into the suprascapular notch, under the scapular superior transverse ligament (or suprascapular ligament). The nerve then runs posteriorly, supplies motor branches to the supraspinatus muscle, and then enters the spinoglenoid notch under the scapular inferior

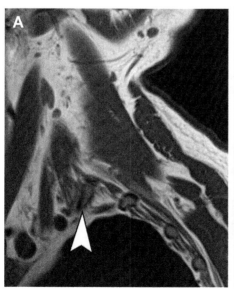

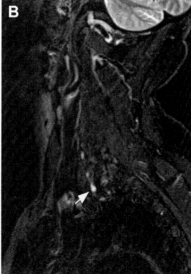

Fig. 13. TOS. Sagittal T1-weighted (*A*) and T2-weighted with fat suppression (*B*) images of the brachial plexus. There is a cervical rib (*arrowhead*) associated with thickening and increased signal of C8 nerve root, indicating neuropathy (*arrow*).

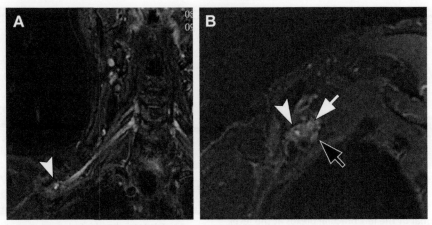

**Fig. 14.** Metastatic involvement of the brachial plexus. A 52-year-old woman with breast cancer. (*A*) Coronal T2-weighted image with fat saturation shows a nodule at the level of the cords. (*B*) Sagittal T2-weighted fat-suppressed image of the brachial plexus shows that the nodule infiltrates the lateral cord (*arrowhead*). The posterior (*white arrow*) and medial (*black arrow*) cords are well demonstrated.

transverse ligament (or spinoglenoid ligament), supplying motor branches to the infraspinatus muscle (**Fig. 18**).

MR is useful in evaluating the course of the nerve and muscle denervation patterns. Entrapment of the nerve at the suprascapular notch, beneath the supraspinatus muscle, may lead to edema and/or atrophy of both the supraspinatus and the infraspinatus muscles. A more distal entrapment at the spinoglenoid notch will result in selective denervation of the infraspinatus (**Fig. 19**).[18] Visualization of the superior transverse ligament and its relationship to the nerve is also possible.[19]

### Quadrilateral space syndrome

Quadrilateral space syndrome (QSS) is a rare condition caused by compression of the axillary nerve and the posterior circumflex artery in the quadrilateral space (**Fig. 20**). The clinical manifestations of this condition may be confusing, and MR is useful in the diagnosis.

Quadrilateral space compression may be static or dynamic. MR findings of QSS include increased teres minor and deltoid muscle signal (on T2-weighted images) and/or fatty atrophy (on T1-weighted images) (**Fig. 21**). Isolated teres minor atrophy can be seen in 3% of all routine MR studies and may be associated with other conditions.[20] MR angiography can also be useful in diagnosing QSS and demonstrating occlusion of the posterior circumflex artery during abduction and external rotation of the arm (**Fig. 22**).[21] Direct visualization of the axillary nerve has been described in MR neurography.[22]

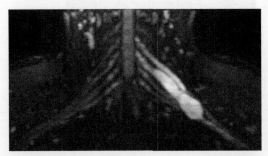

**Fig. 15.** Primary brachial plexus tumor. Coronal MIP reconstruction of DW sequence of the brachial plexus. A plexiform neurofibroma at the left superior trunk.

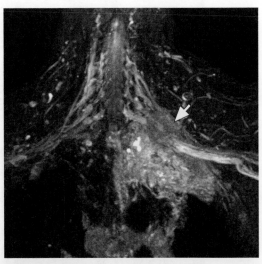

**Fig. 16.** Coronal MIP reconstruction of T2-weighted fat-suppressed acquisition of the brachial plexus demonstrates a Pancoast tumor invading the left brachial plexus (*arrow*).

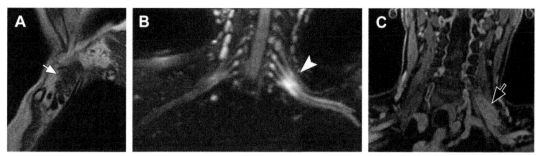

Fig. 17. Actinic involvement of the brachial plexus. A 58 year-old woman with a history of breast cancer underwent radiotherapy for the left breast 3 years ago. (*A*) Sagittal T1-weighted image of the brachial plexus shows diffuse thickening of the brachial plexus at the level of the cords with obliteration of surrounding fat planes (*white arrow*). (*B*) Coronal MIP reconstruction of a DW sequence shows diffuse and homogeneous brachial plexus thickening (*arrowhead*). (*C*) Coronal 3D gradient-echo T1-weighted postcontrast image shows diffuse and homogeneous enhancement of the left brachial plexus (*black arrow*). Surgery was performed in order to rule out metastatic involvement. Actinic lesion was confirmed on pathology.

## Ulnar nerve compression

Ulnar nerve compression is the most common neuropathy at the elbow and is secondary to dynamic or anatomic factors. In the elbow, the most common compression site is the cubital tunnel as a result of decreased volume during elbow flexion.[23] MR findings include increased signal on T2-weighted images, thickening of the nerve, and obliteration of fat tissue surrounding the nerve on T1-weighted images (**Fig. 23**).

Ulnar nerve subluxation is a common feature and is present in up to 16% of asymptomatic individuals. In a minority of the cases, it may cause a compressive neuropathy. Subluxation can be seen on routine MR images; however, elbow flexion allows better visualization of nerve dislocation (**Fig. 24**).[24]

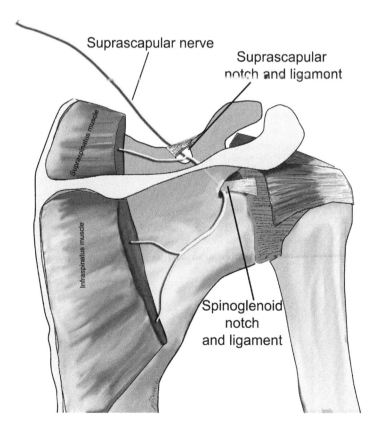

Fig. 18. Suprascapular nerve anatomy and anatomic landmarks, especially with the suprascapular and spinoglenoid notches.

Suprascapular nerve

Suprascapular notch and ligament

Supraspinatus muscle

Infraspinatus muscle

Spinoglenoid notch and ligament

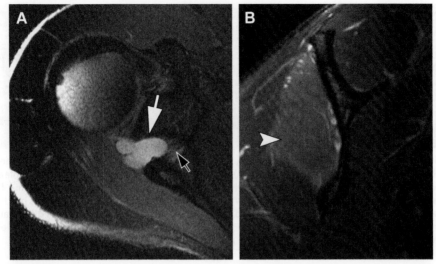

**Fig. 19.** Suprascapular nerve compression. (*A*) Axial T2-weighted image of the shoulder. There is a paralabral cyst at the spinoglenoid notch (*white arrow*) with compression of the suprascapular nerve (*black arrow*). (*B*) Sagittal T2-weighted image with fat suppression shows denervation with edema at the infraspinatus muscle (*arrowhead*).

Ulnar nerve compression can occur at the wrist level. Within Guyon's canal, the ulnar nerve divides into superficial sensory and deep motor branches. On MR, the normal anatomy is well depicted on T1-weighted images, and bifurcation of superficial and deep nerve branches is adequately seen. MR imaging is useful in detecting mass lesions in the course of the ulnar nerve branches (**Fig. 25**). Ulnar nerve signal

and caliber alterations are not well visualized on MR.[25]

### Radial nerve compression
Radial nerve entrapment is the least common type of compression and is frequently associated with trauma. In the arm, the radial nerve can be compressed at the humeral spiral groove as it crosses the lateral intermuscular septum, where

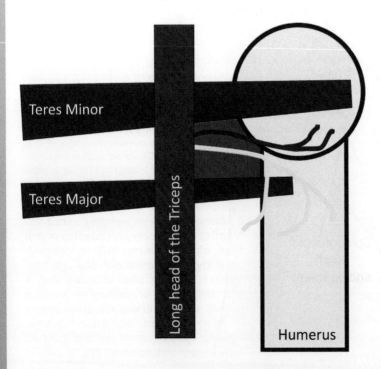

**Fig. 20.** Quadrilateral space (*blue*) and the anatomic landmarks. Exiting the quadrilateral space are the axillary nerve (*yellow*) and the posterior circumflex artery (*red*).

Teres Minor

Teres Major

Long head of the Triceps

Humerus

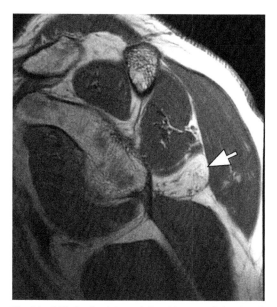

Fig. 21. QSS. Sagittal T1-weighted image of the shoulder. Complete fatty atrophy of the teres minor muscle (*arrow*).

it enters the anterior compartment of the arm. With 3D volumetric sequences, MR neurography is able to depict radial nerve thickening in the lateral intermuscular septum, caliber, and signal abnormalities (**Fig. 26**).[26] At the level of the elbow joint, the radial nerve bifurcates into the superficial radial nerve, a sensory branch, and the posterior interosseous nerve (PIN), a motor branch. The PIN passes under the arcade of Frohse, a fibrous arch present in 35% of individuals and formed by the proximal thickened edge of the superficial head of the supinator muscle, and then travels between the superficial and deep heads of the supinator muscle, which is the most common site of compression of the PIN.[27] Compression of the PIN may lead to a denervation pattern at the muscles innervated by the PIN, namely, the supinator, extensor digitorum communis, extensor digitorum minimi, and extensor carpi ulnaris (**Fig. 27**).[6,28]

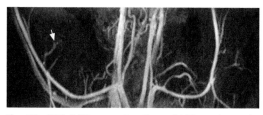

Fig. 22. QSS. MIP reconstruction of MR angiography of the upper limbs in a patient with edema and atrophy of the teres minor muscle at the left side. The normal posterior circumflex artery is seen at the right side (*arrow*) and obliterated at the left side.

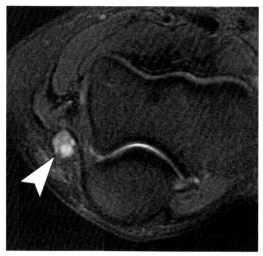

Fig. 23. Ulnar neuropathy. Axial T2-weighted image with fat saturation. Thickening and increased signal of the ulnar nerve with loss of the regular fascicular pattern (*arrowhead*).

## Median nerve compression

The pronator syndrome is a compression of the median nerve at the level of the elbow, usually underneath the lacertus fibrosus, between the superficial (humeral) and deep (ulnar) heads of the pronator teres muscle or at the origin of the flexor digitorum superficialis muscle. The MR findings in the pronator syndrome are related to space-occupying lesions at the course of the nerve and, especially, signal abnormalities and/or atrophy in the flexor pronator muscle group (**Fig. 28**). Recently, intrinsic MR alterations within the median nerve in entrapment syndromes have been described with the use of high-resolution sequences.[29]

Anterior interosseous nerve syndrome is a compression of the anterior interosseous nerve at the forearm. The MR findings are typically related to muscle denervation pattern in the pronator quadratus, flexor digitorum profundus, and flexor pollicis longus muscles (**Fig. 29**). However, signal alterations in the pronator quadratus at fluid-sensitive sequences have been described as frequent and may be a normal finding without clinical significance.[30]

Carpal tunnel syndrome (CTS) is the most common compressive neuropathy of the upper extremity, with a prevalence of 3% in the general population.[31] MR imaging has been shown to be accurate in 90% of the cases and to predict surgical benefit for patients with CTS. The most specific MR signs of CTS are proximal median nerve enlargement, flattening of the median nerve in the carpal tunnel, volar bowing of the flexor

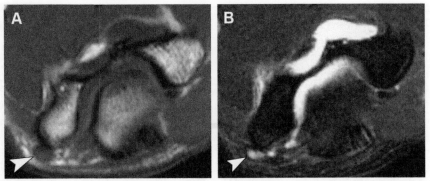

**Fig. 24.** Ulnar nerve subluxation. Axial T1-weighted (*A*) and T2-weighted with fat-suppression (*B*) images of the elbow demonstrate the ulnar nerve at the apex of the medial epicondyle (*arrowheads*), indicating subluxation. There is associated ulnar neuropathy with increased signal and thickening of the nerve.

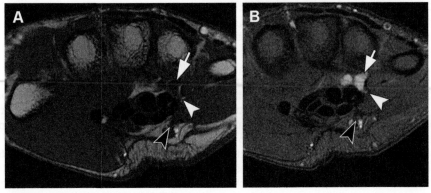

**Fig. 25.** Ulnar nerve entrapment at the wrist. Axial T1-weighted (*A*) and T2-weighted fat-suppressed (*B*) images of the wrist. A cyst (*arrow*) compresses the deep branch of the ulnar nerve (*white arrowhead*). The superficial branch of the ulnar nerve is normal (*black arrowhead*).

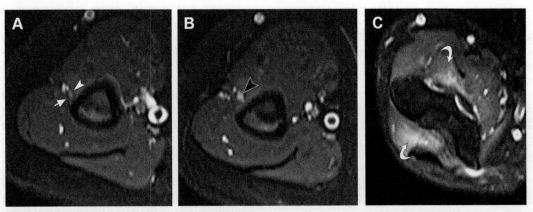

**Fig. 26.** Radial nerve compression at the spiral groove. Axial T2-weighted fat-suppressed images at the level of the humeral spiral groove (*A, B*) and the level of the elbow joint (*C*). In (*A*), the ulnar nerve has normal size and signal (*white arrowhead*) and is starting to cross the lateral intermuscular septum (*arrow*). At a slightly more distal image, there is increased signal and thickening of the radial nerve (*black arrowhead*) and denervation edema of the brachialis and supinator muscles (*curved arrows*).

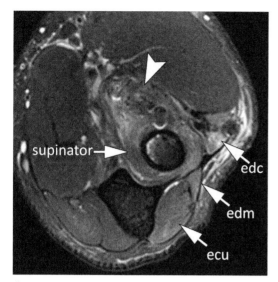

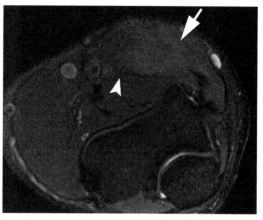

**Fig. 28.** Pronator syndrome. Axial T2-weighted image with fat saturation of the elbow shows edema of the pronator teres muscle (*arrow*). The median nerve is normal at this level (*arrowhead*).

**Fig. 27.** Posterior interosseous nerve entrapment. Axial T2-weighted image with fat saturation demonstrates a postoperative scar tissue at the anterolateral aspect of the elbow (*arrowhead*) with obliteration of the PIN. There is denervation muscle edema of the supinator, extensor carpi ulnaris (ecu), extensor digitorum minimi (edm), and extensor digitorum communis (edc) (*arrows*).

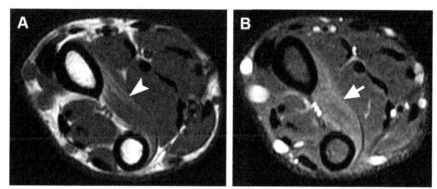

**Fig. 29.** Anterior interosseous nerve syndrome. Axial (*A*) T1-weighted and (*B*) T2-weighted fat-suppressed images at the level of the distal forearm. There is fatty atrophy (*arrowhead*) and edema (*arrow*) of the pronator quadratus muscle.

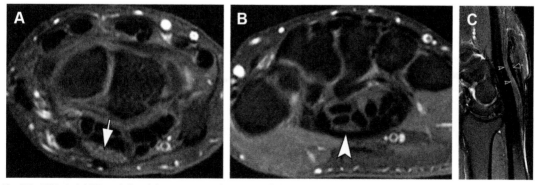

**Fig. 30.** CTS. Axial T2-weighted fat-suppressed images of the wrist at the levels of the pisiform (*A*) and the distal aspect of the carpal tunnel (*B*). Sagittal T2-weighted fat-suppressed image of the wrist (*C*) shows the longitudinal axis of the median nerve. There is proximal enlargement (*white arrow*) and distal flattening (*white arrowhead*) of the median nerve. Note the increased signal and decrease in size with an "hour-glass" appearance of the median nerve at the middle and distal aspects of the carpal tunnel (*black arrowheads*). There is also thickening of the flexor retinaculum (*black arrow*).

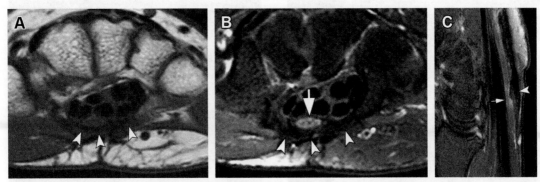

**Fig. 31.** Postoperative CTS. Axial (*A*) T1-weighted and (*B*) T2-weighted fat-suppressed images of the wrist at the level of the distal carpal tunnel. (*C*) Sagittal T2-weighted fat-suppressed image of the wrist shows the longitudinal axis of the median nerve. There is an incomplete flexor retinaculum release with fibrous tissue and thickening (*arrowheads*). The median nerve is flattened with increased signal (*arrows*).

retinaculum, and T2 hypersignal in distal median nerve branches (**Fig. 30**). Isolated T2 hypersignal of the median nerve within the carpal tunnel has been reported to have a lower specificity.[32] Recently, diffusion tensor imaging has been reported in various studies as a potential tool in the diagnosis and evaluation of CTS treated

conservatively.[33] Quantitative analysis is possible in CTS, and fractional anisotropy values of the nerve less than 0.5 are considered abnormal. MR neurography also has an important role in the postsurgical evaluation of CTS, detecting incomplete flexor retinaculum release and signal alterations within the nerve (**Fig. 31**).

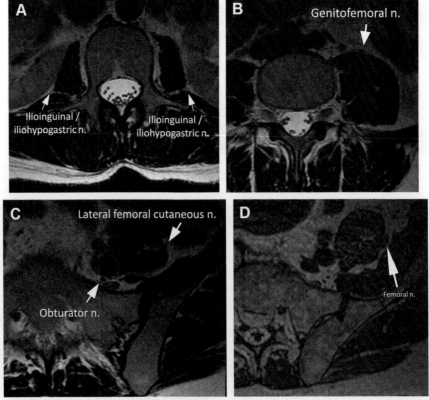

**Fig. 32.** Lumbar plexus MR anatomy. Axial T2-weighted images of the lumbar plexus at the levels of L2 (*A*), L3 (*B*), S1 (*C*), and S1/S2 (*D*) vertebral bodies. The lumbar plexus nerves are depicted in relation to the psoas muscle. n., nerve.

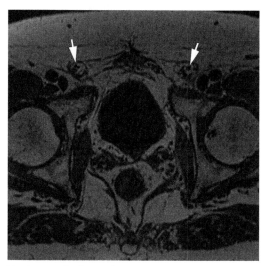

Fig. 33. Genitofemoral nerve. Axial 3D volumetric T1-weighted image at the level of the hips demonstrates the normal genitofemoral nerves within the inguinal canals (*arrows*).

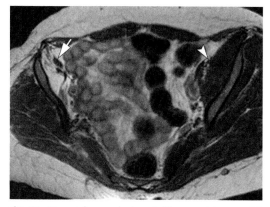

Fig. 34. Femoral nerve lesion. A 44-year-old man with a right femoral nerve iatrogenic injury related to a hip prosthesis surgery. Axial T1-weighted image shows thickening of the right femoral nerve (*arrow*) and complete atrophy of the iliopsoas muscles. The left femoral nerve is normal (*arrowhead*).

## Lumbosacral plexus

The lumbar plexus nerves course around or within the psoas muscle. Axial MR images are useful in visualizing the nerves: the iliohypogastric, ilioinguinal, lateral femoral cutaneous and femoral nerves run lateral to the psoas muscle, whereas the genitofemoral nerve courses anteriorly and the obturator nerve courses posteromedially to this muscle (**Fig. 32**). The sacral plexus forms the sciatic, superior gluteal, inferior gluteal, and pudendal nerves

*The genitofemoral nerve* courses along the anterior margin of the psoas. In men, this nerve enters the inguinal canal. MR neurography demonstrates the nerve in its proximal course along the anterior portion of the psoas muscle and distally within the inguinal canal (**Fig. 33**).

*The femoral nerve* runs along the posterolateral margin of the psoas major and medially to the iliacus muscle. It exits the pelvis under the inguinal ligament laterally to the femoral vessels.

MR imaging is able to demonstrate nerve abnormalities, especially in the intrapelvic location (**Fig. 34**).[34]

*The lateral femoral cutaneous nerve* courses laterally to the psoas muscle, traveling distally along the iliacus muscle to exit the pelvis through or underneath the inguinal ligament at the anterosuperior iliac spine. Entrapment of the lateral femoral cutaneous nerve produces the classic meralgia paresthetica (paresthesia in the proximal and lateral aspect of the thigh). Common causes are tight belts, retroperitoneal tumors, iatrogenic injury in surgeries, and avulsion injury of the sartorius muscle at the anterosuperior iliac spine. MR neurography is useful to visualize nerve thickening and T2 hypersignal (**Fig. 35**).[35]

*The obturator nerve* travels next to the posteromedial aspect of the psoas muscle and exits the pelvis at the obturator foramen. The MR findings include a denervation pattern of the adductor muscles and thickening and increased signal of the nerve (**Fig. 36**).[36]

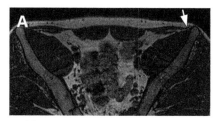
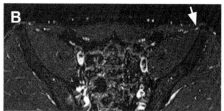

Fig. 35. Lateral femoral cutaneous nerve injury. A 49 year-old man with left meralgia paresthetica. Axial 3D volumetric T1-weighted (*A*) and STIR (*B*) images of the pelvis show the left lateral femoral cutaneous nerve with thickening and increased signal (*arrows*), indicating neuropathy.

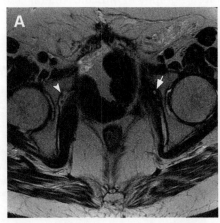
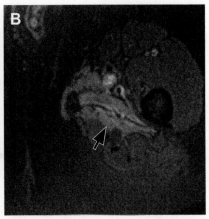

Fig. 36. Obturator neuropathy. Patient with a previous left supra-acetabular fracture 4 years ago develops left obturator neuropathy. (*A*) Axial T2-weighted image shows complete obliteration and fibrous tissue surrounding the left obturator nerve (*white arrow*). The right obturator nerve is normal (*arrowhead*). (*B*) Axial T2-weighted image with fat suppression of the proximal thigh. There is muscle edema in the left adductor muscles (*black arrow*), related to denervation.

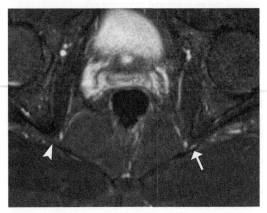

Fig. 37. Pudendal neuropathy. A 36-year-old man with left pudendal nerve symptoms. Axial 3D volumetric STIR image depicts thickening and increased signal of the left pudendal nerve in its course anterior the sacrotuberous ligament (*arrow*). The right pudendal nerve is normal (*arrowhead*).

*Pudendal nerve* compression may occur in association with occupations requiring prolonged sitting and in cyclists, due to repetitive compression by the saddle. The nerve is seen on high-resolution MR neurography as the most posterior structure within the Alcock canal.[37] High-resolution MR techniques allow visualization of nerve abnormalities (**Fig. 37**).

*The sciatic nerve* is composed of a tibial (medial) and a common peroneal (lateral) division. MR findings include an enlarged sciatic nerve with high-signal intensity on fluid-sensitive sequences, similar to the signal intensity of adjacent vessels (**Fig. 38**). It is important to note that mildly increased signal intensity may be a normal finding.[38] Abnormalities in fascicular pattern and obliteration of the fat planes surrounding the nerve are also depicted

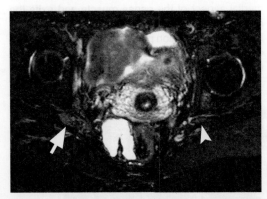

Fig. 38. Sciatic neuropathy. Axial 3D volumetric STIR image of the pelvis. The right sciatic nerve is thickened and with increased signal and loss of the regular fascicular pattern, indicating neuropathy (*arrow*). Note the normal left sciatic nerve (*arrowhead*).

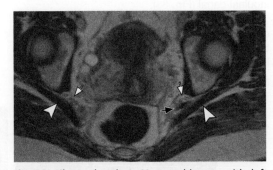

Fig. 39. Fibrous band. A 41-year-old man with left sciatic nerve symptoms. Axial 3D volumetric T1-weighted image of the pelvis demonstrating both sciatic nerves (*white arrows*) and the piriformis muscles (*arrowheads*). There is a thick fibrous band (*black arrow*) posterior to the left sciatic nerve. (*Courtesy of* Dr Denise Tokechi Amaral, São Paulo, Brazil.)

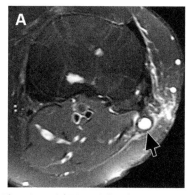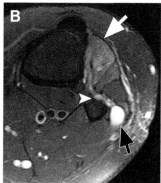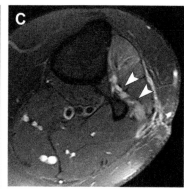

**Fig. 40.** Axial T2-weighted consecutive images (*A–C*) of the left knee with fat suppression. There is a cyst within the common peroneal nerve (*black arrows*), originating from the proximal tibiofibular joint through its articular nerve branch (*arrowheads*). There is denervation edema within the extensor muscles (*white arrow*).

by MR imaging. Muscle denervation pattern may be absent in up to 18% of the cases. In the piriformis syndrome, MR neurography is important to analyze muscle relationships with the sciatic nerve and the presence of anatomic variations and fibrous bands (**Fig. 39**).

### Common peroneal nerve

The peroneal and tibial divisions of the sciatic nerve usually split at the level of the popliteal fossa to form the common peroneal and tibial nerves. The common peroneal nerve is more commonly compressed as it courses by the fibular neck, due to its more superficial location. Intraneural ganglia can develop from the proximal tibiofibular joint into the articular branch of the common peroneal nerve. MR neurography enables visualization of nerve abnormalities like thickening and T2 hypersignal (**Fig. 40**).[39,40]

### Tibial nerve

Nerve compression in the leg and at the tarsal tunnel is more commonly caused by extrinsic space-occupying lesions like cysts, tumors, aneurysms, and ganglia. High-resolution MR neurography can provide valuable information about the tibial nerve.[39]

## SUMMARY

MR neurography is an excellent technique for the evaluation of peripheral nerves. Knowledge of currently available techniques is essential to perform state-of-the-art MR examinations. In order to provide an accurate diagnosis, radiologists must also be familiar with the basic clinical aspects of nerve entrapments and, especially, with anatomic and pathologic aspects related to the nerves.

## REFERENCES

1. Howe FA, Filler AG, Bell BA, et al. Magnetic resonance neurography. Magn Reson Med 1992;28(2): 328–38.
2. Aagaard BD, Maravilla KR, Kliot M. MR neurography. MR imaging of peripheral nerves. Magn Reson Imaging Clin N Am 1998;6(1):179–94.
3. Chhabra A, Flammang A, Padua A, et al. Magnetic resonance neurography: technical considerations. Neuroimaging Clin N Am 2014;24(1):67–78.
4. Takahara T, Hendrikse J, Yamashita T, et al. Diffusion-weighted MR neurography of the brachial plexus: feasibility study. Radiology 2008;249(2): 653–60.
5. Petchprapa CN, Rosenberg ZS, Sconfienza LM, et al. MR Imaging of entrapment neuropathies of the lower extremity. Part 1. The pelvis and hip. Radiographics 2010;30(4):983–1000.
6. Bordalo-Rodrigues M, Rosenberg ZS. MR imaging of entrapment neuropathies at the elbow. Magn Reson Imaging Clin N Am 2004;12(2):247–63, vi.
7. Chhabra A, Ahlawat S, Belzberg A, et al. Peripheral nerve injury grading simplified on MR neurography: as referenced to Seddon and Sunderland classifications. Indian J Radiol Imaging 2014; 24(3):217–24.
8. Chhabra A, Madhuranthakam AJ, Andreisek G. Magnetic resonance neurography: current perspectives and literature review. Eur Radiol 2018;28(2): 698–707.
9. Vanderwerken C, Devries LS. Brachial-plexus injury in multitraumatized patients. Clin Neurol Neurosurg 1993;95:S30–2.
10. Blair DN, Rapoport S, Sostman HD, et al. Normal brachial plexus: MR imaging. Radiology 1987; 165(3):763–7.
11. Dubuisson AS, Kline DG. Brachial plexus injury: a survey of 100 consecutive cases from a single service. Neurosurgery 2002;51(3):673–82.

12. Chen WC, Tsai YH, Weng HH, et al. Value of enhancement technique in 3D-T2-STIR images of the brachial plexus. J Comput Assist Tomogr 2014; 38(3):335–9.

13. Tagliafico A, Succio G, Emanuele Neumaier C, et al. MR imaging of the brachial plexus: comparison between 1.5-T and 3-T MR imaging: preliminary experience. Skeletal Radiol 2011;40(6):717–24.

14. Bilbey JH, Lamond RG, Mattrey RF. MR imaging of disorders of the brachial plexus. J Magn Reson Imaging 1994;4(1):13–8.

15. Somashekar D, Yang LJ, Ibrahim M, et al. High-resolution MRI evaluation of neonatal brachial plexus palsy: a promising alternative to traditional CT myelography. AJNR Am J Neuroradiol 2014;35(6): 1209–13.

16. Demondion X, Bacqueville E, Paul C, et al. Thoracic outlet: assessment with MR imaging in asymptomatic and symptomatic populations. Radiology 2003; 227(2):461–8.

17. Montagna P, Colonna S. Suprascapular neuropathy restricted to the infraspinatus muscle in volleyball players. Acta Neurol Scand 1993;87(3):248–50.

18. Fritz RC, Helms CA, Steinbach LS, et al. Suprascapular nerve entrapment: evaluation with MR imaging. Radiology 1992;182(2):437–44.

19. Simeone FJ, Bredella MA, Chang CY, et al. MRI appearance of the superior transverse scapular ligament. Skeletal Radiol 2015;44(11):1663–9.

20. Sofka CM, Lin J, Feinberg J, et al. Teres minor denervation on routine magnetic resonance imaging of the shoulder. Skeletal Radiol 2004;33(9):514–8.

21. Mochizuki T, Isoda H, Masui T, et al. Occlusion of the posterior humeral circumflex artery: detection with MR angiography in healthy volunteers and in a patient with quadrilateral space syndrome. AJR Am J Roentgenol 1994;163(3):625–7.

22. Salvalaggio A, Cacciavillani M, Gasparotti R, et al. 3D-MR-Neurography of axillary nerve injury: case report of a professional rugby player. Neurol Sci 2016;37(8):1361–2.

23. Chen SH, Tsai TM. Ulnar tunnel syndrome. J Hand Surg Am 2014;39(3):571–9.

24. Patel VV, Heidenreich FP, Bindra RR, et al. Morphologic changes in the ulnar nerve at the elbow with flexion and extension: a magnetic resonance imaging study with 3-dimensional reconstruction. J Shoulder Elbow Surg 1998;7(4):368–74.

25. Bordalo-Rodrigues M, Amin P, Rosenberg ZS. MR imaging of common entrapment neuropathies at the wrist. Magn Reson Imaging Clin N Am 2004; 12(2):265–79, vi.

26. Chhabra A, Deune GE, Murano E, et al. Advanced MR neurography imaging of radial nerve entrapment at the spiral groove: a case report. J Reconstr Microsurg 2012;28(4):263–6.

27. Spinner M. The arcade of Frohse and its relationship to posterior interosseous nerve paralysis. J Bone Joint Surg Br 1968;50(4):809–12.

28. Ferdinand BD, Rosenberg ZS, Schweitzer ME, et al. MR imaging features of radial tunnel syndrome: initial experience. Radiology 2006;240(1): 161–8.

29. Thawait GK, Subhawong TK, Thawait SK, et al. Magnetic resonance neurography of median neuropathies proximal to the carpal tunnel. Skeletal Radiol 2012;41(6):623–32.

30. Gyftopoulos S, Rosenberg ZS, Petchprapa C. Increased MR signal intensity in the pronator quadratus muscle: does it always indicate anterior interosseous neuropathy? AJR Am J Roentgenol 2010; 194(2):490–3.

31. Katz JN, Simmons BP. Clinical practice. Carpal tunnel syndrome. N Engl J Med 2002;346(23):1807–12.

32. Chalian M, Behzadi AH, Williams EH, et al. High-resolution magnetic resonance neurography in upper extremity neuropathy. Neuroimaging Clin N Am 2014;24(1):109–25.

33. Barcelo C, Faruch M, Lapègue F, et al. 3-T MRI with diffusion tensor imaging and tractography of the median nerve. Eur Radiol 2013;23(11):3124–30.

34. Delaney H, Bencardino J, Rosenberg ZS. Magnetic resonance neurography of the pelvis and lumbosacral plexus. Neuroimaging Clin N Am 2014;24(1): 127–50.

35. Chhabra A, Del Grande F, Soldatos T, et al. Meralgia paresthetica: 3-Tesla magnetic resonance neurography. Skeletal Radiol 2013;42(6):803–8.

36. Tipton JS. Obturator neuropathy. Curr Rev Musculoskelet Med 2008;1(3–4):234–7.

37. Chhabra A, McKenna CA, Wadhwa V, et al. 3T magnetic resonance neurography of pudendal nerve with cadaveric dissection correlation. World J Radiol 2016;8(7):700–6.

38. Chhabra A, Chalian M, Soldatos T, et al. 3-T high-resolution MR neurography of sciatic neuropathy. AJR Am J Roentgenol 2012;198(4):W357–64.

39. Donovan A, Rosenberg ZS, Cavalcanti CF. MR imaging of entrapment neuropathies of the lower extremity. Part 2. The knee, leg, ankle, and foot. Radiographics 2010;30(4):1001–19.

40. Chhabra A, Faridian-Aragh N, Chalian M, et al. High-resolution 3-T MR neurography of peroneal neuropathy. Skeletal Radiol 2012;41(3):257–71.

# MR Imaging of Fetal Musculoskeletal Disorders

Heron Werner, MD, PhD[a,b,*], Renata Nogueira, MD, MSc[a,b],
Flávia Paiva Proença Lobo Lopes, MD, PhD[a,b,c]

## KEYWORDS

- Fetal • Musculoskeletal disorders • MR imaging • Imaging

## KEY POINTS

- Ultrasound remains the main imaging technique used during pregnancy to detect fetal malformations.
- MR imaging may provide additional information in the assessment of musculoskeletal disorders.
- Computed tomography scan is used only in specific cases of suspected fetal malformation, particularly those related to the skeleton, because of potential risks associated with fetal exposure to radiation.
- Technological innovations that accompany medical advances have enabled fetal images with improved definition, which help establish accurate diagnoses and contribute toward proper genetic counseling to parents during the prenatal period.

## INTRODUCTION

During fetal development, the musculoskeletal system may be affected by several insults, of which the most common are the skeletal dysplasias (or osteochondrodysplasias),[1-3] a genetically heterogeneous group of more than 350 distinct disorders. The main challenge in detecting such diseases during pregnancy is to differentiate known lethal disorders from nonlethal ones.[1,3] Skeletal dysplasias affect approximately 2 in 10,000 live births and are lethal in approximately 50% of the affected infants.[4] This condition may occur alone or in association with genetic syndromes, and its prenatal diagnosis is essential for proper genetic counseling, prognosis, and postnatal management.[1,3]

Prenatal diagnosis of skeletal disorders remains challenging.[4] Ultrasound (US) may detect some of these disorders but the findings may not be pathognomonic of a specific condition.[1,3] MR imaging plays an important role as a complementary tool in the evaluation of cartilage and muscle.[4]

Computed tomography (CT) scans with 3-dimensional (D) reconstruction may also be used in the evaluation of fetal dysplasia.[5,6] The main advantages of 3D US over CT are lower cost and easier accessibility; however, 3D US is an operator-dependent method and is influenced by the volume of amniotic fluid

Disclosure Statement: The authors have nothing to disclose.
[a] Radiology Department, Clínica de Diagnóstico por Imagem (CDPI)/DASA, Avenida das Américas, 4666, sala 301B, Centro Médico BarraShopping, CDPI, Barra da Tijuca, Rio de Janeiro, RJ CEP: 22640-102, Brazil; [b] Radiology Department, Alta Excelência Diagnóstica/DASA, Avenida das Américas, 4666, sala 301B, Centro Médico BarraShopping, CDPI, Barra da Tijuca, Rio de Janeiro, RJ CEP: 22640-102, Brazil; [c] Radiology Department, Federal University of Rio de Janeiro (UFRJ), Rua Rodolpho Paulo Rocco, 255, Cidade Universitária, Ilha do Fundão, Rio de Janeiro, RJ CEP: 21941-913, Brazil
* Corresponding author. Av Carlos Peixoto, 80/401, Botafogo, RJ CEP: 22290-090, Brazil.
*E-mail address:* heronwerner@hotmail.com

Magn Reson Imaging Clin N Am 26 (2018) 631–644
https://doi.org/10.1016/j.mric.2018.06.011

and the position of the fetus. In contrast, CT with 3D reconstruction has the ability to assess the entire fetal skeleton with a higher resolution but has the disadvantage of involving ionizing radiation, even when the doses are below the modulated dose of 3 mili Gray (which is similar to the dose used in conventional fetal radiology).

Recently, the use of multidetector CT for fetal evaluation has gained popularity in the prenatal diagnosis of severe skeletal dysplasias.[6–8] The ability of this method to delineate details of the entire fetal skeleton ensures an accurate prenatal diagnosis. Cassart and colleagues[6] studied a variety of skeletal dysplasias. 3D CT had a better diagnostic yield than did US. Both imaging techniques were useful in the management of fetal dysplasia but US was a useful screening test and 3D CT was a valuable complementary diagnostic tool.

Nevertheless, fetal CT remains controversial under the principle of protection by the use of radiation that is as low as reasonably possible (ALARA).[6]

Several studies have evaluated skeletal dysplasias using fetal CT.[5,6] However, only a few studies have evaluated the safety of the amount of radiation involved in this diagnostic technique in a large cohort, showing no correlation between the occurrence of malformations and fetal CT performed during pregnancy.[6]

The main purpose of fetal MR imaging is to complement an examination performed by an expert US operator.[9] The paradigm that MR imaging is blind to bones is changing with the emergence of ultrafast imaging techniques and new sequences. The use of the conventional sequence T2 and other new sequences has been recommended in the evaluation of skeletal malformations in locations other than the spine. MR imaging has been established as a useful second-line tool for fetal imaging. Fetal movement artifacts have become less problematic, and improved imaging quality provides an increasing number of potential indications for fetal MR imaging, including skeletal evaluation.[10–12] In the presence of adverse situations, such as increased maternal body mass index or oligohydramnios, fetal MR imaging can add information and establish diagnoses that are not otherwise possible with US.[7,13] This contributes to appropriate perinatal management and allows the referral of the newborn to a tertiary center staffed with a multidisciplinary team, thereby reducing perinatal morbidity and mortality.

In addition to the assessment of skeletal dysplasias, MR imaging may contribute to the evaluation of other pathologic conditions, such as limb defects and neuromuscular disorders.

Several congenital disorders may result in limb reduction defects, such as developmental errors, ischemic insults, or even amputations (eg, those occurring in the amniotic band sequence spectrum), primary vascular insults, teratogens, and chromosomal abnormalities. Amniotic bands may lead to loss of any body part, and a precise evaluation of the entire fetus is essential to identify the severity of eventual constrictions and enable prompt treatment or counseling.[1,3]

A precise diagnosis of reduced fetal movement is always challenging. Reduced fetal movement may be caused, for example, by neuromuscular disorders. When the reduced fetal movement occurs with the extremities in a fixed position or with contractures, it is called arthrogryposis multiplex congenita and may be associated with a variety of etiologic factors. The main differential diagnoses of reduced fetal movement include multiple pterygium syndrome, fetal akinesia syndrome, myopathy, and maternal myasthenia gravis.[4]

Even though US can easily evaluate fetal movement, MR imaging may be recommended instead to assess the fetal neural axis to identify possible causes of generalized hypotonia or contractures.[4]

Several studies have emphasized the benefits of MR imaging in the evaluation of congenital anomalies in the fetal brain and lungs, as well as complex syndromes.[7,8,13] However, few studies have demonstrated the contribution of MR imaging in the diagnosis of fetal skeletal abnormalities.[2,5,6,14,15]

Some studies have evaluated the use of 3D virtual models and additive manufacturing (AM) in general medicine and fetal medicine.[16,17] The main outcomes were the possibility of creating 3D models from 3D US, MR imaging, or CT images, separately and in various combinations.[18–22]

AM is the automatic, layer-by-layer construction of physical models using solid free-form fabrication. The first AM techniques were used in the late 1980s to produce models and prototypes. The use of AM in the biomedical sector has increased steadily over the past decade. Different uses have been reported widely in the medical literature but little has been published on its application to pregnancy.[20,21]

The aim of this article is to describe the main findings in musculoskeletal disorders occurring during the prenatal period.

## MR IMAGING PROTOCOLS

According to the guidelines of the International Society of Ultrasound in Obstetrics and Gynecology (ISUOG),[23] fetal MR imaging performed without contrast is considered generally safe and not associated with known adverse fetal effects at any moment during pregnancy. However, MR imaging is not recommended in the first trimester of pregnancy to avoid, or at least minimize, potential teratogenic or harmful effects on both the fetus and mother.[13,24] In several studies using 1.5-T MR imaging during pregnancy, no side effects have been described.[23]

Usually, MR imaging is performed as a complementary diagnostic method when skeletal and other congenital anomalies are identified on previous US examinations performed by expert operators. Skeletal anomalies occur alone or in association with chromosomal defects and are diagnosed prenatally using imaging methods and genetic testing.[25,26] These procedures allow appropriate parental counseling in regard to the disease's prognosis, natural history, and risk of recurrence in future pregnancies. The management of pregnancies involving skeletal anomalies depends on 3 factors: gestational age at diagnosis, disease severity, and parental decision. When a skeletal anomaly is detected, a careful evaluation of the entire fetus should be performed to identify other associated anomalies. The presence or absence of findings on MR imaging can help identify whether the problem is isolated or associated with other anomalies, which is a major contribution of fetal MR imaging. Multiplanar reconstructed MR imaging images allow a complete fetal evaluation and contribute to determining the origin of the anomaly and the characteristics of the fetal skeleton (**Fig. 1**).

MR imaging examinations should be performed on a 1.5-T scanner at gestational age greater than 22 weeks and must be conducted by a multidisciplinary team. Use of a 3.0-T scanner can also be considered. The patient is placed in the supine and/or left lateral position (whichever is more comfortable) (**Fig. 2**), and a surface coil is placed on the patient's abdomen. The routine protocol follows the sequence of the protocol proposed for 3D MR imaging reconstructions.

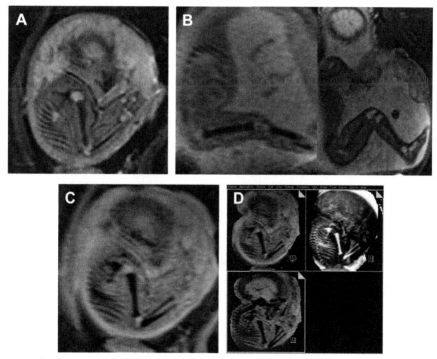

Fig. 1. A 27-week fetus with oligohydramnios. Sagittal oblique T2 weighted echo-planar image. The skeleton and the cartilage appear hypointense and hyperintense, respectively (*A, B*). T2-weighted 3D flash sequence. Compared with the surrounding tissue, the bones and cartilage appear hypointense and hyperintense (although less hyperintense than in the echo-planar image sequence) (*C*). Same fetus: magnetic resonance perfusion (MPR) (*upper left*), volume rendering (VRT) (*upper right*), and minimal intensity projection (MInIP) (*lower left*) (*D*).

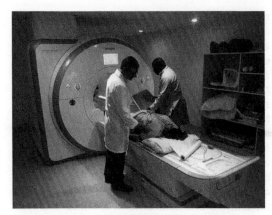

Fig. 2. Preparation for fetal MR imaging scan.

For evaluation of possible congenital anomalies, T1-weighted and T2-weighted sequences should be performed. Additional sequences are mandatory in cases of musculoskeletal disorders. These sequences include echo-planar imaging (EPI), thick-slab T2-weighted sequences, dynamic steady-state free precession (SSFP) sequences, T2-weighted half-Fourier single-shot turbo spin echo (HASTE) sequences, true fast imaging with SSFP (trueFISP; or 3D trueFISP [3D TRUFI]), and volumetric interpolated breath-hold examination (VIBE) modified.

T2-weighted HASTE evaluates the fetal anatomy, especially the fetal brain and organs with a high percentage of water.[16]

Ossification centers can be identified at 12 weeks of gestation; however, it is only at approximately 27 to 29 weeks that the definition of the fetal skeleton becomes more evident.[6] EPI sequences can provide additional anatomic information about the bones and are mainly indicated to evaluate the fetal bone and skeletal development. Bones are hypointense structures and their cartilaginous epiphyses appear as hyperintense areas. However, the use of EPI has major limitations due to this method's low spatial resolution. Of note, the sequence parameters must be modified according to the gestational period because the distinction between bone and muscle becomes less conspicuous with advancing pregnancy. Despite few studies, image reconstruction of the skeleton, in the authors' experiences, allows the identification of defects in long fetal bones with an optimal resolution to establish a definitive diagnosis.

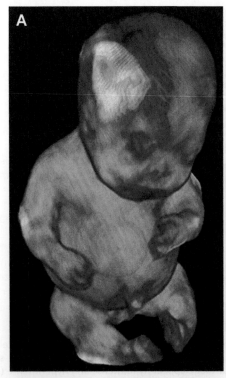
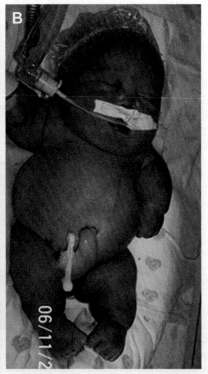

Fig. 3. Three-dimensional MR imaging reconstruction of a trueFISP sequence in a 27-week fetus with achondrogenesis (A). Postnatal view (B).

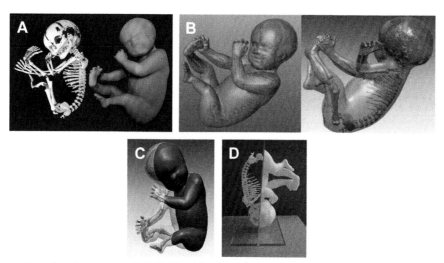

**Fig. 4.** Three-dimensional reconstruction obtained by CT and MR imaging (trueFISP sequence): physical model, skeletal and surface, respectively (*A*) and virtual model (*B*). Imaging fusion obtained from CT and MR imaging: virtual model (*C*) and physical model (*D*).

Nemec and colleagues[7] assessed the fetal skeleton using other MR imaging sequences, including EPI, thick-slab T2-weighted, and dynamic SSFP sequences; however, in assessing the entire fetal skeleton, these sequences offer no advantage over the VIBE sequence. MR imaging using the VIBE sequence shows advantages over 3D US in assessing parts of the fetal body but depends on the position of the fetus.

Thick-slab T2-weighted sequences enable a 3D image of the fetus, yielding more easily recognizable anomalies on a single image. Thus, these sequences may be useful in cases of clubfeet, limb deformities, and arthrogryposis. These sequences may also represent an alternative to 3D US because they provide a shine-through effect to other organs. Thick-slab heavily T2-weighted cine sequences may also assess neuromuscular

**Table 1**
**Protocol of the T1-weighted and thick-slab sequences**

| Sequence | T1-Weighted | Thick-Slab |
|---|---|---|
| Type | — | T2-weighted |
| Scan time | 20 s | 5 s |
| Res (mm³) | 0.7 × 0.7 × 4.5 mm | 0.8 × 0.8 × 50 mm |
| TR (ms) | 264 | 4500 |
| TE (ms) | 2.38/5.08 | 754 |
| FOV (mm) | 300 | 100/350 |
| Slices | 30 | 1 |
| Gap | 0.9 mm | 25 mm |
| Average | 1 | 1 |
| Concatenations | 1 | 1 |
| Flip angle | 70 | 180 |
| Slice thickness | 4.5 mm | 50 |
| Bandwidth | 440 | No |

*Abbreviations:* FOV, field of view; Res, resolution; TE, echo time; TR, repetition time.

**Table 2**
**Protocol of the T2-weighted half-Fourier single-shot turbo spin echo and 3-dimensonal true fast imaging with steady-state free precession sequences**

| Sequence | T2-Weighted HASTE | 3D TRUFI |
|---|---|---|
| Scan time | 18 s | 22 s |
| Res (mm³) | 1.1 × 1.1 × 4.0 mm | 1.0 × 1.0 × 1.0 |
| TR (ms) | 1000 | 3.16 |
| TE (ms) | 140 | 1.4 |
| FOV (mm) | 1340 | 380 |
| Slices | 24 | 160 |
| Gap | 0.8 mm | 0 |
| Average | 1 | 1 |
| Concatenations | 1 | 1 |
| Flip angle | 180 | 55 |
| Slice thickness | 4.0 | 1–4 |
| Bandwidth | 710 | No |

*Abbreviations:* FOV, field of view; Res, resolution; TE, echo time; TR, repetition time.

**Table 3**
**Fetal skeletal MR imaging protocol**

| Sequence | 2D EPSE | VIBE Modified |
|---|---|---|
| Type | EPI | GRE |
| Scan time | 27 s | 21 s |
| Res (mm³) | 1.7 × 1.7 × 3.5 | 2 × 2 × 2 |
| TR (ms) | 2280 | 11.1 |
| TE (ms) | 46 | 9.53 |
| FOV (mm) | 300 | 380 |
| Slices | 24 | 60 |
| Gap | 0 | 0 |
| Average | 8 | 1 |
| Concatenations | 1 | 1 |
| Flip angle | 90 | 4 |
| Slice thickness | 3.5 | 2 |
| Bandwidth | 1050 | 475 |
| ETL | 46 | N/A |

Abbreviations: EPSE, echo planar spin echo; ETL, echo train length; GRE, gradient echo.

disorders because they can detect decreased fetal movement.

Dynamic SSFP sequences are also able to evaluate fetal movement because they can acquire 4 to 6 images per second and may be a complementary tool to US in the diagnosis of movement disorders or extremity malformations. However, the lack of quantitative information is the main limitation of this method. Although US remains superior in detecting movement disorders, dynamic MR imaging sequences in combination with morphology may be performed to discriminate transient mispositioning from an actual musculoskeletal or nervous disorder.

When spine anomalies are observed on fetal US, MR imaging is considered the image of choice to complement the evaluation because it may provide additional information in fetuses with spina bifida. Due to its advanced resolution, MR imaging may determine the type of spinal dysraphism, providing the exact delineation of the cord and the interface between the

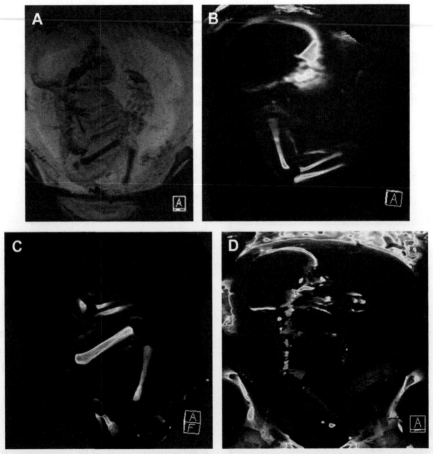

**Fig. 5.** A 35-week fetus with platyspondyly. T2-weighted 3D flash sequence (sagittal view). Femur and tibia can be clearly identified (A). T2-weighted 3D flash sequence. Humerus, ulna, and radius can be clearly identified (B). T2-weighted 3D flash sequence. Femur and tibia can be clearly identified (C). T2-weighted 3D flash sequence. Note the presence of platyspondyly of the vertebral bodies (D).

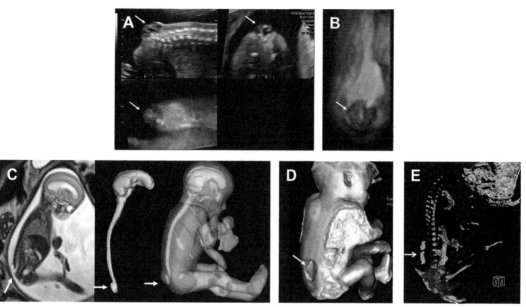

Fig. 6. 26-week fetus with Arnold-Chiari II malformation. US (*multiplanar view*) (*A*) with 3D reconstruction shows meningocele (*arrows*) (*B*). Sagittal T2 (*left*) with 3D reconstruction also shows meningocele (*center and right*) (*arrows*) (*C, D*). Sagittal T2-weighted 3D flash sequence (28 weeks) after endoscopic fetal surgery for correction of meningocele in a case of Arnold-Chiari II malformation. Note the presence of the patch (*arrow*) (*E*).

cerebrospinal fluid and the extradural space.[5] Additionally, MR imaging may be able to detect changes in muscle thickness, atrophy, and contour, and may be helpful in the diagnosis of neuromuscular disorders.[4]

Assessment with 3D TRUFI allows for both multiplanar and 3D evaluation through reconstructions in the workstation. This method is useful for adequate anatomic and pathologic evaluation of all systems. The parameters for 3D TRUFI are

TR/TE = 3.16/1.4 and isotropic voxel = 1.5 × 1.5 × 1.5 mm

This is with an acquisition time of 23 seconds and 96 slices (TR/TE where TR is repetition time and TR is echo time) (**Figs. 3** and **4**).

Unlike other sequences already published,[10,19] which only display parts of the skeleton, the VIBE sequence allows complete visualization of the fetal skeleton. A previously described sequence that allowed a full 3D evaluation, the T2-weighted thick-slab,[10] differs in the sense that a single

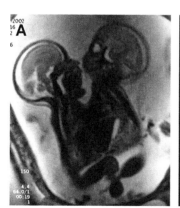
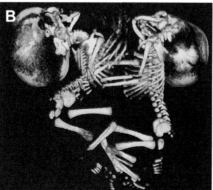
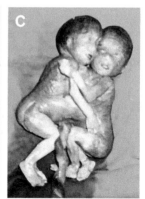

Fig. 7. Thoracoomphalopagus conjoined twins. MR imaging at 28 weeks of gestation (*A*). CT at 32 weeks (*B*) and postnatal at 35 weeks (*C*).

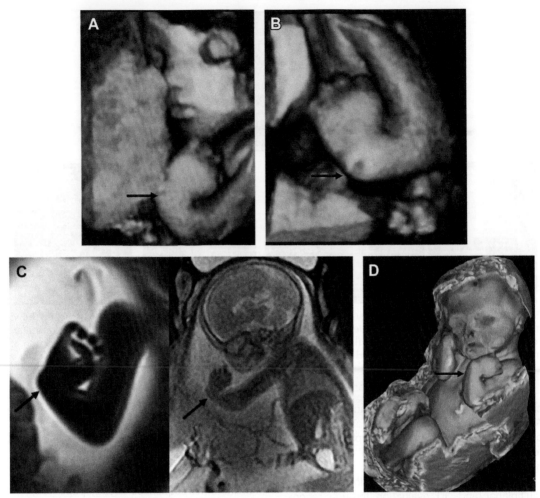

**Fig. 8.** Bilateral club hands (*arrows*) at 28 weeks of gestation. 3D US (*A, B*), sagittal T2 (*left and right*) (*C*), and 3D MR imaging (*D*). Note that in MR imaging we can see the whole body.

acquisition is performed in 1 second and the image is reproduced by simulating a 3D evaluation (**Table 1**). However, the VIBE-modified sequence performs a true 3D analysis and has some advantages over CT and 3D US in the evaluation of the entire skeleton: it is not limited by excess adipose tissue, oligohydramnios, or fetal movement, as observed with US images; and does not involve exposure to ionizing radiation, as in CT evaluations.[6,10,20]

Tables 2 and 3 summarize the parameters related to T2-weighted HASTE, 3D TRUFI, EPI, and VIBE-modified sequences.

The inclusion of the reconstructed sequence to evaluate the fetal skeleton does not substantially affect the duration of the examination because the estimated mean duration of these sequences is 23 seconds and the mean duration of the examination is 30 minutes.[21] Therefore, the inclusion of these sequences would not increase the eventual discomfort to the patient caused by different positions required to perform the examination (**Figs. 5–18**).

## SUMMARY

US imaging remains invaluable in fetal medicine and will not be replaced by fetal MR imaging, which can be used as a complementary tool. The authors believe that a detailed evaluation of the fetal skeleton using 3D reconstructions performed after image acquisition using a VIBE MR imaging sequence allows a full evaluation of the fetal skeleton. This MR imaging sequence has the advantage of being operator-independent but has poor accuracy in the evaluation of fetal extremities. Improvements in these sequences should be the focus of future studies.

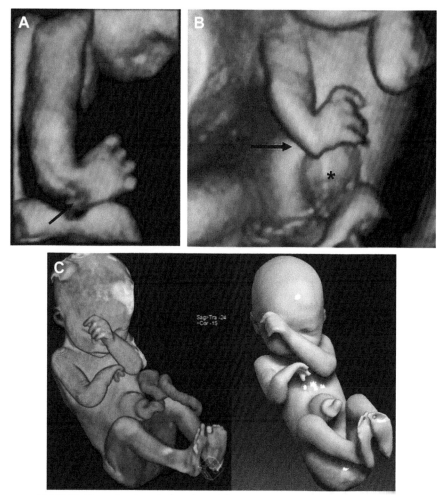

**Fig. 9.** Radial clubhand at 29 weeks of gestation. 3D US show clearly the clubhand (*arrow*) (*A*). 3D US show club-hand (*arrow*) and omphalocele (*asterisk*) (*B*). Virtual (*left*) and physical (*right*) models obtained by MR imaging (*C*).

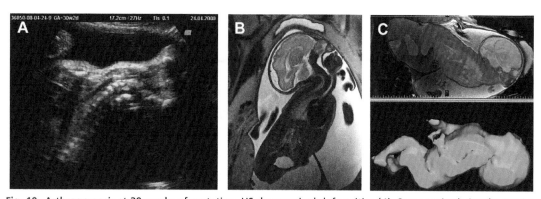

**Fig. 10.** Arthrogryposis at 29 weeks of gestation. US shows spinal deformities (*A*). Same sagittal view by MR im-aging in T2 weighted sequences (*B*). 3D reconstruction obtained by MR imaging (*above and below*) (*C*).

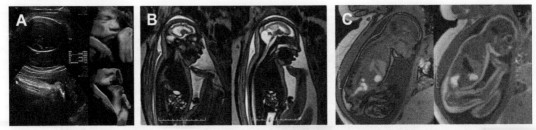

Fig. 11. Arthrogryposis in a 31-week fetus with Zika virus. 2D (*left*) and 3D US (*right*) show joint contractures (*A*). Sagittal T2 shows microcephaly and joint contractures (*B*). Same sagittal view in T1 weighted sequences (*C*).

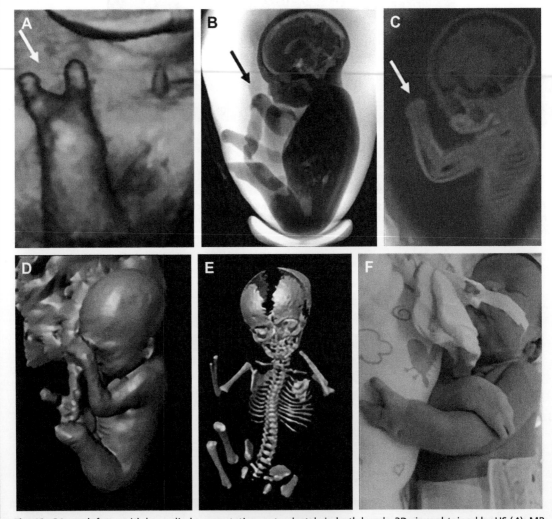

Fig. 12. 31-week fetus with lower limbs amputation, ectrodactyly in both hands. 3D view obtained by US (*A*), MR Imaging (*B, C*), 3D reconstruction by MRI (*D*) and CT (*E*). Postnatal (*F*).

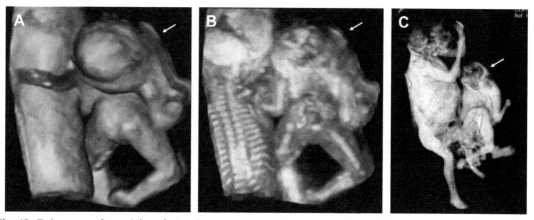

**Fig. 13.** Twin reversed arterial perfusion (TRAP) sequence at 27 weeks of gestation. It occurs 1% of monochorionic twin pregnancies. The normal twin (pump twin) drives blood through both fetuses. The upper structures of the body are not well-visualized in the TRAP fetus (*arrows*). 3D US (*A*) with bone reconstructions (*B*). 3D MR imaging (*C*).

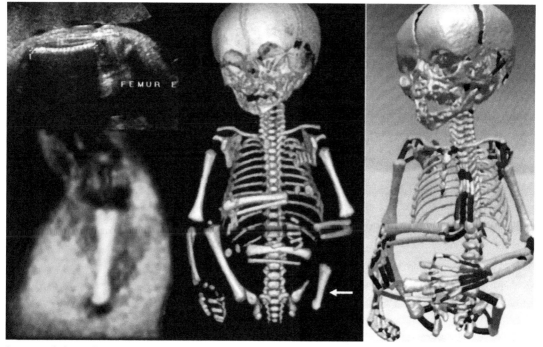

**Fig. 14.** Left femur hypoplasia (34 weeks of gestation). US with 3D reconstruction (*left*) and 3D CT reconstruction (*center and right*). The left femur can be easily visualized (*arrow*).

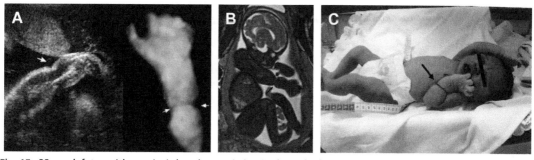

**Fig. 15.** 32-week fetus with amniotic band constriction in the right forearm (*arrows*). US (*left*) with 3D reconstruction (*right*) (*A*). Sagittal T2-weighted (*B*). Postnatal view (*C*).

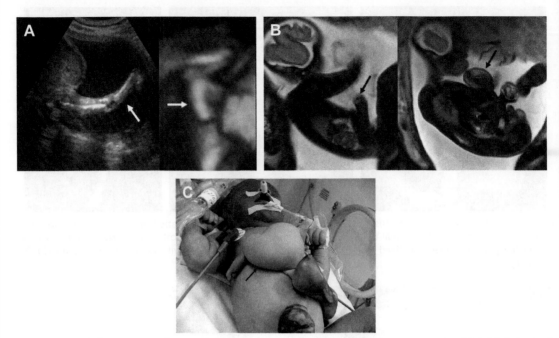

**Fig. 16.** 28-week fetus. Note rudimentary extra arm (*arrows*). US (*left*) with 3D reconstruction (*right*) (*A*). Sagittal T2-weighted (*B*) and postnatal view (*C*).

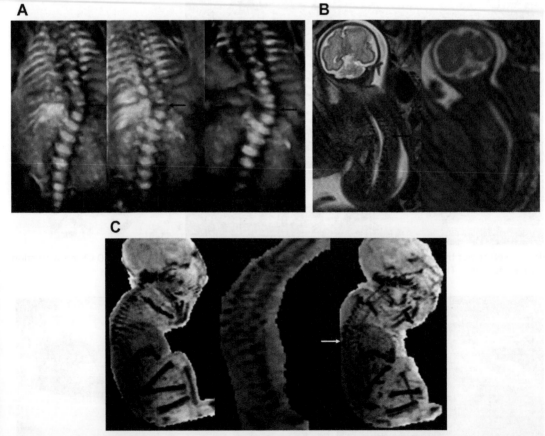

**Fig. 17.** 31-week fetus with alteration of the vertebral axis with angulation in the lumbar transition with the convexity to the right. Malformation of the vertebral bodies can be observed (*arrows*). 3D US (*A*). Sagittal T2-weighted (*B*) and sagittal VIBE-modified (*C*).

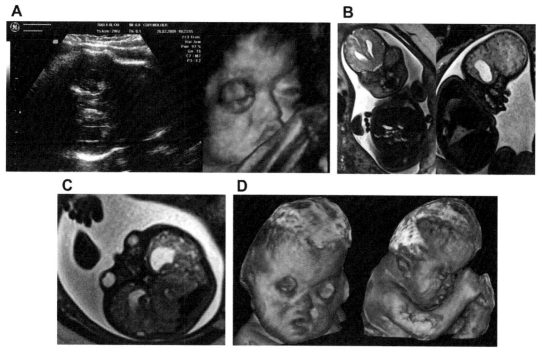

Fig. 18. 28-week fetus with craniosynostosis. US (*left*) with 3D reconstruction (*right*) (*A*). Coronal (*left*) and sagittal (*right*) T2-weighted (*B*). Note hypertelorism in axial T2-weighted (*C*) and 3D MR imaging (*D*).

## REFERENCES

1. Hall CM. International nosology and classification of constitutional disorders of bone (2001). Am J Med Genet 2002;113(1):65–77.

2. Morcuende JA, Weinstein SL. Developmental skeletal anomalies. Birth Defects Res C Embryo Today 2003;69(2):197–207.

3. Superti-Furga A, Unger S. Nosology and classification of genetic skeletal disorders: 2006 revision. Am J Med Genet A 2007;143A(1):1–18.

4. Dighe M, Fligner C, Cheng E, et al. Fetal skeletal dysplasia: an approach to diagnosis with illustrative cases. Radiographics 2008;28(4):1061–77.

5. Ciasca ES, Peixoto-Filho FM, Daltro P, et al. Prenatal diagnosis of proximal femoral focal deficiency combining ultrasound and computer tomography. Adv Comput Tomogr 2013;2:102–6.

6. Cassart M, Massez A, Cos T, et al. Contribution of three-dimensional computed tomography in the assessment of fetal skeletal dysplasia. Ultrasound Obstet Gynecol 2007;29(5):537–43.

7. Nemec U, Nemec SF, Krakow D, et al. The skeleton and musculature on foetal MRI. Insights Imaging 2011;2(3):309–18.

8. Salomon LJ, Garel C. Magnetic resonance imaging examination of the fetal brain. Ultrasound Obstet Gynecol 2007;30(7):1019–32.

9. Saleem SN. Fetal MRI: an approach to practice: a review. J Adv Res 2014;5(5):507–23.

10. Perrone A, Savelli S, Maggi C, et al. Magnetic resonance imaging versus ultrasonography in fetal pathology. Radiol Med 2008;113(2):225–41.

11. Santos XM, Papanna R, Johnson A, et al. The use of combined ultrasound and magnetic resonance imaging in the detection of fetal anomalies. Prenat Diagn 2010;30(5):402–7.

12. Krupa K, Bekiesinska-Figatowska M. Artifacts in magnetic resonance imaging. Pol J Radiol 2015; 80:93–106.

13. Breysem L, Bosmans H, Dymarkowski S, et al. The value of fast MR imaging as an adjunct to ultrasound in prenatal diagnosis. Eur Radiol 2003;13(7): 1538–48.

14. Kubik-Huch RA, Huisman TA, Wisser J, et al. Ultrafast MR imaging of the fetus. AJR Am J Roentgenol 2000;174(6):1599–606.

15. Krakow D, Lachman RS, Rimoin DL. Guidelines for the prenatal diagnosis of fetal skeletal dysplasias. Genet Med 2009;11(2):127–33.

16. Armillotta A, Bonhoeffer P, Dubini G, et al. Use of rapid prototyping models in the planning of percutaneous pulmonary valve stent implantation. Proc Inst Mech Eng H 2007;221:407–16.

17. Robiony M, Salvo I, Costa F, et al. Virtual reality surgical planning for maxillofacial distraction osteogenesis: the role of reverse engineering rapid prototyping and cooperative work. J Oral Maxillofac Surg 2007;65:1198–208.

18. Werner H, dos Santos JR, Fontes R, et al. Additive manufacturing models of fetuses built from three-dimensional ultrasound, magnetic resonance imaging and computed tomography scan data. Ultrasound Obstet Gynecol 2010;36(3): 355–61.

19. Werner H, Rolo LC, Araujo Junior E, et al. Manufacturing models of fetal malformations built from 3-dimensional ultrasound, magnetic resonance imaging, and computed tomography scan data. Ultrasound Q 2014;30(1):69–75.

20. Werner H, Lopes dos Santos JR, Ribeiro G, et al. Combination of ultrasound, magnetic resonance imaging and virtual reality technologies to generate immersive three-dimensional fetal images. Ultrasound Obstet Gynecol 2017;50:271–3.

21. Werner H Jr, Santos JL, Belmonte S, et al. Applicability of three dimensional imaging techniques in fetal medicine. Radiol Bras 2016;49: 281–7.

22. Santos JL, Werner H, Fontes R, et al. Additive manufactured models of fetuses built from 3D ultrasound, magnetic resonance imaging and computed tomography scan data. In: Hoque ME, editor. Rapid prototyping technology: principles and functional requirements. Rijeka (Croatia): InTech; 2011. p. 179–92.

23. Prayer D, Malinger G, Brugger PC, et al. ISUOG practice guidelines: performance of fetal magnetic resonance imaging. Ultrasound Obstet Gynecol 2017;49(5):671–80.

24. Frates MC, Kumar AJ, Benson CB, et al. Fetal anomalies: comparison of MR imaging and US for diagnosis. Radiology 2004;232(2):398–404.

25. Warman ML, Cormier-Daire V, Hall C, et al. Nosology and classification of genetic skeletal disorders: 2010 revision. Am J Med Genet A 2011; 155A(5):943–68.

26. Robinson AJ, Blaser S, Vladimirov A, et al. Foetal "black bone" MRI: utility in assessment of the foetal spine. Br J Radiol 2015;88(1046):20140496.

# MR Imaging at Rio 2016 Olympic and Paralympic Games: Report of Experience Using State-of-the-Art 3.0-T and 1.5-T Wide-Bore MR Imaging Scanners in High-Performance Athletes

Rômulo Domingues, MD[a,b,*], Bruno Hassel, MD[a,b],
João Grangeiro Neto, MD, MS[c],
Flávia Paiva Proença Lobo Lopes, MD, PhD[a,b,d]

## KEYWORDS

• Olympic games • Paralympic games • MR imaging • Imaging • Ultimate technology

## KEY POINTS

- The imaging center must have the most advanced diagnostic equipment to attend the athletes as it plays a critical role in the diagnosis and management of sports injuries and disorders.
- Wide-bore MRI has as a major advantage the possibility of offering a comfortable experience to the athletes, particularly tall, large or paralympic athletes.
- Trained personnel and the best imaging technology available are essential during the entire event for better athlete evaluation.
- A specific workflow must be planned to allow for quick and precise diagnoses, helping athletes to resume their competitive mode as quickly as possible.
- Each event experience is helpful in planning future Olympic and Paralympic Games.

## INTRODUCTION

The first official Olympic game was in 1896, and it was held in Athens, Greece, in April of that year. This was officially recognized as the first international Olympic Games held in modern history. By that time, an international organization was created to plan all the games' environment (from competitions to health care planning): the International Olympic Committee (IOC). The IOC was created by Pierre de Coubertin, and since then, the IOC has been in charge of these events.[1,2] The first international Paralympic Games started

Disclosure Statement: The authors have nothing to disclose.
[a] Radiology Department - Clínica de Diagnóstico por Imagem (CDPI)/DASA, Avenida das Américas, 4666, sala 301B, Centro Médico BarraShopping, CDPI, Barra da Tijuca, Rio de Janeiro, RJ CEP: 22640-102, Brazil; [b] Radiology Department - Alta Excelência Diagnóstica/DASA, Avenida das Américas, 4666, sala 301B, Centro Médico BarraShopping, CDPI, Barra da Tijuca, Rio de Janeiro, RJ CEP: 22640-102, Brazil; [c] Sports Trauma Group at Instituto Nacional de Traumato-Ortopedia, Rua Carlos Goes, 375, sala 502, Leblon, Rio de Janeiro, RJ CEP: 22440-040, Brazil; [d] Radiology Department - Federal University of Rio de Janeiro (UFRJ), Rua Rodolpho Paulo Rocco, 255 - Cidade Universitária - Ilha do Fundão, Rio de Janeiro, RJ CEP: 21941-913, Brazil
* Corresponding author. Avenida das Américas, 4666, sala 301B - Centro Médico BarraShopping, Clínica de Diagnóstico por Imagem (CDPI) - Barra da Tijuca, Rio de Janeiro, RJ CEP: 22640-102, Brazil.
E-mail address: romulodom6@gmail.com

64 years later and was held in Rome, Italy, and featured 400 athletes from 23 countries.[3,4]

Because of the complexity of the games, the IOC observed the need of more specialized medical services for the athletes and their respective delegations during the games. To the authors' knowledge, Haid[1] was the first author to describe the experience of the medical services during the winter Olympic Games that took place in 1964 in Innsbruck, Austria. By that time, there were no imaging facilities inside the polyclinics, likely causing a delay in treatment for athletes.[1,2,5]

In 2010, at the Winter Olympic Games that took place in Vancouver, Canada, an ambitious imaging facility was planned at the Olympic and Paralympic Village.[6-9] It was the first time in the modern history of such events that diagnostic imaging played such a huge role. All 4 radiology modalities– digital radiography, ultrasound, computed tomography (CT), and MRI were provided to the athletes and their delegations. Portable ultrasound units at or near the field of play were also available. Another advantage of these portable devices is the relatively small size (of a laptop).[6-10]

At the London Olympic and Paralympic Games, the imaging center was the first to have 3-T wide-bore MRI scanners in such events, plus a 1.5-T wide-bore MRI scanner, Discovery 750 HD 64 slice CT scanner, 2 Logic E9 ultrasound units and an XR656 wireless digital radiograph system.[11-15]

Planning for medical care including imaging facilities in Rio 2016 Olympic Games began several years before the opening ceremonies, like in other countries.[2,3,9,13] In Rio de Janeiro, Brazil, the planning started in 2009 after Rio's election to be the first South American city ever selected to host the Olympic Games. Besides all the planning for the Olympic Games, a special effort was made to evaluate and understand probable medical needs of paralympic athletes who have different disabilities.[14-16]

The Rio 2016 Olympic and Paralympic Games involved 11,274 elite athletes from 206 different countries and a team of 10 stateless refugees.[2,17-20] The Olympic Games took place between Aug. 5 and Aug. 21, and the Paralympic Games occurred between Sept. 7 and Sept. 18.[2,3] A major challenge for the IOC and the local committee was to offer the best environment with the most advanced diagnostic equipment for the extremely select population of athletes.[11,12,19] An imaging center with ultimate technology was established in the Polyclinic at the Athletes' Village, situated close to the main Olympic Village in Barra da Tijuca, Rio de Janeiro, in order to manage the diverse diagnostic needs of the athletes. The IOC sponsor General Electric (GE) Healthcare was directly involved with Brazilian authorities and the medical team to provide ultimate imaging equipment and pave the way for the use of electronic medical records (EMRs), which had never been used before at the Olympic or Paralympic Games.

The clinical services were offered between 7 a.m. and 11 p.m. during the Olympic and Paralympic Games, and from 9 a.m. to 6 p.m. before the Olympic Games and between the Olympic and Paralympic Games. The Olympic Village was open from July 25 to Aug. 28 during the Olympic Games (a total of 34 days) and from Aug. 31 to Sept. 21 during the Paralympic Games (22 days). During both games, radiologists and technicians alternated between 2 shifts a day (3 radiologists and 3 technicians per shift) to a total of 204 and 132 shifts during the Olympic and Paralympic Games, respectively.

The imaging center was constructed in the polyclinic (**Fig. 1**), a 3500 $m^2$ health care facility located within the Olympic Village. The imaging center (**Fig. 2**) was equipped with a digital radiograph system (Discovery XR656 Advanced Digital Radiography System, GE Healthcare, Brazil) (**Fig. 3**), an ultrasound machine (Logiq E9, GE Healthcare, Milwaukee, Wisconsin) (**Fig. 4**), and 1.5-T (Optima MR450w, GE Medical Systems Incorporated, Waukesha, Wisconsin) and 3.0-T (Discovery MR750w, GE Healthcare, Milwaukee) (**Fig. 5**) wide-bore MRI systems.

The imaging center also featured a completely digital system with state-of-the-art technology and a paperless and filmless environment, allowing a high-quality level of service. GE Healthcare provided the information and technology solution, which comprised RIS/PACS (**Fig. 6**), 4 workstations, and EMRs. This was the first time that EMRs were used in the Olympics, as previously described. Dual-monitor workstations and voice recognition systems integrated with GE Healthcare RIS/PACS were used for reading and reporting the imaging tests. The use of EMRs emerged as a major advantage, as it enabled physicians to link each athlete's diagnosis and treatment and maintain a digital record for improved follow-up. A teleradiology station was also available for examinations obtained at soccer venues.

The clinical staff comprised renowned physicians with extensive experience in their fields; this allowed a differential health care service to be offered at a single place in a dedicated on-site medical facility similar to that of the 2012 London Olympic and Paralympic Games.[11,12] The objective of this approach was to manage internally most health care issues related to the

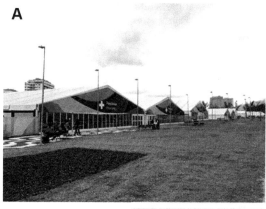
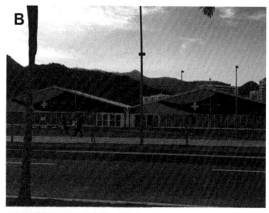
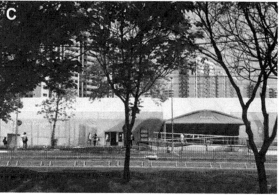

Fig. 1. (*A, B*) Outside views of the polyclinic, located within the Olympic Village in Barra da Tijuca, Rio de Janeiro. The imaging center was constructed inside the polyclinic. (*C*) Outside view of the village main entrance.

games. Life-threatening emergencies and severe trauma were referred to a nearby hospital, also in Barra da Tijuca, Rio de Janeiro, where interventional procedures were performed. Similar to other Olympic and Paralympic events, most of the injuries were managed at the polyclinics, and few patients had to be transferred to the hospital. Based on previous experiences in Olympic Games and on the limited number of CT examinations performed in London (107 in total),[11,12] CT scanners were forgone in the imaging center; this decision was also based on the proximity of the center to the referral hospital and resulted in a cost reduction of $1,472,000.

The peak demand of the facility occurred around the final events, when the Athletes' Village was at its busiest. Additionally, 2 major peaks were observed, the first on day 5 and the second on day 12.[1,2,18–20]

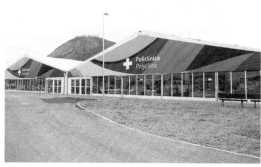

Fig. 2. Outside view of the imaging center of Rio 2016 Olympic and Paralympic Games.

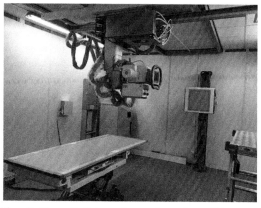

Fig. 3. The digital radiograph system (Discovery XR656 Advanced Digital Radiography System, GE Healthcare, Brazil) in the imaging center.

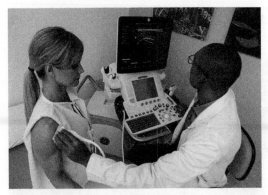

**Fig. 4.** The ultrasound machine (Logiq E9, GE Healthcare, Milwaukee, WI) used inside the imaging center during Olympic and Paralympic Games. (Used with permission of GE Healthcare.)

At the polyclinic, as previously reported,[11,12] most consultations were related to musculoskeletal manifestations, but a sizable proportion was also related to dental and ophthalmologic complaints, as observed in prior Olympic and Paralympic Games.

The demand for MRI was also substantial, probably because this method is usually not available in countries with limited resources.[18,19]

*Staff*

All radiologists and technicians had volunteered for the job. Twenty-six musculoskeletal radiologists and 26 technicians offered their services for the Olympic Games, while 16 musculoskeletal radiologists and 16 technicians volunteered during the Paralympic Games. All musculoskeletal radiologists had at least 10 years of experience and were responsible for reporting all radiological examinations.

The radiologists at the imaging center verified the tests requests and spoke with the athletes and physicians of the Olympic commissions to ensure that the test to be performed was the most appropriate and focused on the individual's diagnosis, thus avoiding prolonged examination.

The reports were generally bilingual (Portuguese and English) and were issued within 1 hour of the examination.

Overall, there were 1540 diagnostic investigations performed at the imaging center during the Olympic Games and 629 during the Paralympic Games: 893 MRI tests (58%), 178 (11.5%) diagnostic ultrasounds, and 469 (30.5%) radiographic examinations during the Olympic Games, and 400 MRI tests (63.6%), 33 diagnostic ultrasounds (5.2%), and 196 radiographic examinations (31.2%), respectively, during the Paralympic Games.[18–20] Compared with the 2012 London Summer Games, there were 6.94% more MRI scans during the 2016 Rio Olympic Games and 57.5% more MRI scans during the Paralympic Games.

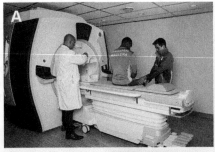
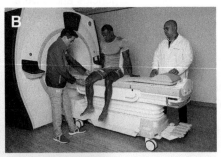
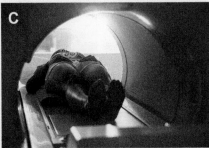

**Fig. 5.** Magnetic Resonance Systems (*A, B*) 3.0-T Discovery MR750w (GE Healthcare, Milwaukee, WI) and (*C*) 1.5-T Optima MR450w (GE Medical Systems Inc, Waukesha, WI) wide-bore MRI systems equipped with 32 independent and simultaneous receiver channels and dedicated coils to knee, ankle/foot, wrist, and shoulder. The maximum weight allowed for acquisition and vertical movement of the table is 227 kg, allowing examinations in large patients and also for disabled patients. (Image *courtesy of* GE Healthcare.)

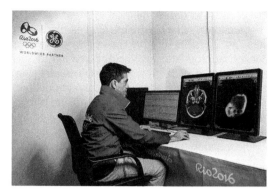

Fig. 6. GE Healthcare RIS/PACS system.

The most common imaging sites evaluated during the Olympic Games were the knees, lumbar spine, ankles, and shoulders, and during the Paralympic Games, the most common sites were the knees, shoulders, and lumbar spine (in this order). The results showed that 1101 injuries occurred in 718 of the 11,274 Olympic athletes.[18–20]

Most examinations done during the Games were performed on athletes, and the preference was given to those who were still competing.

## Ultrasound

The latest generation available of Ultrasound equipment was used (see **Fig. 4**) and also a portable handheld ultrasound (Vscan, GE Healthcare, Milwaukee, WI) (**Fig. 7**). The main advantage of the ultrasound equipment used is the possibility to detect minimal superficial pathologies such as tendinopathy, tenosynovitis, tendon tears, muscle lesions, bursitis, and plantar fascial injury, allowing the physicians and athletes to be informed about the appropriate time to resume physical activity and return to the competition.[19] Ultrasound is recognized as an operator-dependent imaging method; therefore, it must be performed by specialized personnel, especially in the case of high-performance athletes.

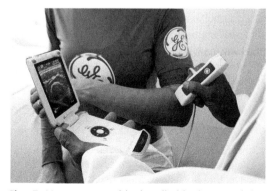

Fig. 7. Vscan a portable handheld ultrasound (GE Healthcare, Milwaukee, WI)

In superficial lesions, ultrasound was often used as a first-line investigation; however, MRI was further performed in some cases for improved morphologic assessment and grading, because the improved information obtained impacted the management plan.[18,19]

Another advantage of ultrasound imaging in radiology units, such as the one set at the Olympic Games, is that it is a fast examination that can be performed without the requirement of complex structures. Additionally, there is no risk to the patient or discomfort during the acquisition.[19]

## Radiographs

The Discovery XR656 Advanced Digital Radiography System (see **Fig. 3**) used is a digital radiographic imaging system that provides excellent image quality and advanced clinical applications. The Discovery XR656 is designed to handle standard 2-dimensional examinations and advanced radiographic applications using GE's wireless flat panel digital detector.

During the Olympic Games, 304 radiographs were performed, mostly because of musculoskeletal lesions. From those 138 were for lower limb, 92 for upper limb, 34 for spine injuries; additionally, there were 23 Chest radiographs, 1 to evaluate abdominal pain, 9 for pelvic complaint, and the remaining examinations were for other investigations. Besides other clinical complaints, the major objective of the radiographs was to evaluate possible fractures.[18–20]

## MR Imaging

MRI was the method of radiological investigation most widely used during both games. Similar to the 2012 London Olympic Games, it was essential to have 2 MRI scanners at the imaging center, as they facilitated the scanning dynamic, especially during busy hours.[1,11,12,19] MRI provides excellent lesion detection and localization. The images are anatomic and clearly visualized by both health care professionals and patients alike.[19]

MRI equipment used during the games consisted wide-bore systems with bright inner lighting and flared gantry, offering a comfortable experience to the patients (**Fig. 8**), and flexibility in positioning individuals requiring extra space.[11,13,16]

Both 1.5-T Optima MR450w and 3.0-T Discovery MR750w wide-bore MRI systems have the ability to perform high-resolution images, which are essential for musculoskeletal evaluation. Small-structure examinations were performed in the 3.0-T MRI to push the limits in terms of obtaining higher resolution and better contrast-to-noise ratio.

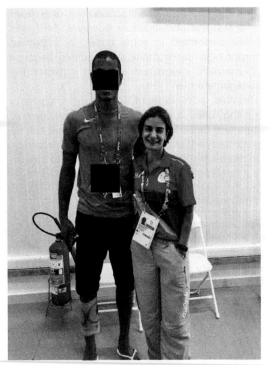

environment to detect minimal injuries, and efficient workflow is key in maintaining as many athletes as possible on the competition. In this manner, appropriate planning and staffing for imaging services at large-scale events is essential to provide for a safe and successful competition.

The authors' imaging center was able to offer a wide variety of state-of-the-art imaging options for proper diagnosis and follow-up of all injured athletes, and to predict with precision the amount of time required for the athletes to return to the sport.

Olympic athletes have an Olympic cycle, in which they prepare and dedicate their lives to their sports modality. In order to produce expressive results, these athletes push themselves to their physical limits, which is precisely when lesions emerge. Therefore, an extremely orchestrated structure is required to help these athletes in returning to their competitive mode as quickly as possible. The Rio 2016 Olympic Games featured a center of diagnostic excellence with the best professionals in their areas, and state-of-the-art equipment in all areas in order to offer the best imaging diagnostic tools.

Despite the immense challenge imposed on all professionals involved, this was an extraordinary experience for everyone, and the authors hope their experience is helpful in the planning of future Olympic and Paralympic Games.

**Fig. 8.** Example of a very tall athlete side by side with one of the radiologists, that was submitted to a MRI due to lower limb injury. The exams were performed in the Discovery MR750w (GE Healthcare, Milwaukee, WI), a 3.0-T, wide-bore MRI system providing a comfortable experience.

The examinations were carried out in less than 15 minutes, and no enhanced contrast was used in accordance with the IOC regulations. Patients requiring contrast were directed to the referral hospital.

## Main Limitations and Future Recommendations

In the imaging center, the authors were expecting to attend athletes with injuries related to sports practice and trauma, but were surprised with the number of examinations performed in members of the Olympic Committees who had preexisting conditions unrelated to the Olympic cycle.

During the events, especially in their beginning, there was a great shortage of volunteers in the administrative area, like receptionists, which resulted in an overload of work to radiologists and technicians.

## SUMMARY

Imaging diagnosis is crucial in major international sports events featuring elite athletes. Availability of trained personnel and the latest available technology is essential in providing the best

## REFERENCES

1. 1896 Summer Olympics. Available at: https://en. wikipedia.org/wiki/1896_Summer_Olympics. Accessed April 20, 2018.
2. Jogos Olímpicos de Verão de 2016 [2016 Summer Olympic Games]. Available at: https://pt.wikipedia. org/wiki/Jogos_Ol%C3%ADmpicos_de_Ver%C3% A3o_de_2016. Accessed March 7, 2018.
3. Paralympics - history of the movement. Available at: https://www.paralympic.org/the-ipc/history-of-the-movement. Accessed April 20, 2018.
4. Summer Paralympic Games. Available at: https:// en.wikipedia.org/wiki/Summer_Paralympic_Games. Accessed March 7, 2018.
5. Haid B. Medical care at winter Olympic Games. Logistics. JAMA 1972;221(9):990–2.
6. Eaton SB, Woodfin BA, Askew JL, et al. The polyclinic at the 1996 Atlanta Olympic Village. Med J Aust 1997;167:599–602.
7. Ljungqvist A, Jenoure P, Engebretsen L, et al. The International Olympic Committee (IOC) consensus statement on periodic health evaluation of elite athletes. Br J Sports Med 2009;43:631–43.
8. Oberladstaetter J, Kamelger FS, Rosenberger R, et al. Planning of traumatological hospital resources

for a major winter sporting event as illustrated by the 2005 Winter Universiad. Arch Orthop Trauma Surg 2009;129:359–62.

9. Reeser JC, Willick S, Elstad M. Medical services provided at the Olympic Village polyclinic during the 2002 Salt Lake City Winter Games. WMJ 2003; 102(4):20–5.

10. Dapeng J, Xiaowan Z, Tunon C. Overview of health-care services for the games. In: Dapeng J, Ljungqvist A, Troedsson H, editors. The health legacy of the 2008 Beijing Olympic Games: Successes and Recommendations. Manila (Philippines): World Health Organization Western Pacific Region. Available at: https://stillmed.olympic.org/Documents/Commissions_PDFfiles/Medical_commission/The_Health_Legacy_of_the_2008_Beijing_Olympic_Games.pdf. Accessed April 20, 2018.

11. Bethapudi S, Campbell RS, O'Connor P. Perspective on imaging services at the London 2012 Olympic and Paralympic Games. Skeletal Radiol 2014; 43(9):1201–3.

12. Bethapudi S, Budgett R, Engebretsen L, et al. Imaging at London 2012 summer Olympic Games: analysis of demand and distribution of workload. Br J Sports Med 2013;47(13):850–6.

13. Bethapudi S, Campbell RS, Budgett R, et al. Imaging services at the Paralympic Games London 2012: analysis of demand and distribution of workload. Br J Sports Med 2015;49(1):20–4.

14. National Health Service. Health Service planning and delivery (no. two in a series of four reports). London (United Kingdom): National Health Service; 2012.

15. Blank C, Schamasch P, Engebretsen L, et al. Medical services at the first Winter Youth Olympic Games 2012 in Innsbruck/Austria. Br J Sports Med 2012;46: 1048–54.

16. Taunton J, Wilkinson M, Celebrini R, et al. Paralympic medical services for the 2010 paralympic winter games. Clin J Sport Med 2012;22(1): 10–20.

17. Kononovas K, Black G, Taylor J, et al. Improving Olympic health services: what are the common health care planning issues? Prehosp Disaster Med 2014;29(6):623–8.

18. Guermazi A, Hayashi D, Jarraya M, et al. Sports injuries at the Rio de Janeiro 2016 Summer Olympics: use of diagnostic imaging services. Radiology 2018; 26:171510.

19. Crema MD, Jarraya M, Engebretsen L, et al. Imaging-detected acute muscle injuries in athletes participating in the Rio de Janeiro 2016 Summer Olympic Games. Br J Sports Med 2018;52(7): 460–4.

20. Soligard T, Steffen K, Palmer D, et al. Sports injury and Illness incidence in the Rio de Janeiro 2016 Olympic Summer Games: a prospective study of 11274 athletes from 207 countries. Br J Sports Med 2017;51(17):1265–71.

| 1. Publication Title | 2. Publication Number | | 3. Filing Date |
|---|---|---|---|
| MAGNETIC RESONANCE IMAGING CLINICS OF NORTH AMERICA | 0 1 1 – 9 0 9 | | 9/18/2018 |

| 4. Issue Frequency | 5. Number of Issues Published Annually | 6. Annual Subscription Price |
|---|---|---|
| FEB, MAY, AJG, NOV | 4 | $394.00 |

7. Complete Mailing Address of Known Office of Publication (Not printer) (Street, city, county, state, and ZIP+4®)

ELSEVIER INC.
230 Park Avenue, Suite 800
New York, NY 10169

Contact Person
STEPHEN R. BUSHING

Telephone (Include area code)
215-239-3688

8. Complete Mailing Address of Headquarters or General Business Office of Publisher (Not printer)

ELSEVIER INC.
230 Park Avenue, Suite 800
New York, NY 10169

9. Full Names and Complete Mailing Addresses of Publisher, Editor, and Managing Editor (Do not leave blank)

Publisher (Name and complete mailing address)

TAYLOR E BALL, ELSEVIER INC.
1600 JOHN F KENNEDY BLVD. SUITE 1800
PHILADELPHIA, PA 19103-2899

Editor (Name and complete mailing address)

JOHN VASSALLO, ELSEVIER INC.
1600 JOHN F KENNEDY BLVD. SUITE 1800
PHILADELPHIA, PA 19103-2899

Managing Editor (Name and complete mailing address)

PATRICK MANLEY, ELSEVIER INC.
1600 JOHN F KENNEDY BLVD. SUITE 1800
PHILADELPHIA, PA 19103-2899

10. Owner (Do not leave blank. If the publication is owned by a corporation, give the name and address of the corporation immediately followed by the names and addresses of all stockholders owning or holding 1 percent or more of the total amount of stock. If not owned by a corporation, give the names and addresses of the individual owners. If owned by a partnership or other unincorporated firm, give its name and address as well as those of each individual owner. If the publication is published by a nonprofit organization, give its name and address.)

| Full Name | Complete Mailing Address |
|---|---|
| WHOLLY OWNED SUBSIDIARY OF REED/ELSEVIER, US HOLDINGS | 1600 JOHN F KENNEDY BLVD. SUITE 1800 PHILADELPHIA, PA 19103-2899 |
| | |
| | |
| | |

11. Known Bondholders, Mortgagees, and Other Security Holders Owning or Holding 1 Percent or More of Total Amount of Bonds, Mortgages, or Other Securities. If none, check box. ▶ ☐ None

| Full Name | Complete Mailing Address |
|---|---|
| N/A | |

12. Tax Status (For completion by nonprofit organizations authorized to mail at nonprofit rates) (Check one)
The purpose, function, and nonprofit status of this organization and the exempt status for federal income tax purposes:
☒ Has Not Changed During Preceding 12 Months
☐ Has Changed During Preceding 12 Months (Publisher must submit explanation of change with this statement)

PS Form **3526**, July 2014 [Page 1 of 4 (see instructions page 4)] PSN: 7530-01-000-9931  PRIVACY NOTICE: See our privacy policy on www.usps.com.

| 13. Publication Title | | | 14. Issue Date for Circulation Data Below |
|---|---|---|---|
| MAGNETIC RESONANCE IMAGING CLINICS OF NORTH AMERICA | | | MAY 2018 |

| 15. Extent and Nature of Circulation | | Average No. Copies Each Issue During Preceding 12 Months | No. Copies of Single Issue Published Nearest to Filing Date |
|---|---|---|---|
| a. Total Number of Copies (Net press run) | | 345 | 511 |
| b. Paid Circulation (By Mail and Outside the Mail) | (1) Mailed Outside-County Paid Subscriptions Stated on PS Form 3541 (Include paid distribution above nominal rate, advertiser's proof copies, and exchange copies) | 244 | 343 |
| | (2) Mailed In-County Paid Subscriptions Stated on PS Form 3541 (Include paid distribution above nominal rate, advertiser's proof copies, and exchange copies) | 0 | 0 |
| | (3) Paid Distribution Outside the Mails Including Sales Through Dealers and Carriers, Street Vendors, Counter Sales, and Other Paid Distribution Outside USPS® | 64 | 96 |
| | (4) Paid Distribution by Other Classes of Mail Through the USPS (e.g., First-Class Mail®) | 0 | 0 |
| c. Total Paid Distribution (Sum of 15b (1), (2), (3), and (4)) | ▶ | 308 | 439 |
| d. Free or Nominal Rate Distribution (By Mail and Outside the Mail) | (1) Free or Nominal Rate Outside-County Copies included on PS Form 3541 | 37 | 72 |
| | (2) Free or Nominal Rate In-County Copies Included on PS Form 3541 | 0 | 0 |
| | (3) Free or Nominal Rate Copies Mailed at Other Classes Through the USPS (e.g., First-Class Mail) | 0 | 0 |
| | (4) Free or Nominal Rate Distribution Outside the Mail (Carriers or other means) | 0 | 0 |
| e. Total Free or Nominal Rate Distribution (Sum of 15d (1), (2), (3) and (4)) | ▶ | 37 | 72 |
| f. Total Distribution (Sum of 15c and 15e) | ▶ | 345 | 511 |
| g. Copies not Distributed (See instructions to Publishers #4 (page #3)) | ▶ | 0 | 0 |
| h. Total (Sum of 15f and g) | ▶ | 345 | 511 |
| i. Percent Paid (15c divided by 15f times 100) | ▶ | 89.28% | 85.91% |

* If you are claiming electronic copies, go to line 16 on page 3. If you are not claiming electronic copies, skip to line 17 on page 3.

| 16. Electronic Copy Circulation | | Average No. Copies Each Issue During Preceding 12 Months | No. Copies of Single Issue Published Nearest to Filing Date |
|---|---|---|---|
| a. Paid Electronic Copies | ▶ | 0 | 0 |
| b. Total Paid Print Copies (Line 15c) + Paid Electronic Copies (Line 16a) | ▶ | 308 | 439 |
| c. Total Print Distribution (Line 15f) + Paid Electronic Copies (Line 16a) | ▶ | 345 | 511 |
| d. Percent Paid (Both Print & Electronic Copies) (16b divided by 16c × 100) | ▶ | 89.28% | 85.91% |

☒ I certify that 50% of all my distributed copies (electronic and print) are paid above a nominal price.

17. Publication of Statement of Ownership
☒ If the publication is a general publication, publication of this statement is required. Will be printed in the NOVEMBER 2018 issue of this publication. ☐ Publication not required.

18. Signature and Title of Editor, Publisher, Business Manager, or Owner

*Stephen R. Bushing* Date 9/18/2018

STEPHEN R. BUSHING - INVENTORY DISTRIBUTION CONTROL MANAGER

I certify that all information furnished on this form is true and complete. I understand that anyone who furnishes false or misleading information on this form or who omits material or information requested on the form may be subject to criminal sanctions (including fines and imprisonment) and/or civil sanctions (including civil penalties).

PS Form **3526**, July 2014 (Page 3 of 4)  PRIVACY NOTICE: See our privacy policy on www.usps.com

Printed and bound by CPI Group (UK) Ltd, Croydon, CR0 4YY

15/05/2025

01872230-0001